Sinusitis: An Issue of Otolaryngology Clinics

Sinusitis: An Issue of Otolaryngology Clinics

Editor: Kara Stanley

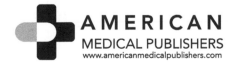

AMERICAN
MEDICAL PUBLISHERS
www.americanmedicalpublishers.com

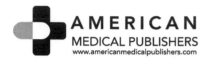

Cataloging-in-Publication Data

Sinusitis : an issue of otolaryngology clinics / edited by Kara Stanley.
    p. cm.
Includes bibliographical references and index.
ISBN 978-1-63927-414-7
1. Sinusitis. 2. Paranasal sinuses--Diseases. 3. Otolaryngology. 4. Otolaryngologists--Guidebooks. I. Stanley, Kara.
RF425 .S56 2021
616.212--dc23

American Medical Publishers,
41 Flatbush Avenue,
1st Floor, New York,
NY 11217, USA

ISBN 978-1-63927-414-7 (Hardback)

Contents

Preface

The purpose of the book is to provide a glimpse into the dynamics and to present opinions and studies of some of the scientists engaged in the development of new ideas in the field from very different standpoints. This book will prove useful to students and researchers owing to its high content quality.

The inflammation of the mucous membrane which lines the sinuses is referred to as sinusitis. It is also known as a sinus infection. The most common symptoms of sinusitis include a plugged nose, facial pain and thick nasal mucous. It may also exhibit other symptoms such as fever, headache, sore throat, cough and poor sense of smell. It is caused due to infections in the respiratory tract, allergies and air pollution. It can also be caused due to structural problems in the nose. People suffering from respiratory diseases like asthma, cystic fibrosis or having poor immune function tend to experience long term sinusitis. Bacterial and viral sinusitis are distinguished by watchful waiting in the initial period, however, a CT scan is used to diagnose chronic sinusitis. Pain killers such as naproxen, nasal steroids and nasal irrigation are used to minimize the effects of its symptoms. The treatment of sinusitis ranges from using antibiotics in acute disease, to surgery in people facing chronic sinusitis. This book contains some path-breaking studies on sinusitis. Those in search of information to further their knowledge will be greatly assisted by this book. This book will serve as a valuable source of reference for graduate and post graduate students.

At the end, I would like to appreciate all the efforts made by the authors in completing their chapters professionally. I express my deepest gratitude to all of them for contributing to this book by sharing their valuable works. A special thanks to my family and friends for their constant support in this journey.

Editor

Chronic Rhinosinusitis and Obstructive Sleep Apnea: CPAP Reservoir Bacterial Colonization Is Not Associated with Sinus Culture Positivity

Rosa B. Lipin [1], Anita Deshpande [1], Sarah K. Wise [1], John M. DelGaudio [1] and Zara M. Patel [2,*

[1] Department of Otolaryngology—Head and Neck Surgery, Emory University School of Medicine, Atlanta, GA 30308, USA; rosa.bene.lipin@emory.edu (R.B.L.); asdeshp@emory.edu (A.D.); skmille@emory.edu (S.K.W.); jdelgau@emory.edu (J.M.D.)

[2] Department of Otolaryngology—Head and Neck Surgery, Stanford University School of Medicine, Stanford, CA 94305, USA

* Correspondence: zpatel@ohns.stanford.edu

Academic Editors: Claudina A. Pérez Novo and César Picado

Abstract: Chronic rhinosinusitis (CRS) and obstructive sleep apnea (OSA) are both highly prevalent chronic diseases in the United States. Association between culture positivity of CPAP machines and sinus samples has not been studied in patients with both disease states. Our objective was to compare the microbes present in the sinus cavities and CPAP reservoirs of patients with both CRS and OSA. Patients from an academic tertiary care Rhinology practice were identified with both CRS and OSA and enrolled prospectively. Inclusion criteria included age over 18 years; diagnosis of OSA by sleep study; regular CPAP use; and an active diagnosis of CRS. Exclusion criteria included treatment with antibiotics or cleaning of the CPAP reservoir in the month prior. Cultures were taken from participants' sinus cavities and CPAP reservoirs and resulting microbial growth was compared. The most common organisms on CPAP culture were *Enterobacter cloacae* and *Acinetobacter baumanii*, whereas the most common on sinus culture were *Staphyloccoccus aureus* and *Pseudomonas aeruginosa*. Microbial growth from the sinus cavities and the CPAP reservoirs were not concordant in any of our patients. There is no association between bacterial colonization of the CPAP reservoir and the sinus cavities of those with CRS and OSA based on microbiologic cultures.

Keywords: chronic rhinosinusitis (CRS); obstructive sleep apnea (OSA); continuous positive airway pressure (CPAP); unified upper airway; bacterial colonization; microbial culture

1. Introduction

Chronic rhinosinusitis (CRS) is an end result of over 12 weeks of symptoms from underlying inflammation of the lining of the paranasal cavities, leading to over 18.3 million office visits a year [1]. Patients with CRS see primary care providers twice as much as those without the disease, and are five times more likely to be prescribed antibiotics [2]. The presentation of this disease can be highly variable, and the etiology remains poorly understood. The pathophysiology is likely multi-factorial, involving infectious agents, innate and adaptive immune responses, and other host and environmental factors [3]. As there is currently no standardized therapy for CRS, patients are managed using a combination of strategies, including systemic and topical corticosteroids, antimicrobial agents, intranasal saline, immune modulators, and endoscopic sinus surgery [4].

Obstructive sleep apnea (OSA) is another common chronic disease, found in 9%–26% of middle aged adults and characterized by the presence of five or more episodes of complete (apnea) or partial (hypopnea) airflow obstruction per hour while asleep [5]. Untreated OSA is thought to contribute

$3.4 billion annually to U.S. health care costs [6]. The gold standard treatment for this condition is continuous positive airway pressure (CPAP), which functions to splint the upper airway open during both inspiration and expiration, and thus counteracts the structural airway abnormalities leading to collapse during sleep [5]. Unfortunately, the use of CPAP may lead to upper airway dryness and nasal congestion, side effects which may compromise patient compliance and satisfaction [7]. Heated humidification has been shown to yield higher compliance, increased satisfaction, feeling more refreshed on awakening, and greater comfort as opposed to using CPAP without humidity [7,8]. However, Sanner *et al.* found that users of CPAP with humidification experienced an increased rate of upper airway infection compared to OSA patients utilizing non-CPAP therapies, with a significantly higher rate observed in patients who cleaned their devices inadequately [9].

The association between OSA and CRS has not been extensively studied. Chin *et al.* administered the chronic sinusitis survey (CSS) to OSA patients who were regular CPAP users and analyzed the relationship between CPAP reservoir culture positivity and CRS symptomatology based on CSS scores, finding no association between the two [10]. Of note, this group excluded patients with a known history of CRS, thus leaving a gap in our knowledge about how CPAP culture positivity may affect this subgroup of patients.

To our knowledge, no studies to date have examined the association between microbes present in the sinonasal cavities and CPAP machine reservoirs of patients with known diagnoses of both CRS and OSA. In this study, we first set out to establish the rate of CPAP reservoir culture positivity in patients with CRS. In addition, we aimed to compare bacterial culture results from sinonasal cavities and CPAP reservoirs of patients with both OSA and CRS to determine if an association existed.

2. Materials and Methods

After approval was obtained from the Institutional Review Board, study participants were identified at an academic tertiary care Rhinology practice using ICD-9 codes for obstructive sleep apnea and chronic rhinosinusitis. Patients were either contacted on the phone or met with a research assistant in clinic to determine if they met the inclusion criteria: age over 18 years, diagnosis of OSA by polysomnography, regular CPAP use (meaning use of the machine all night, every night and waking up with the machine still on and attached in correct postion), and an active diagnosis of CRS (not symptomatically controlled, with objective evidence via CT and/or nasal endoscopy of CRS). Exclusion criteria were: treatment with antibiotics or cleaning of the CPAP reservoir in the month prior to enrollment. If participants met criteria and were interested in participation they were prospectively enrolled in the study, gave written informed consent, and had cultures taken from their sinonasal cavities. If the patients had not been operated on in the past, the culture was taken from the middle meatus. If they had been operated on, a culture was taken directly from the diseased sinus. If participants were able to bring their CPAP reservoirs in, cultures were taken from the hydration chambers of the machines at that time as well. Otherwise, patients were given a culture swab with instructions on how to culture their CPAP reservoirs and return the swab for laboratory testing.

Both sets of swabs from each patient were cultured and results of speciation were recorded. Swabs were transported in Amies gel medium, appropriate for both aerobic and anaerobic growth. Resulting microbial growth from sinonasal cavity samples for each patient were compared to microbial growth from that individual's CPAP reservoir. Cultures were reported in a standard 1+ through 4+ fashion based on the common practice of cultures being inoculated onto media using a sterile loop that sequentially dilutes the specimen from the first area or quadrant of the medium to the last area or quadrant. Results are then reported depending on which areas or quadrants demonstrate bacterial growth with 4+ showing bacterial growth even with the most dilute concentration of specimen. Specimens were processed on the day of submission.

3. Results

Ten patients meeting inclusion criteria were enrolled in the study and nine had both sinonasal and CPAP reservoir samples obtained. Of these nine patients remaining at the conclusion of the study, seven (78%) were male and two (22%) were female. Mean age was 52 (range, 39–68 years), and four (44%) had undergone endoscopic sinus surgery in the past. All patients had undergone multiple courses of antibiotics previously (although none in the month leading up to the culture), including amoxicillin, amoxicillin with clavulanate, levofloxacin, ciprofloxacin, cephalexin, and doxycycline. All patients who had previously undergone sinus surgery had already been on CPAP prior to that intervention and continued to use it after the surgery.

The final culture results for the nine patients with both sets of samples taken are listed in Table 1. All nine CPAP reservoir samples displayed culture positivity. The most common organisms on CPAP culture were *Enterobacter cloacae*, *Acinetobacter baumanii*, *Candida parapsilosis*, and *Brevidimonas diminuta*. All sinus cultures were also positive, but with differing organisms. The most common on sinus culture were *Staphyloccoccus aureus*, *Staphlococcus epidermidis*, and *Pseudomonas aeruginosa*. Speciation of microbial growth from sinonasal samples was not associated with CPAP reservoir growth in any of the nine study participants.

Table 1. CPAP reservoir and sinonasal culture results.

Patient	CPAP Reservoir Culture	Sinonasal Sample
1	1+ *Enterobacter cloacae* 3+ *Burkholderia cepacia complex* 1+ *Staphylococcus coagulase negative* 1+ *Candida parapsilosis* 1+ *Rhodotorula mucilaginosa*	1+ *Staphylococcus aureus*
2	2+ *Enterobacter cloacae* 2+ *Brevundimonas diminuta*	2+ *Staphylococcus aureus* 1+ *Staphylococcus epidermidis*
3	1+ *Trichosporon asahii* 1+ *Serratia marascens*	4+ *Pseudomonas*
4	1+ *Acinetobacter baumanii*	2+ *Staphylococcus aureus*
5	2+ *Acinetobacter baumanii*	2+ *Staphylococcus aureus* 1+ *Staphylococcus epidermidis*
6	2+ *Candida parapsilosis*	2+ *Pseudomonas* 1+ *Staphylococcus epidermidis*
7	2+ *Enterobacter cloacae* 1+ *Brevundimonas diminuta*	2+ *Citrobacter koseri*
8	2+ *Enterobacter cloacae* 1+ *Acinetobacter baumanii*	2+ *Pneumococcus*
9	1+ *Enterobacter cloacae*	2+ *Staphylococcus aureus* 1+ *Pseudomonas*

4. Discussion

Though cultures of all CPAP machine reservoirs tested in our study produced bacterial growth, we found no association between bacterial colonization of the CPAP reservoir and the sinus cavities of patients with both CRS and OSA. This finding reflects that observed by Chin *et al.* with one major exception. Whereas Chin *et al.* found culture positivity in only 48.6% of CPAP reservoirs, we witnessed this phenomenon in 100% of our samples, albeit our sample size was small [10]. This finding lends evidence to the theory that the warm, moist environment of CPAP machine reservoirs is conducive to bacterial growth, but this microbial proliferation does not appear to have clinical relevance in relation to CRS.

In our study, the three most commonly observed microorganisms on sinus culture were *Staphyloccoccus aureus*, *Staphlococcus epidermidis*, and *Pseudomonas aeruginosa*. This finding is concordant with prior studies showing that the most common bacterial isolates in CRS patients undergoing endoscopic sinus surgery are coagulase-negative *Staphlococcus*, gram-negative rods, and *Staphylococcus aureus* [11,12]. Chin *et al.* found that the most commonly cultured organisms from CPAP reservoirs were gram-negative rods [10]. Consistent with the Chin study, three of the four most commonly cultured organisms from our study participants' CPAP reservoir samples (*Enterobacter cloacae*, *Acinetobacter baumanii*, and *Brevidimonas diminuta*) are classified as gram-negative rods.

The small sample size of our study is an important limitation. Although we cannot make any statistically significant conclusions regarding our data and results, our findings are certainly interesting, as no patient displayed any association between microbial growth cultured from their sinonasal samples and CPAP reservoirs. Our observations are similar to those of Lee *et al.*, who found that culture positivity of nasal irrigation bottle and fluid was not related to higher infection rates following endoscopic sinus surgery [13].

Another important limitation of this study stems from the growing knowledge we have of the sinus microbiome. Recent studies have shown a vast and diverse array of bacteria living within both normal and diseased sinuses, with many of these organisms not regularly identified on microbial culture [14–16]. Whether or not the bacteria found in the CPAP cultures may have joined this larger, less readily measurable population is unknown. The cost of PCR and other advanced techniques has generally limited full examination of the microbiome to research environments, and clinicians still rely heavily on culture results to drive therapy. In this study we chose to limit our investigation to the tool most commonly used clinically to search for bacterial growth, but certainly further study using those other tools may demonstrate more subtle additions or changes to the microbial environment of the sinuses in these patients.

Although we did not observe a direct association between microbial growth in CPAP reservoirs and sinonasal samples, proper care and cleaning of CPAP reservoirs should be emphasized to patients diagnosed with OSA, as prior evidence has shown that this population experiences an increased rate of upper airway infections [10]. As the development and perpetuation of CRS is still poorly understood, it may be possible that microbial growth from CPAP machines still plays a role in the etiology of CRS, perhaps by altering innate and/or adaptive immune response prior to the development of CRS. Additionally, given the subtypes of CRS and their varied responses to different therapies, we support the continued investigation of infectious sources for CRS symptoms, including culturing sinonasal samples and tailoring antibiotic choice to speciation and sensitivity results.

To our knowledge, this is the first study to examine the association between microbes present in the sinus cavities and CPAP machine reservoirs of patients with known diagnoses of both CRS and OSA. We found that culture results from both sinonasal and CPAP reservoir samples reflected data published in the literature about which microbes are most typical in these settings, lending credibility to our study despite its small sample size. We conclude it is unlikely, in OSA patients suffering CRS symptoms, that the bacteria growing in their CPAP machine is leading to the development or perpetuation of their CRS.

5. Conclusions

We found no association between microbial culture of the CPAP reservoirs and the sinus cavities of patients with dual diagnoses of CRS and OSA. Further study looking more deeply into the microbiome with enhanced tools for measuring bacterial growth may further our knowledge of this subset of patients.

Acknowledgments: Rosa Lipin: No financial disclosures; Anita Deshpande: No financial disclosures; Sarah Wise: Greer Laboratories—Scientific Advisory Board, Genentech, Research funding; John DelGaudio: No financial disclosures; Zara Patel: No financial disclosures.

Author Contributions: Z.M.P. and R.B.L. conceived and designed the study; R.B.L. and A.D. performed the study; Z.M.P., R.B.L. and A.D. analyzed the data; S.K.W. and J.M.D. contributed patients and played a major role in editing of the manuscript; Z.M.P. wrote the manuscript; R.B.L., Z.M.P., A.D., S.K.W. and J.M.D. all contributed to revising and editing of the manuscript.

Conflicts of Interest: The authors declare no conflict of interest.

References

1. Rosenfeld, R.M.; Piccirillo, J.F.; Chandrasekhar, S.S.; Brook, I.; Kumar, K.A.; Kramper, M.; Orlandi, R.R.; Palmer, J.N.; Patel, Z.M.; Peters, A.; *et al*. Clinical practice guideline (update) adult sinusitis. *Otolaryngol. Head Neck Surg.* **2015**, *152*, 1–39. [CrossRef] [PubMed]

2. Ray, N.; Baraniuk, J.; Thamer, M. Healthcare expenditures for sinusitis in 1996: Contributions of asthma, rhinitis, and other airway disorders. *J. Allergy Clin. Immunol.* **1999**, *103*, 408–414. [CrossRef]

3. Manes, R.; Bhatra, P. Etiology, diagnosis and management of chronic rhinosinusitis. *Expert Rev. Anti. Infect. Ther.* **2013**, *11*, 25–35. [CrossRef] [PubMed]

4. Cain, R.; Lal, D. Update on the management of chronic rhinosinusitis. *Infect. Drug Resist.* **2013**, *6*, 1–14. [PubMed]

5. Basner, R. Continuous positive airway pressure for obstructive sleep apnea. *N. Engl. J. Med.* **2007**, *17*, 1751–1758. [CrossRef] [PubMed]

6. Kapur, V.; Blough, D.K.; Sandblom, R.E.; Hert, R.; de Maine, J.B.; Sullivan, S.D.; Psaty, B.M. The medical cost of undiagnosed sleep apnea. *Sleep* **1999**, *22*, 749–755. [PubMed]

7. Massie, C.A.; Hart, R.W.; Peralez, K.; Richards, G.N. Effects of humidification on nasal symptoms and compliance in sleep apnea patients using continuous positive airway pressure. *Chest* **1999**, *116*, 403–408. [CrossRef] [PubMed]

8. Wiest, G.H.; Lehnert, G.; Brück, W.M.; Meyer, M.; Hahn, E.G.; Ficker, J.H. A heated humidifier reduces upper airway dryness during continuous positive airway pressure therapy. *Respir. Med.* **1999**, *93*, 21–26. [CrossRef]

9. Sanner, B.M.; Fluerenbrock, N.; Kleiber-Imbeck, A.; Mueller, J.B.; Zidek, W. Effect of continuous positive airway pressure therapy on infectious complication in patients with obstructive sleep apnea syndrome. *Respiration* **2001**, *68*, 483–487. [CrossRef] [PubMed]

10. Chin, C.J.; George, C.; Lannigan, R.; Rotenberg, B.W. Association CPAP bacterial colonization with chronic rhinosinusitis. *J. Clin. Sleep Med.* **2013**, *9*, 747–750. [CrossRef] [PubMed]

11. Nadel, D.; Lanza, D.; Kennedy, D. Endoscopically guided cultures in chronic sinusitis. *Am. J. Rhinol.* **1998**, *12*, 233–241. [CrossRef] [PubMed]

12. Kingdom, T.; Swain, R. The microbiology and antimicrobial resistancepatterns in chronic rhinosinusitis. *Am. J. Otolaryngol.* **2004**, *25*, 323–328. [CrossRef] [PubMed]

13. Lee, J.M.; Nayak, J.V.; Doghramji, L.L.; Welch, K.C.; Chiu, A.G. Assessing the risk of irrigation bottle and fluid contamination after endoscopic sinus surgery. *Am. J. Rhinol. Allergy* **2010**, *24*, 197–199. [CrossRef] [PubMed]

14. Ramakrishnan, V.R.; Feazel, L.M.; Gitomer, S.A.; Ir, D.; Robertson, C.E.; Frank, D.N. The microbiome of the middle meatus in healthy adults. *PLoS ONE* **2013**, *8*, e85507. [CrossRef] [PubMed]

15. Hauser, L.J.; Feazel, L.M.; Ir, D.; Fang, R.; Wagner, B.D.; Robertson, C.E.; Frank, D.N.; Ramakrishnan, V.R. Sinus culture poorly predicts resident microbiota. *Int. Forum Allergy Rhinol.* **2015**, *5*, 3–9. [CrossRef] [PubMed]

16. Ramakrishnan, V.R.; Hauser, L.J.; Feazel, L.M.; Ir, D.; Robertson, C.E.; Frank, D.N. Sinus microbiota varies among chronic rhinosinusitis phenotypes and predicts surgical outcomes. *J. Allergy Clin. Immunol.* **2015**, *136*, 334–342. [PubMed]

2

Sinusitis and Respiratory Disease at Pediatric Age

Francisco Muñoz-López [1,2]

[1]   Pediatric Immunology Center, Barcelona 08028, Spain

[2]   Former Head of the Department of Pediatric Immunoallergology, Hospital Clinic, Faculty of Medicine, University of Barcelona, Barcelona 08028, Spain; 5314fml@comb.cat

Academic Editor: César Picado

Abstract: Here, we present a review of the development of paranasal sinuses and pathologies associated to them, allergic and/or infectious sinusitis, in children. A review of 200 medical records of children and adolescents affected with respiratory disease is carried out. 66 patients (33%) were diagnosed with sinusitis, six of which did not present any other respiratory processes. Of the remainder, association with rhinitis, asthma, or wheezy bronchitis, and one case with immune deficiency, was found. Other associated pathologies, such as cystic fibrosis, bronchiectasis, and other processes described as associated with sinusitis, were not detected in any case.

Keywords: sinusitis; rhinitis; asthma; wheezy bronchitis; children; adolescents

1. Introduction

The first step in the study of any child with repeated respiratory processes, either in the upper airways or the tracheobronchial tree, is to ascertain the state of the paranasal sinuses. The examination should be carried out at a very early age, even from the first year in which the maxillary sinuses are sufficiently developed to be seen on a properly executed radiological examination, in which signs of inflammation that might be responsible for recurrent clinical picture may be evident.

Nearly two-thirds of children with recurrent spastic bronchopaties suffer from sinusitis; this occurs at a rate approximately equal in children with extrinsic bronchial asthma to those with wheezy bronchitis.

It is well known that the paranasal sinuses are not fully developed during infancy, but evolve during childhood, with a time line that differs among the various sinus pairs. This asynchrony conditions their pathology and special features in childhood.

The maxillary sinuses are already visible in the 3rd–4th month of intrauterine life, as well as the ethmoidal sinuses, as an out-pouching of the mucous membrane of the nasal meatus, reaching $7 \times 4 \times 4$ mm in size at birth, with an annual increase of about 2 mm high and 3 mm in the anteroposterior direction. With these measures, the maxillary sinuses are already radiologically visible from the second year of age, just like the ethmoidal sinuses, and are susceptible to an early disease, while the frontal sinuses evolve more slowly and it is not until 3–6 years of age that their image can be seen [1,2]. The maxillary sinus communicates with the nasal cavity through a small hole, through which the mucus secretion produced by various glands drains.

Due to this early development, the maxillary sinuses together with the ethmoidal sinuses are susceptible to sickness more often in younger children, with a clear net predominance of the former given their anatomical location. They share symptoms common to many diverse processes that must be taken into consideration in the differential diagnosis.

Maxillary sinusitis can be a single entity of infectious cause, but we must not forget that the mucosa of the sinuses is part of the lining of the entire respiratory tree and therefore often coincides with rhinitis (rhinosinusitis) or with asthma, having found that up to 73% of children between 2 and 6 years of age with allergic pathology can suffer from long-evolution maxillary sinusitis [3,4].

2. Symptomatology

The symptoms of sinusitis in children, mostly of the maxillary location, are essentially different from those found in adults. They are not so intense or severe, but manifests themselves with a latent focus, often because of recurrence of infectious processes of the upper respiratory tract and even the bronchial tree. For this reason, the discovery of sinusitis in children is often the result of a routine examination carried out in cases of bronchial or recurrent infection of the upper airways or of persistent and nocturnal cough [5–7].

The more specific symptoms include persistent rhinorrhea, which, if unilateral and accompanied by mucus-pus, indicates the possibility of bacterial sinusitis. If it is bilateral and accompanied by mucus fluid, it may correspond to allergic rhinosinupathy.

Nocturnal cough, sometimes afflicting these children, may be caused by sinus secretion that drains more easily from the cavity with the lateral or supine decubitus adopted during sleep.

Unlike in adults, headache in children is exceptional because frontal sinusitis is more common in the former.

Ethmoidal sinusitis, which may affect the infant, results in palpebral edema, particularly affecting the lower eyelid unilaterally. It is very typically due to its paranasal location.

General symptoms include paleness, anemia, and anorexia, common signs of any long-term infection, such as sinusitis. These symptoms that go with repeated respiratory infections should lead to an investigation of a possible sinupathy.

Symptoms rarely resemble those found in adults. They are characterized by intensity and are further evidence of local symptoms, particularly with respect to the classic painful points; this occurs more in older children, except in ethmoid sinusitis, which can affect the infant, as we already mentioned, appearing with obvious intensity and signs of severity [8].

3. Diagnosis

Due to its frequency, prolonged coughing would raise suspicion of maxillary sinusitis, which is confirmed by viewing an image of the sinuses. Traditionally, radiology has been enough to get demonstrative images with a classic Waters' occipito-mental projection or other positions, even in very young children. More recently, other less risky techniques, such as computed tomography or magnetic resonance imaging, have been introduced. High-definition computed tomography (CT) scans allow for tomographic slices in coronal and axial direction, which display in great detail and at the same time, both the bone structure and the soft tissue, including the sinusal mucosa. However, a study of 134 patients by radiology (Water' projection) and CT demonstrate that plain radiography has a sensitivity of 68% and a specificity of 87%. In definitive, this and other studies show that the diagnostic performances of Waters' projection are able to maintain a role for radiography in the diagnosis. On the other hand, magnetic resonance imaging provides data in three dimensions, offering very valuable information in doubtful cases, being especially useful for viewing ethmoidal and sphenoidal sinuses [9–13].

Despite the advantages of these techniques, the need to sedate young children, and economic reasons, make radiology has not lost ground, except when images are not enough to provide demonstration. Images show the thickening of the mucosa, the total or partial opacification of the sinus, liquid levels, mucous, and, more rarely, polyps or calcifications corresponding to other pathological facts. After appropriate treatment, it is advisable to check the disappearance of pathological signs previously observed.

Although some allergic children may suffer from allergic sinusitis several times (recurrent sinusitis), given this circumstance, it is necessary to ensure that there is no other diseases, as sinusitis may accompany various pathological processes that are only occasionally expressed by this local pathology. This can occur with selective IgA deficiency, also present in a large number of allergic patients (1/200 *vs.* 1/700 in the general population), and with transient hypogammaglobulinemia in childhood, which is usually compensated within five years of age. Other immunodeficiencies have a wider expression with serious infections of various localizations [14,15].

Another process to be considered is cystic fibrosis, in which it is common that both sinuses are filled by the increased viscosity of secretions, sometimes associated with polyposis. Other processes are rarer, such as Kartagener syndrome in which sinupathy is one of its features along with the situs inversus, bronchiectasis, and cilia immobility. In other clinical profiles, such as primary ciliary dyskinesia, polyposis, and alpha-1-antitrypsin, maxillary sinuses may be equally affected [16,17].

Consequently, given the high frequency of maxillary sinusitis in children with cough, bronchitis, or asthma, it is advisable to include paranasal sinuses X-rays in the diagnostic routine of these processes [4].

4. Clinical Study

In a review of 200 children, all with respiratory symptoms, we selected a total of 66 seen when they were aged between 15 months and 14 years and 7 months, and all were diagnosed with sinusitis (33%). In 30 of them, this was caused by an allergy. In 16 others, it was due to infection. The remaining 20 had mixed or uncertain origins. Only 6 of them showed no association with other respiratory processes (tracheobronchitis, asthma, wheezy bronchitis). In another 5, different allergic diseases (eczema, urticaria, food, medicament) were found, and only one patient was diagnosed with immunodeficiency, data collected in Table 1. The table also shows the number of patients whose serum variations of the various immunoglobulins were found, without a direct relationship of their variations of the three types of sinusitis mentioned above, except for those of allergic cause ($\uparrow$ IgE). In 9 cases, the levels were normal.

Table 1. Clinical and immunological study.

Family Precedent of Atopy: Parents, Grandparents	Age at Diagnosis	Other Respiratory Processes			Other Allergic Processes	Immuno-Deficiency	Immunoglobulins			
		Rhinitis	Asthma	Wheezing			IgE	IgG	IgM	IgA
34 cases	15 months–14 years/7 months	34	40	15	5	1	$\uparrow$ 50	$\uparrow$ 16 $\downarrow$ 13	$\uparrow$ 31 $\downarrow$ 0	$\uparrow$ 12 $\downarrow$ 5

For none of the patients was family history of respiratory processes listed as associated with sinusitis (cystic fibrosis, *etc.*), so the possible hereditary factor thereof was discarded.

In a previous study of 100 medical records of children under 18 years old visited consecutively, with symptoms suggestive of asthma, rhinitis, or other respiratory conditions (bronchopaties) mentioned above, it was found that 38% of them suffered from sinusitis, either as an exclusive process or linked to other respiratory disorders processes, as summarized in Table 2 [18].

Table 2. Summary of the study of 100 clinical cases.

	Preschool	School	Adolescent	Total
Rhinitis only	0	20	10	30
Asthma only	9	8	1	18
Asthma and rhinosinusitis	7	4	7	18
Bronchopathy only	11	3	0	14
Bronchopathy and rhinosinusitis	4	5	0	9
Rinosinusitis only	8	2	1	11
Total sinusitis (%)	**19 (48.7)**	**11 (26.1)**	**8 (42.1)**	**100**
Total sinusitis: 38%				

5. Conclusions

In both studies, the high incidence of sinusitis in children is confirmed. It was predominant in smaller children—as the sole condition in some of them; in others, with rhinitis, asthma, or other respiratory conditions—but in none was found the existence of other processes that have been linked to the existence of sinupathy, such as the aforementioned bronchiectasis, cystic fibrosis, Kartagener syndrome, *etc*. Nevertheless, we have seen partial deficits of some immunoglobulins, which could facilitate the infectious cause of sinusitis.

In short, the high frequency of sinusitis, alone or linked to other respiratory conditions, requires appropriate testing. Radiology is the easiest and sometimes sufficient; however, if necessary, other techniques mentioned (computed tomography or magnetic resonance imaging) could be used in all children who present symptoms suggestive of sinusitis.

Conflicts of Interest: The author declares no conflict of interest.

References

1. Adibelli, Z.H.; Songu, M.; Adibelli, H. Paranasal sinus development in children: A magnetic resonance imaging analysis. *Am. J. Rhinol. Allergy* **2011**, *25*, 30–35. [CrossRef] [PubMed]
2. Shah, R.K.; Dhingra, K.; Carter, B.L.; Rebeiz, E.E. Paranasal sinus development: A radiographic study. *Laryngoscope* **2003**, *113*, 205–209. [CrossRef] [PubMed]
3. Nguyen, K.L.; Corbet, M.L.; García, D.P.; Eberly, S.M.; Massey, E.N.; Le, H.T.; Shearer, L.T.; Karibo, J.M.; Pence, H.L. Chronic sinusitis among pediatric patients with chronic respiratory complaints. *J. Allergy Clin. Immunol.* **1993**, *92*, 824–830. [CrossRef]
4. Bachert, C.; Patou, J.; van Cauwenberge, P. The role of sinus disease in asthma. *Curr. Opin. Allergy Clin. Immunol.* **2006**, *6*, 29–36. [CrossRef] [PubMed]
5. McQuillan, L.; Crane, L.A.; Kempe, A. Diagnosis and management of acute sinusitis by pediatricians. *Pediatrics* **2009**, *123*, 193–198. [CrossRef] [PubMed]
6. Esposito, S.; Bosis, S.; Bellasio, M.; Proncipi, N. From clinical practice to guidelines; how to recognize rhinosinusitis in children. *Pediatr. Allergy Immunol.* **2007**, *18* (Suppl. S18), 53–55. [CrossRef] [PubMed]
7. Marseglia, G.L.; Castellazzi, A.M.; Licari, A.; Marseglia, A.; Leone, M.; Pagella, F.; Ciprandi, G.; Klersy, C. Inflammation of paranasal sinuses: The clinical pattern is age-dependent. *Pediatr. Allergy Immunol.* **2007**, *18* (Suppl. S18), 10–12. [CrossRef] [PubMed]
8. Kashani, S.; Carr, T.F.; Grammer, L.C.; Schleimer, R.P.; Hulse, K.E.; Kato, A.; Kern, R.C.; Conley, D.B.; Chandra, R.K.; Tan, B.K.; *et al.* Clinical characteristics of adults with chronic rhinosinusitis and specific antibody deficiency. *J. Allergy Clin. Immunol. Pract.* **2015**, *3*, 236–242. [CrossRef] [PubMed]
9. Kolawole, S.; Okuyemi, M.D.; Terance, T. Tsue. Radiologic imaging in the management of sinusitis. *Am. Fam. Phys.* **2002**, *10*, 1882–1886.
10. Triulzi, F.; Zipoli, S. Imaging techniques in the diagnosis and management of rhinosinusitis in children. *Pediatr. Allergy Immunol.* **2007**, *18* (Suppl. S18), 46–49. [CrossRef] [PubMed]
11. Leo, G.; Triulzi, F.; Consonni, D.; Cazzavillan, A.; Incorvaia, C. Reappraising the role of radiography in thr diagnosis of chronic rhinosinusitis. *Rhinology* **2009**, *47*, 271–274. [PubMed]
12. Konen, E.; Faibel, M.; Kleinbaum, Y.; Wolf, M.; Lusky, A.; Hoffman, C.; Eyal, A.; Tadmor, R. The value of the occipital (Waters') view in diagnosis of sinusitis: A comparative study with computed tomography. *Clin. Radiol.* **2000**, *55*, 856–860. [CrossRef] [PubMed]
13. Diament, M.J. The diagnosis of sinusitis in infants and children X-ray, computed tomography and magnetic resonance imaging. *J. Allergy Clin. Immunol.* **1992**, *90*, 442–444. [CrossRef]
14. Costa Carvalho, B.T.; Tiemi Nagao, A.; Arslanian, C.; Carneiro Sampaio, M.M.S.; Naspitz, C.H.K.; Sorensen, R.U.; Solé, D. Immunological evaluation of allergic respirtory children with recurrent sinusitis. *Pediatr. Allergy Immunol.* **2005**, *16*, 534–538. [CrossRef] [PubMed]
15. Guilemany, J.M.; Mullol, J.; Picado, C. Relaciones entre rinosinusitis y bronquiectasias. *Arch. Bronconeumol.* **2006**, *42*, 135–140. [CrossRef] [PubMed]

16. Antunes, J.; Fernandes, A.; Miguel-Borrego, L.; Leiria-Pinto, P.; Cavaco, J. Cystic fibrosis, atopy asthma and ABPA. *Allergol. Immunopathol.* **2010**, *38*, 278–284. [CrossRef] [PubMed]

17. Berdon, W.E.; Willi, U. Situs inversus, bronchiectasis and sinusitis its relation to immotile cilia history of the diseases and their discovers—Manes Kartagener and Bjorn Afzelius. *Pediatr. Rinol.* **2004**, *34*, 38–42.

18. Muñoz-López, F. Sinusitis asociada a patología respiratoria alérgica. *Rev. Esp. Pediatr.* **2012**, *69*, 74–78.

3

Are Chronic Rhinosinusitis and Paranasal Sinus Pneumatization Related?

Michael J. Marino [1], Charles A. Riley [1], Eric L. Wu [1], Jacqueline E. Weinstein [1] and Edward D. McCoul [1,2,3,*]

[1]   Department of Otolaryngology-Head and Neck Surgery, Tulane University School of Medicine, New Orleans, LA 70112, USA; mike.j.marino@gmail.com (M.J.M); criley2@tulane.edu (C.A.R.); ewu2@tulane.edu (E.L.W.); jacquelinecaputi@gmail.com (J.E.W.)

[2]   Department of Otorhinolaryngology, Ochsner Clinic Foundation, New Orleans, LA 70121, USA

[3]   Ochsner Clinical School, University of Queensland School of Medicine, New Orleans, LA 70121, USA

*   Correspondence: emccoul@gmail.com

Academic Editor: César Picado

Abstract: The relationship between paranasal sinus pneumatization and chronic rhinosinusitis (CRS) without cystic fibrosis is not well understood. Previous investigations have confirmed sinus hypoplasia in cystic fibrosis (CF) patients. This study compares paranasal sinus pneumatization of CRS patients to unaffected controls to determine if there is an analogous effect to that seen in CF. 591 sinus computed tomography (CT) scans, comprised of 303 adolescents (age 13–18) and 288 adults (age > 18), were analyzed for Lund-MacKay and Assessment of Pneumatization of the Paranasal Sinuses (APPS) scores. The APPS score is validated for measuring the extent of sinus pneumatization. A diagnosis of CRS and CRS phenotype was determined from the medical record. The mean APPS score for patients with a diagnosis of CRS was 10.61 ($n = 111$) compared to 9.62 ($n = 448$) for unaffected controls ($p = 0.001$). This was significant in adult ($p = 0.021$) and adolescent subgroups ($p = 0.035$). Sinus pneumatization did not differ according to CRS phenotype ($p = 0.699$). This suggests that there is not analogous anatomical sinus variation between CRS and CF, and that the mechanisms underlying sinus hypoplasia in CF may not be universal in patients with other types of sinus inflammation.

Keywords: pneumatization; paranasal sinuses; computed tomography; chronic rhinosinusitis; cystic fibrosis

1. Introduction

The relationship of paranasal sinus pneumatization with chronic rhinosinusitis (CRS) has been incompletely studied. Among cystic fibrosis (CF) patients, for whom sinus mucosal inflammation is nearly universal [1,2], sinus hypoplasia is well documented [2–6]. Because of these findings in CF, it has been suggested that mucosal disease and infection may lead to arrested sinus development [6–8]. Previous studies using radiographic instruments have been successful at differentiating sinus hypoplasia in CF [3–5], but have not been able to discern a difference in CRS without CF from unaffected controls [4,6].

Studying paranasal sinus pneumatization in CRS has been hindered by the lack of a validated measure for sinus pneumatization. The instruments used to discern sinus hypoplasia in previous studies of CF patients are incompletely validated for use in a general population of sinus computed tomography (CT) scans [3–5]. Furthermore, volumetric or dimensional analysis of sinus CT tends to be too cumbersome for the large populations that may be necessary to detect small differences [6]. The Assessment of Pneumatization of the Paranasal Sinuses (APPS) score was recently validated for evaluating the extent of sinus pneumatization [9,10]. The APPS score evaluates for the presence of nine anatomic variants bilaterally (Table 1, Figure 1), and can be used for clinician assessment of paranasal sinus pneumatization. This method of determining the extent of sinus pneumatization has not been previously applied to CF or CRS patients.

Table 1. APPS Score Items.

Item	Anatomic Variant
1	Maxillary floor inferior to nasal floor
2	Supraorbital cell (Air cell superior to anterior ethmoid artery)
3	Middle turbinate concha bullosa presen
4	Frontal sinus present
5	Superior frontal sinus wall superior to supraorbital rim
6	Lateral frontal sinus wall lateral to medial edge of globe
7	Lateral frontal sinus wall lateral to mid-pupillary line
8	Lateral sphenoid sinus wall lateral to V_2-VN line
9	Anterior clinoid process pneumatized

APPS = Assessment of Pneumatization of the Paranasal Sinuses; V_2 = Maxillary nerve canal; VN = Vidian nerve canal.

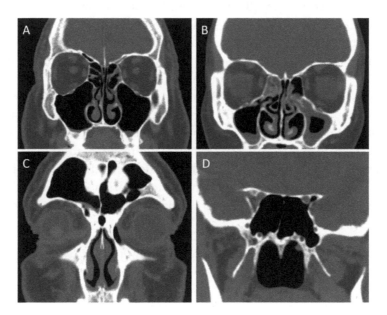

Figure 1. The nine APPS parameters are demonstrated in these radiographic examples. (**A**) The bilateral maxillary floor is pneumatized inferior to the nasal floor and the bilateral supraorbital cell is present superior to the anterior ethmoid artery; (**B**) Bilateral concha bullosa is present; (**C**) The bilateral frontal sinuses are present, superior to the supraorbital rim, and lateral to both the medial edge of the globe and midpupillary line; (**D**) The left anterior clinoid process is pneumatized and there is pneumatization lateral to a line drawn from the maxillary nerve canal to the Vidian nerve canal on the left. APPS: Assessment of Pneumatization of the Paranasal Sinuses.

The purpose of this study was to apply the APPS score to a large population of CRS patients and healthy controls in order to determine if paranasal sinus pneumatization differs between these two groups. Understanding sinus pneumatization in CRS patients might help to understand if sinus disease and anatomy are related in a generalizable way.

2. Materials and Methods

Sinus and maxillofacial CT scans performed at the Ochsner Clinic Foundation were considered for inclusion in the study. An adolescent cohort ($n = 303$), defined as patients age 13–18 at the date of service, was assembled from all CT scans performed between 1 January 2010 and 31 December 2014. Only scans with axial and coronal orientations available were included. A similarly-sized cohort of adults (n = 288), defined as patients over 18 years of age, was assembled for all sinus and maxillofacial CT scans acquired from 6 July 2015 to 6 August 2015. All CT scans were evaluated for APPS and Lund-Mackay scores. A diagnosis of CRS or CF, as determined by the treating physician, was then retrospectively gathered from the medical record for each scored CT scan. CRS phenotype was also determined and recorded as chronic rhinosinusitis with nasal polyposis (CRSwNP), chronic rhinosinusitis without nasal polyposis (CRSsNP), or allergic fungal rhinosinusitis (AFRS). The diagnosis of CRS or CF was assigned independent of Lund-MacKay score. Patients without a diagnosis of CRS or CF were included in the unaffected control group. CT scans in the control group were typically acquired for the evaluation of facial trauma without positive findings, or as part of the diagnostic workup to rule out CRS in the primary care setting. Radiographic scoring and diagnostic information were stored in a secure, web-based Research Electronic Data Capture (REDCap) database (version 6.6.2, REDCap, Nashville, TN, USA) for management and analysis [11].

The CRS and CF groups were compared to the unaffected control group for both APPS and Lund-Mackay scores. Subgroup analysis was then performed for each comparison within both the adolescent and adult subgroups. Separate analysis was conducted within the CRS population for patients with a Lund-Mackay score ≥3, while the control population was limited to individuals with a Lund-Mackay score <3. This value was selected for restricting the two groups since it has previously been described as the incidental score [12,13]. The incidental score was determined from patients without sinonasal disorders or facial skeletal trauma [12,13], and reflects the degree of sinus opacification that may be encountered in healthy subjects. Continuous variables were analyzed using two-sample independent t-tests. One-way analysis of variance was used when more than two groups were compared simultaneously. p-values less than 0.05 were considered significant. Statistical analysis was performed using SAS software (version 9.3, SAS Institute Inc., Cary, NC, USA). The study was approved by the Institutional Research Board of the Ochsner Clinic Foundation.

3. Results

Demographic data for the total study population and each of the subgroups is presented in Table 2. There were no significant age differences between the CRS cohort and the control group for the total study population, or for the adult and adolescent subgroups. The CF cohort was significantly younger than controls within the adult subgroup ($p < 0.001$), but there were no statistical age differences in the total study population or the adolescent subgroup. There were no significant gender differences between the CRS group and controls for the total study population or within the adolescent subgroup. The adult subgroup, however, had significantly more males in the CRS population compared to controls ($p = 0.004$). No significant gender differences were found between the CF cohort and controls for the total study population, or within the adult and adolescent subgroups. APPS scores in the entire study group were normally distributed with a mean score of 9.47 and standard deviation of 3.43. Therefore 95% of all scores were between 3 and 16.

APPS scores were significantly higher for CRS patients compared to unaffected controls, and this effect was preserved within both the adult and adolescent subgroups (Table 3). When the CRS group was restricted to patients with a Lund-Mackay score ≥3 and the control group was restricted to Lund-Mackay scores <3, the CRS group again had a higher mean APPS score (Table 4). This result reached significance in the adult and adolescent subgroups. According to the normal distribution of APPS scores, the mean CRS score was in the 63rd percentile of all subjects. Subgroup analysis by CRS phenotype did not reveal any statistical difference of sinus pneumatization between patients with CRSwNP, CRSsNP, and AFRS, a finding that was consistent among adults and adolescents (Table 5). CF patients were found to have decreased sinus pneumatization by the APPS score when compared to healthy controls (Table 6). Subgroup analysis of adults and adolescents was also significant for sinus hypoplasia in the CF group. The mean APPS score in CF patients was in the 4th percentile of all subjects. As expected, Lund-Mackay scores were higher in the CRS and CF groups compared to unaffected control patients (Tables 3 and 6).

Table 2. Demographic Characteristics of Study Population.

Subjects	Unaffected Controls	CRS	CF	Total
Total Study Patients	448	111	32	591
Mean Age ± SD	32.42 + 22.77	36.96 ± 22.13	26.28 ± 10.33	32.94 ± 22.26
Males	224 (50.0%)	64 (57.7%)	17 (53.1%)	305 (51.6%)
Females	224 (50.0%)	47 (42.3%)	15 (46.9%)	286 (48.4%)
Adolescent Patients	247	47	9	303
Mean Age ± SD	15.82 ± 1.41	15.96 ± 1.43	15.56 ± 1.42	15.83 ± 1.41
Males	145 (58.7%)	26 (55.3%)	4 (44.4%)	175 (57.8%)
Females	102 (41.3%)	21 (44.7%)	5 (55.6%)	128 (42.2%)
Adult Patients	201	64	23	288
Mean Age ± SD	52.81 ± 19.97	52.39 ± 16.80	30.48 ± 9.17	50.93 ± 19.56
Males	79 (39.3%)	38 (59.4%)	13 (56.5%)	130 (45.1%)
Females	122 (60.7%)	26 (40.6%)	10 (43.5%)	158 (54.9%)

CRS = Chronic rhinosinusitis without cystic fibrosis; CF = Cystic fibrosis; SD = Standard deviation.

Table 3. APPS and LMS in the CRS population.

Subjects	Unaffected Controls	CRS	p-Value
APPS (All Patients) ± SD	9.62 ± 3.19	10.61 ± 2.76	0.001
LMS (All Patients) ± SD	2.15 ± 2.51	6.28 ± 5.14	<0.001
APPS (Adolescents) ± SD	9.57 ± 3.24	10.66 ± 3.13	0.035
LMS (Adolescents) ± SD	2.09 ± 2.52	6.09 ± 5.13	<0.001
APPS (Adults) ± SD	9.69 ± 3.14	10.58 ± 2.48	0.021
LMS (Adults) ± SD	2.22 ± 2.51	6.42 ± 5.18	<0.001

CRS = Chronic rhinosinusitis without cystic fibrosis; APPS = Assessment of Pneumatization of the Paranasal Sinuses score; LMS = Lund-Mackay score; SD = Standard deviation.

Table 4. APPS between study groups restricted by LMS.

Subjects	Unaffected Controls with LMS < 3	CRS with LMS ≥ 3	p-Value
APPS (All Patients) ± SD	9.23 ± 3.24 ($n = 304$)	10.79 ± 2.66 ($n = 84$)	<0.001
APPS (Adolescents) ± SD	9.21 ± 3.26 ($n = 169$)	10.68 ± 3.36 ($n = 34$)	0.018
APPS (Adults) ± SD	9.25 ± 3.22 ($n = 135$)	10.86 ± 2.09 ($n = 50$)	<0.001

CRS = Chronic rhinosinusitis without cystic fibrosis; APPS = Assessment of Pneumatization of the Paranasal Sinuses score; LMS = Lund-Mackay score; SD = Standard deviation.

Table 5. APPS by CRS Phenotype.

Subjects	CRSwNP	CRSsNP	AFRS	p-Value
APPS (All Patients) ± SD	10.29 ± 1.96 ($n = 35$)	10.77 ± 3.13 ($n = 71$)	10.60 ± 2.07 ($n = 5$)	0.699
APPS (Adolescents) ± SD	9.86 ± 2.30 ($n = 13$)	10.97 ± 3.37 ($n = 34$)	$n = 0$	0.277
APPS (Adults) ± SD	10.56 ± 1.74 ($n = 22$)	10.59 ± 2.92 ($n = 37$)	10.60 ± 2.07 ($n = 5$)	1.000

APPS = Assessment of Pneumatization of the Paranasal Sinuses score; CRS = Chronic rhinosinusitis; CRSwNP = Chronic rhinosinusitis with nasal polyposis; CRSsNP = Chronic rhinosinusitis without nasal polyposis; AFRS = Allergic fungal rhinosinusitis; SD = Standard deviation.

Table 6. APPS and LMS in the CF population.

Subjects	Unaffected Controls	CF	p-Value
APPS (All Patients) ± SD	9.62 ± 3.19	3.50 ± 2.92	<0.001
LMS (All Patients) ± SD	2.15 ± 2.51	12.44 ± 3.87	<0.001
APPS (Adolescents) ± SD	9.57 ± 3.24	4.00 ± 2.92	<0.001
LMS (Adolescents) ± SD	2.09 ± 2.52	13.22 ± 3.49	<0.001
APPS (Adults) ± SD	9.69 ± 3.14	3.30 ± 2.96	<0.001
LMS (Adults) ± SD	2.22 ± 2.51	12.13 ± 4.04	<0.001

CF = Cystic fibrosis; APPS = Assessment of Pneumatization of the Paranasal Sinuses score; LMS = Lund-Mackay score; SD = Standard deviation.

4. Discussion

There appears to be wide variation in paranasal sinus anatomy [14,15], but the cause for these differences and their impact on sinonasal disease is unclear. CF is associated with sinus hypoplasia [2–5], and is frequently associated with chronic sinus disease [1,2]. This raises the relevant question of whether the relationship between sinus pneumatization and mucosal disease can applied as a generalization. This remains incompletely resolved because paranasal sinus pneumatization has been difficult to quantify. Furthermore, while sinus hypoplasia tends to be dramatic in CF, anatomical differences in other disease processes may be more subtle.

Previous studies indicate that while sinus hypoplasia is present in CF, this effect may be independent of mucosal disease. A porcine model of CF indicated that impaired sinus development was present in utero, prior to clinical sinus disease [2]. Woodworth et al. found that CF patients with homozygous delta F508 mutations had more pronounced underdevelopment of the paranasal sinuses compared to patients with other mutations of the cystic fibrosis transmembrane conductance regulator (CFTR) gene [3]. Delta F508 homozygosity has also been associated with increased, rather than impaired, temporal bone pneumatization [4]. Overall, these findings suggest that mucosal disease is not a sufficient condition alone to explain impaired paranasal sinus development, and genetic abnormalities may underlie sinus hypoplasia.

The role of decreased paranasal sinus pneumatization in the development of CRS is also unclear. Kim et al. found that CRS patients had similar paranasal sinus pneumatization compared to healthy controls, although CF patients demonstrated impaired sinus development [6]. That study, however, was restricted to volumetric and dimensional analysis of the maxillary sinus in children and adolescents, age 4 to 17. In a study of frontal sinus coronal CT, Meyer et al. indicated that the presence of frontal cells was associated with middle turbinate concha bullosa and hyperpneumatizion of the frontal sinus [16]. Frontal cells were also found to be associated with increased frontal sinus mucosal thickening [16]. Alternatively, there have been reports of decreased maxillary sinus volume in patients with CRS [17,18]. These studies, however, did not measure the volumes of the other paranasal sinuses or did not find differences outside of the maxillary sinus. On the whole, sinus hypoplasia does not appear to be a universal factor in the development of sinusitis.

In the present study, CRS is associated with increased paranasal sinus pneumatization compared to unaffected controls. This further supports other work suggesting that mucosal disease may not be a sufficient condition for the development of sinus hypoplasia [2–4]. Our findings also indicate that impaired sinus pneumatization is not a universal factor in the development of sinusitis, and is consistent with some previous studies of CRS patients [6,16]. Paranasal sinus pneumatization was not different between CRS phenotypes (Table 5). The finding of increased pneumatization does not appear to be restricted to patients with CRSwNP and AFRS where expansile disease might lead to bony remodeling. The novel approach used to quantify paranasal sinus pneumatization, however, distinguishes this study from prior work. Because the APPS score can be performed quickly, this was applied to a large population in order to detect subtle differences between CRS patients and healthy controls. The APPS score is also a comprehensive instrument of variations affecting each of the four paired paranasal sinuses, and is validated for rater reliability. Previous studies have been limited to individual anatomical variations [16], or volumetric and dimensional analysis of individual sinuses [6,17,18]. Finally, the APPS score simultaneously estimates total paranasal sinus volume, and lower scores are indicative of impaired development globally [10].

A limitation of this study is that the diagnosis of CRS was discerned retrospectively. Because numerous practitioners, with differing qualifications across a large health system, made the diagnosis, there was likely some degree of inconsistency. While CT findings alone are not diagnostic for CRS, 144 patients who did not have a diagnosis of CRS were found to have Lund-Mackay scores ≥3. Conversely, 27 patients who were diagnosed with CRS had Lund-Mackay scores <3. Nevertheless, the APPS score has only been validated recently and could be easily applied to an existing population for initial impressions on paranasal sinus pneumatization in CRS. The findings were also consistent in a subgroup of patients with both a diagnosis of CRS and radiographic evidence of disease, compared to a cohort without a diagnosis of CRS and no radiographic evidence of disease. Future studies would benefit from a cross-sectional or prospective design for assigning the diagnosis of CRS, and restricting the assignment of that diagnosis to a single physician or group of physicians with advanced training in rhinology. Furthermore, future study would benefit from more sophisticated classification of CRS, rather than the somewhat simplistic delineation of phenotypes according to CRSwNP, CRSsNP, and AFRS. Severe Chronic Upper Airway Disease (SCUAD) has been described to highlight that complex pathophysiological mechanisms contribute to sinonasal mucosal inflammatory disease [19]. Observed anatomical differences may be a manifestation of disease categorization that is only recently being acknowledged. Another limitation of this study is that in the adult subgroup there were significantly more males than females in the CRS group compared to the control population (Table 2). This may confound the finding that CRS patients have increased sinus pneumatization, since this might be attributable to male gender. The result, however, was reproducible in the adolescent subgroup and total study population, in which there were no significant differences in gender between the CRS population and unaffected patients.

5. Conclusions

Paranasal sinus anatomy in patients with CRS, particularly those without CF, has been incompletely studied. CRS is found to be associated with increased paranasal sinus pneumatization compared to unaffected controls when assessed with a comprehensive and validated clinical metric. This is opposite the pneumatization patterns detected in patients with CF. Therefore, it does not seem that generalizable conclusions can be made about the relationship between inflammatory mucosal disease and paranasal sinus pneumatization.

Acknowledgments: The authors thank Martha Gastanaduy, BA, MPH, for biostatistical consultation.

Author Contributions: Michael J. Marino, study design, data collection, statistical analysis, drafting, final approval, accountability for all aspects of the work; Charles A. Riley, study design, data collection, drafting, final approval, accountability for all aspects of the work; Jacqueline E. Weinstein and Eric L. Wu, data collection, drafting, final approval, accountability for all aspects of the work; Edward D. McCoul, study design, revision, final approval, accountability for all aspects of the work.

Conflicts of Interest: The authors declare no conflict of interest.

References

1. Wine, J.J.; King, V.V.; Lewiston, N.J. Method for rapid evaluation of topically applied agents to cystic fibrosis airways. *Am. J. Physiol.* **1991**, *261*, L218–L221. [PubMed]
2. Chang, E.H.; Pezzulo, A.A.; Meyerholz, D.K.; Potash, A.E.; Wallen, T.J.; Reznikov, L.R.; Sieren, J.C.; Karp, P.H.; Ernst, S.; Moninger, T.O.; et al. Sinus hypoplasia precedes sinus infection in a porcine model of cystic fibrosis. *Laryngoscope* **2012**, *122*, 1898–1905. [CrossRef] [PubMed]
3. Woodworth, B.A.; Ahn, C.; Flume, P.A.; Schlosser, R.J. The delta F508 mutation in cystic fibrosis and impact on sinus development. *Am. J. Rhinol.* **2007**, *21*, 122–127. [CrossRef] [PubMed]

4. Seifert, C.M.; Harvey, R.J.; Matthews, J.W.; Meyer, T.A.; Ahn, C.; Woodworth, B.A.; Schlosser, R.J. Temporal bone pneumatization and its relationship to paranasal sinus development in cystic fibrosis. *Rhinology* **2010**, *48*, 233–238. [CrossRef] [PubMed]

5. Eggesbo, H.B.; Sovik, S.; Dolvik, S.; Eiklid, K.; Kolmannskog, F. Proposal of a CT scoring system of the paranasal sinuses in diagnosing cystic fibrosis. *Eur. Radiol.* **2003**, *13*, 1451–1460. [PubMed]

6. Kim, H.J.; Friedman, E.M.; Sulek, M.; Duncan, N.O.; McCluggage, C. Paranasal sinus development in chronic sinusitis, cystic fibrosis, and normal comparison population: A computed tomography correlation study. *Am. J. Rhinol.* **1997**, *11*, 275–281. [CrossRef] [PubMed]

7. King, V.V. Upper airway disease, sinusitis, and polyposis. *Clin. Rev. Allergy* **1991**, *9*, 143–157. [PubMed]

8. Jeong, J.H.; Hwang, P.H.; Do-Yeon, C.; Joo, N.S.; Wine, J.J. Secretion rates of human nasal submucosal glands from patients with chronic rhinosinusitis or cystic fibrosis. *Am. J. Rhinol. Allergy* **2015**, *29*, 334–338. [CrossRef] [PubMed]

9. Marino, M.J.; Weinstein, J.E.; Riley, C.A.; Levy, J.M.; Emerson, N.A.; McCoul, E.D. Assessment of pneumatization of the paranasal sinuses: A comprehensive and validated metric. *Int. Forum. Allergy Rhinol.* **2016**, *4*, 429–436. [CrossRef] [PubMed]

10. Marino, M.J.; Riley, C.A.; Kessler, R.H.; McCoul, E.D. Clinician assessment of paranasal sinus pneumatization is correlated with total sinus volume. *Int. Forum. Allergy Rhinol.* **2016**, *6*, 1088–1093. [CrossRef] [PubMed]

11. Harris, P.A.; Taylor, R.; Thielke, R.; Payne, J.; Gonzalez, N.; Conde, J.G. Research electronic data capture (REDCap): A metadata-driven methodology and workflow process for providing translational research informatics support. *J. Biomed. Inform.* **2009**, *42*, 377–381. [CrossRef] [PubMed]

12. Ashraf, N.; Bhattacharyya, N. Determination of the "incidental" Lund score for the staing of chronic rhinosinusitis. *Otolaryngol. Head Neck Surg.* **2001**, *125*, 483–486. [PubMed]

13. Hill, M.; Bhattacharyya, N.; Hall, T.R.; Lufkin, R.; Shapiro, N.L. Incidental paranasal sinus imaging abnormalities and the normal Lund score in children. *Otolaryngol. Head Neck Surg.* **2004**, *130*, 171–175. [CrossRef] [PubMed]

14. Emirzeoglu, M.; Sahin, B.; Bilgic, S.; Celebi, M.; Uzun, A. Volumetric evaluation of the paranasal sinuses in normal subjects using computer tomography images: A stereoglogical study. *Auris Nasus Larynx* **2007**, *34*, 191–195. [CrossRef] [PubMed]

15. Selcuk, O.T.; Erol, B.; Renda, L.; Osma, U.; Eyigor, H.; Gunsoy, B.; Yagci, B.; Yılmaz, D. Do climate and altitude affect paranasal sinus volume? *J. Cranio-Maxillofac. Surg.* **2015**, *43*, 1059–1064. [CrossRef] [PubMed]

16. Meyer, T.K.; Kocak, M.; Smith, M.M.; Smith, T.L. Coronal computed tomography analysis of frontal cells. *Am. J. Rhinol.* **2003**, *17*, 163–168. [PubMed]

17. Cho, S.H.; Kim, T.H.; Kim, K.R.; Lee, J.M.; Lee, D.K.; Kim, J.H.; Im, J.J.; Park, C.J.; Hwang, K.G. Factors for maxillary sinus volume and craniofacial anatomical features in adults with chronic rhinosinusitis. *Arch. Otolaryngol. Head Neck Surg.* **2010**, *136*, 610–615. [CrossRef] [PubMed]

18. Kim, H.Y.; Kim, M.B.; Dhong, H.J.; Jung, Y.G.; Min, J.Y.; Chung, S.K.; Lee, H.J.; Chung, S.C.; Ryu, N.G. Changes of maxillary sinus volume and bony thickness of the paranasal sinuses in longstanding pediatric chronic rhinosinusitis. *Int. J. Pediatr. Otorhinolaryngol.* **2008**, *72*, 103–108. [CrossRef] [PubMed]

19. Prokopakis, E.P.; Vlastos, I.M.; Ferguson, B.J.; Scadding, G.; Kawauchi, H.; Georgalas, C.; Papadopoulos, N.; Hellings, P.W. SCUAD and chronic rhinosinusitis. Reinforcing hypothesis driven research in difficulty cases. *Rhinology* **2013**, *52*, 3–8.

4

Contralateral Orbital Mucocele as a Complication of Unilateral Nasal Polyposis

Angélica Bermúdez [1], Amit S. Patel [2] and Edward D. McCoul [1,2,3,*]

[1] Department of Otorhinolaryngology, Ochsner Clinic Foundation, New Orelans, LA 70121, USA; angebermudez@hotmail.com

[2] Department of Otolaryngology, Tulane University School of Medicine, New Orleans, LA 70112, USA; apatel9525@gmail.com

[3] Ochsner Clinical School, University of Queensland School of Medicine, New Orleans, LA 70121, USA

* Correspondence: emccoul@gmail.com

Academic Editor: César Picado

Abstract: Mucocele is a rare complication of chronic rhinosinusitis that typically presents with delayed diagnosis and results in local erosion. We present the case of a symptomatic orbital mucocele arising from contralateral sinus disease that crossed the midline upon diversion by the effect of prior trauma. Effective treatment was provided by combined endoscopic surgery and external drainage.

Keywords: mucocele; chronic rhinosinusitis; facial trauma; orbit; endoscopic sinus surgery

1. Introduction

Mucocele formation is an uncommon complication of chronic rhinosinusitis. While benign, considerable morbidity can result from local erosion, and the insidious clinical course often results in delayed diagnosis [1]. Facial trauma may be a predisposing yet obscure factor in mucocele development [2]. We present an unusual case in which disruption by prior trauma led to diversion of mucus from occult sinus disease into adjacent sinus cavities and orbital mucocele formation.

2. Case Report

A 76-year-old female presented to the outpatient otolaryngology clinic with a four year history of gradually progressive right periorbital swelling with associated diplopia upon upward gaze. She noted intermittent mild pain in the bilateral frontal regions for several years, which had been evaluated at several different institutions without intervention. She had not received any prior sinonasal imaging. She denied sinonasal symptoms including nasal obstruction or rhinorrhea. She had a remote history of prior nasal fractures and right orbital injury over 50 years prior, for which she did not receive treatment. The patient had no previous sinonasal surgeries or procedures.

Physical examination revealed a compressible, mildly tender, fluctuant mass within the soft tissues of the right superior orbit with prominent inferior displacement of the right globe. Nasal endoscopy revealed polyposis in the left middle meatus, with a normal appearance on the right (Figure 1). Computerized tomography (CT) imaging of the sinuses displayed a cystic mass lateral to the right frontal sinus, with complete opacification of both frontal sinuses, as well as the left maxillary sinus and left anterior ethmoid cells (Figure 2). The sphenoid sinuses, right ethmoid sinus, and right maxillary sinus were clear. Magnetic-resonance imaging (MRI) of the orbits confirmed the presence of a mucus-filled extra-axial mass compressing the right globe. Ophthalmologic evaluation was within normal limits, with the exception of hypoglobus.

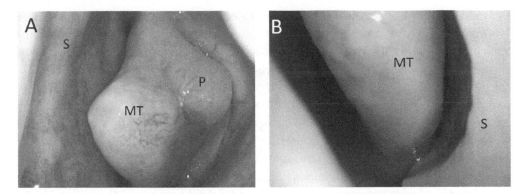

Figure 1. (**A**) Endoscopic view of the left middle turbinate and surrounding polyposis; (**B**) Endoscopic view of the normal-appearing right middle turbinate. MT: middle turbinate; P: polyp; S: septum.

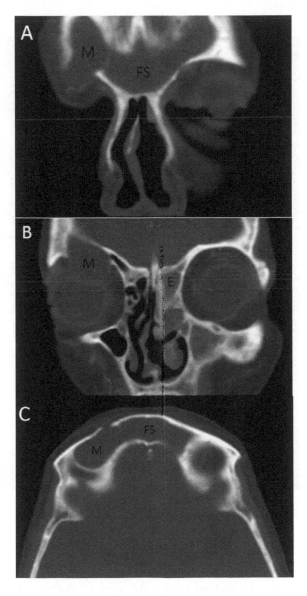

Figure 2. (**A**) Coronal computerized tomography (CT) imaging of the sinuses showing a right orbital mucocele (M) with complete opacification of the frontal sinuses (FS) extending across midline; (**B**) Coronal CT showing left-sided ethmoid polyposis (E) and opacification with clear right-sided sinuses; (**C**) Axial CT showing the absence of a frontal intersinus septum.

The patient underwent surgical treatment via a combined external and endoscopic approach. This was motivated by preoperative imaging studies, which indicated a mucocele that occupied a separate compartment which may not be adequately decompressed by frontal sinusotomy. The mucocele was drained via a right brow incision with release of purulent mucus (Figure 3A). Endoscopic visualization of the mucocele cavity revealed a pinpoint communication with the lateral wall of the frontal sinus (Figure 3B). Bilateral endoscopic frontal sinus exploration with Draf IIB sinusotomy was performed with a 70-degree endoscope and non-powered instrumentation. This revealed a common frontal sinus cavity filled with purulent material, in which the intersinus septum between right and left frontal sinuses was absent. The right frontal ostium could not be identified, whereas the left frontal ostium was occluded by polyposis. Intraoperative electromagnetic image-guided navigation (Medtronic, Minneapolis, MN, USA) was used to confirm the location of the frontal ostia and ensure completeness of the procedure. Left-sided ethmoidectomy and maxillary antrostomy with polypectomy was also performed. Pathologic evaluation was consistent with benign polyposis and chronic sinusitis.

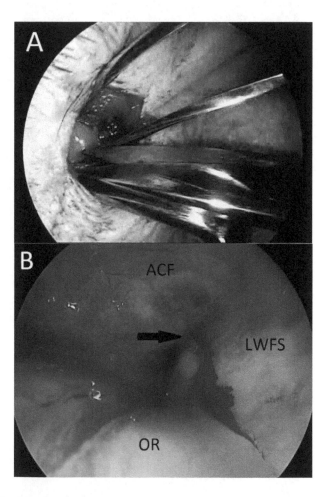

Figure 3. (**A**) Brow incision with encapsulated purulence visible within; (**B**) Endoscopic view of the mucocele lumen showing the communication with the right frontal sinus (arrow). ACF: anterior cranial fossa; LWFS: lateral wall of right frontal sinus; OR: orbital roof.

The patient tolerated the procedure well. At four weeks postoperatively, her vision had normalized with resolution of diplopia and no residual swelling (Figure 4). After one year she remained asymptomatic with full healing of the surgical site and common frontal cavity (Figure 5).

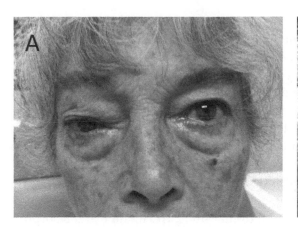
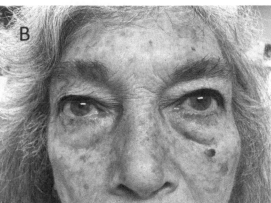

Figure 4. External appearance showing resolution of right eye hypoglobus. (**A**) Preoperative; (**B**) One month postoperative.

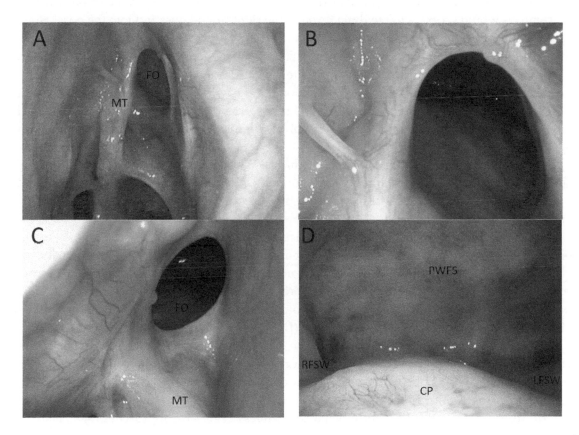

Figure 5. (**A**) Endoscopic appearance with a 0-degree endoscope showing the healed left frontoethmoidectomy without recurrent polyposis; (**B**) Closer view of frontal ostium; (**C**) Endoscopic appearance of the healed right frontal sinus ostium; (**D**) Intraluminal view with 45-degree endoscope advanced into frontal sinus showing the healed contiguous frontal sinus. FO: frontal ostium; MT: middle turbinate remnant; CP: cribiform plate; LFSW: left frontal sinus wall; RFSW: right frontal sinus wall; PWFS: posterior frontal sinus wall.

3. Discussion

Longstanding disruption of a paranasal sinus outflow tract can lead to inadequate mucus clearance and mucocele formation. These epithelium-lined cysts are locally erosive due to pressure exerted on surrounding bony structures. Mucocele is an uncommon occurrence, and is usually seen as a complication of prior sinus surgery. Other contributing factors include mucosal atopy, polyposis, neoplasia, and chronic rhinosinusitis. A history of trauma is occasionally elicited in patients with a sinus mucocele, often years or decades after the injury [3]. Mucocele that occurs in the frontal sinus may erode inferiorly into the orbit, producing orbital edema, diplopia, ptosis, enophthalmos, hypoglobus, or retro-orbital pain [4]. Sinonasal symptoms are typically absent. The differential diagnosis includes orbital cellulitis, abscess, orbital pseudotumor, thyroid ophthalmopathy, and lacrimal gland neoplasm.

The present case is instructive in multiple respects. First, although a mucocele typically arises adjacent to a diseased sinus, in this case the mucocele occurred contralateral to the site of sinus disease. Polyposis represents a subtype of chronic rhinosinusitis which is often bilateral, though may also be unilateral. In this case, polyposis and marked sinus inflammation were present in the left ethmoid sinus, whereas the right ethmoid sinus was completely normal. The polyposis on the left produced obstruction of mucus in the left frontal sinus, which is presumed over the course of time to have eroded the inter-sinus septum to allow extension into the right frontal sinus. Attenuation and resorption of bone may be observed in the setting of chronic sinusitis, in which chemical mediators of inflammation activate local osteoclastic activity [5–7].

Secondly, in the presence of normal sinus anatomy, the crossover of mucus from left to right frontal sinuses would be expected to drain through the right frontal duct and into the nose. However, the prior history of right orbital and nasal trauma contributed to obstruction of the right frontal duct, so that retrograde drainage could not occur. The resulting mucus accumulation instead eroded through the lateral wall of the right frontal sinus to create a mucocele above the right orbit, which in turn eroded inferiorly into the orbit. Thirdly, the prolonged delay in diagnosis was most likely enabled by a delay in obtaining imaging of the orbit and sinuses. Irrespective of history of trauma, unilateral swelling around the face or eye that does not resolve with medical therapy should be evaluated with imaging studies.

Sinus CT is the preferred modality for the diagnosis of mucocele [8]. However, derangements of sinus drainage are often not appreciated on imaging, since the bony laminae may lie oblique to the plane of the image slices. MRI is necessary to rule out other possible pathologies, including meningoencephalocele [4].

Definitive treatment of a mucocele is surgical, which may include trephination, osteoplastic flap, endoscopic sinusotomy, or a combination of approaches, depending on the location and size of the lesion. The goals of treatment are to assure complete removal of mucus and prevent recurrence. Contemporary practice favors an endoscopic approach to frontal sinusotomy, with open approaches reserved for specific cases with unfavorable anatomy, scarring, and disease in the far lateral extent of the frontal sinus [9]. Simple frontal sinusotomy (Draf I, Draf IIA) may provide initial drainage, but may have unclear benefit for long-term ventilation. Extended unilateral frontal sinusotomy (Draf IIB) has been shown to effectively treat frontal sinus mucocele without the potential risk of more aggressive frontal approaches [10]. Endoscopic modified Lothrop procedure (Draf III) is the most aggressive endoscopic approach, and is appropriate for cases of bilateral mucocele with hyperostosis where long-term frontal sinus patency is not anticipated from less aggressive approaches [9].

4. Conclusions

Normal drainage of the paranasal sinuses can be disrupted by facial trauma leading to mucocele formation. A mucocele may be locally erosive and involve intraorbital structures. A high index of suspicion is appropriate for the patient with unilateral eye swelling, even in the absence of sinonasal symptoms.

Author Contributions: Angélica Bermúdez, study design, data collection, drafting, final approval, accountability for all aspects of the work; Amit S. Patel, data collection, revision, final approval, accountability for all aspects of the work; Edward D. McCoul, study design, revision, final approval, accountability for all aspects of the work.

Conflicts of Interest: The authors have no financial or proprietary interest in the subject matter of this manuscript.

References

1. Natvig, K.; Larsen, T.E. Mucocele of the paranasal sinuses. *J. Laryngol. Otol.* **1978**, *92*, 1075–1082. [CrossRef] [PubMed]
2. Tailor, R.; Obi, E.; Burns, J.; Sampath, R.; Durrani, O.M.; Ford, R. Fronto-orbital mucocele and orbital involvement in occult obstructive frontal sinus disease. *Br. J. Ophthalmol.* **2016**, *100*, 525–530. [CrossRef] [PubMed]
3. Metzinger, S.E.; Metzinger, R.C. Complications of Frontal Sinus Fractures. *Craniomaxillofac Trauma Reconstr.* **2009**, *2*, 27–34. [CrossRef] [PubMed]
4. Borkar, S.; Tripathi, A.K.; Satyarthee, G.; Sharma, B.S.; Mahapatra, A.K. Frontal Mucocele Presenting with Forehead Subcutaneous Mass: An Unusual Presentation. *Turk. Neurosurg.* **2008**, *18*, 200–203. [PubMed]
5. Rejowski, J.E.; Caldarelli, D.D.; Campanella, R.S.; Penn, R.D. Nasal polyps causing bone destruction and blindness. *Otolaryngol. Head Neck Surg.* **1982**, *90*, 505–506. [CrossRef] [PubMed]
6. Jung, J.Y.; Chole, R.A. Bone resorption in chronic otitis media: The role of the osteoclast. *ORL J. Otorhinolaryngol. Relat. Spec.* **2002**, *64*, 95–107. [CrossRef] [PubMed]
7. Everts, V.; de Vries, T.J.; Helfrich, M.H. Osteoclast heterogeneity: Lessons from osteopetrosis and inflammatory conditions. *Biochim. Biophys. Acta* **2009**, *1792*, 757–765. [CrossRef] [PubMed]
8. Rao, V.M.; Sharma, D.; Madan, A. Imaging of frontal sinus disease: Concepts, interpretation, and technology. *Otolaryngol. Clin. N. Am.* **2001**, *34*, 23–39. [CrossRef]
9. Courson, A.M.; Stankiewicz, J.A.; Lal, D. Contemporary management of frontal sinus mucoceles: A meta-analysis. *Laryngoscope* **2014**, *124*, 378–386. [CrossRef] [PubMed]
10. Turner, J.H.; Vaezeafshar, R.; Hwang, P.H. Indications and outcomes for Draf IIB frontal sinus surgery. *Am. J. Rhinol. Allergy* **2016**, *30*, 70–73. [CrossRef] [PubMed]

5

A Systematic Review of the Treatment of Chronic Rhinosinusitis in Adults with Primary Ciliary Dyskinesia

Jacob P. Brunner [1], Charles A. Riley [1] and Edward D. McCoul [1,2,3,*]

[1] Department of Otolaryngology—Head and Neck Surgery, Tulane University School of Medicine, New Orleans, LA 70112, USA; jbrunner@tulane.edu (J.P.B.); rileycaf@gmail.com (C.A.R.)
[2] Department of Otorhinolaryngology, Ochsner Clinic Foundation, New Orleans, LA 70121, USA
[3] Ochsner Clinical School, University of Queensland School of Medicine, New Orleans, LA 70121, USA
* Correspondence: emccoul@gmail.com

Academic Editor: César Picado

Abstract: Background: Primary ciliary dyskinesia (PCD) may be an underlying factor in some cases of refractory chronic rhinosinusitis (CRS). However, clinical management of this condition is not well defined. This systematic review examines the available evidence for the diagnosis and management of CRS in adults with PCD. Methods: A systematic review was conducted according to the Preferred Reporting Items for Systematic Reviews and Meta-Analysis (PRISMA) guidelines. Pubmed, EMBASE, and Cochrane database were queried for studies pertinent to treatment of PCD in adults. Two investigators performed eligibility assessment for inclusion or exclusion in a standardized manner. Results: Of the 278 articles identified, six studies met the criteria for analysis. These studies had a predominately low level of evidence. Medical therapy included oral antibiotics and nasal saline rinses. Endoscopic sinus surgery (ESS) was described in three of six studies. Outcomes measures were limited and included non-validated questionnaires, subjective reporting of CRS symptoms, and decreased preciptins against pseudomonas following ESS. Recommendation for a standardized therapeutic strategy was not possible with the available literature. Conclusion: A paucity of evidence is available to guide the treatment of PCD in the adult population. Further prospective studies are needed to determine the optimal diagnostic and management strategy for this condition.

Keywords: primary ciliary dyskinesia; kartagener's syndrome; chronic rhinosinusitis

1. Introduction

Primary ciliary dyskinesia (PCD) is a heterogeneous disorder of ciliary ultrastructure resulting in decreased mucociliary clearance. Ciliary immotility and defective ciliary ultrastructure were initially described by Afzelius in 1976 [1], with subsequent studies demonstrating uncoordinated or ineffective ciliary beat. These ciliary abnormalities result in chronic oto-sino-pulmonary disease including bronchiectasis, rhinitis, sinusitis, bronchitis, pneumonia, and chronic otitis media [2]. The triad of situs inversus, bronchiectasis, and rhinosinusitis, known as Kartagener's syndrome, occurs in approximately 50% of patients with PCD [2,3]. A rare disorder, PCD is thought to have an incidence of 1 per 10,000 to 20,000 births, though, current diagnostic and screening tests such as nasal nitric oxide, ciliary electron microscopy, molecular genetic panels, and ciliary motility studies are often difficult to interpret outside of highly skilled PCD centers [4–6].

Symptoms often begin shortly after birth and are chronic in duration. Sino-nasal symptoms vary but it is estimated that chronic rhinosinusitis (CRS) affects over 50% of patients with PCD, with 15%–40% suffering from nasal polyposis [7,8]. Symptoms of CRS in PCD may be debilitating, as patients suffer from purulent nasal secretions and pansinusitis. Sinusitis may be missed in children due to lack of radiographic imaging [9]. Worsening pulmonary function and respiratory compromise may occur, with bronchiectasis appearing in nearly all adults. The findings of bronchiectasis with chronic sinusitis may be the most identifiable features in an adult with PCD without childhood diagnosis [6].

The treatment of CRS in adults with PCD is difficult given disparate literature and rare incidence of the disease. Adults with PCD are at high risk for pulmonary complications including bronchiectasis and aggressive treatment and monitoring may be necessary. Medical and surgical therapies may be utilized, but outcomes are poorly defined. Recent review on the management of CRS in children with PCD demonstrated similar challenges [10]. A systematic review was performed to evaluate the existing literature on the treatment and outcomes of CRS in adults with PCD.

2. Materials and Methods

A comprehensive, qualitative systematic review of English-language literature was conducted to investigate treatment of CRS in adults with PCD. A search was performed using Pubmed, EMBASE, and Cochrane CENTRAL database. Inclusion criteria for the literature search were defined using the Population, Intervention, Control, Outcome, Study Design (PICOS; Table 1) approach. Search was performed using the Preferred Reporting Items for Systematic Reviews and Meta-Analyses (PRISMA) literature selection process [11]. The initial search included combined key terms and exploded Medical Subject Headings (MeSH) terms. MeSH terms addressed included: primary ciliary dyskinesia, Kartagener's syndrome, sinusitis, rhinitis, rhinosinusitis, functional endoscopic sinus surgery, and functional endoscopic sinus surgery (FESS).

Table 1. Population, Intervention, Control, Outcome, Study Design (PICOS) Inclusion Criteria.

Population	Adult (>18 Years Old) Men and Women
Intervention	Treatment of sinusitis in primary ciliary dyskinesia (PCD)
Control	No comparison group
Outcome	Results of treatment i.e., improvement or worsening of symptoms
Study Design	Case Report, Case Series, Cross-Sectional, Retrospective Cohort, Prospective Single-Arm Trial

Two investigators performed eligibility assessment for inclusion or exclusion in a standardized manner. Studies were included if they contained findings related to the medical or surgical treatment of CRS in adults with PCD. Duplicate records, review articles, articles without an abstract, and non-English articles were removed. Full text articles were reviewed and excluded if they contained pediatric patients only, if the article was unrelated to treatment of sinusitis in PCD, or lacked original patient data.

Data gathered from each article included study design, setting, type of therapy for CRS (medical or surgical), and treatment outcomes. Studies were assessed for bias by examining each study for design, source of patient data collection, and author's stated purpose for the study. Information collected from each article also included year of publication, authors, country of origin, patient population, and number of patients included. Findings were analyzed qualitatively for intervention, outcome assessment, results, and limitations. The level of evidence was determined according to guidelines defined by the Center for Evidence Base Medicine (CEBM) to provide an estimate of the strength of study design [12]. PRISMA guidelines were used for systematic literature review as seen in Figure 1.

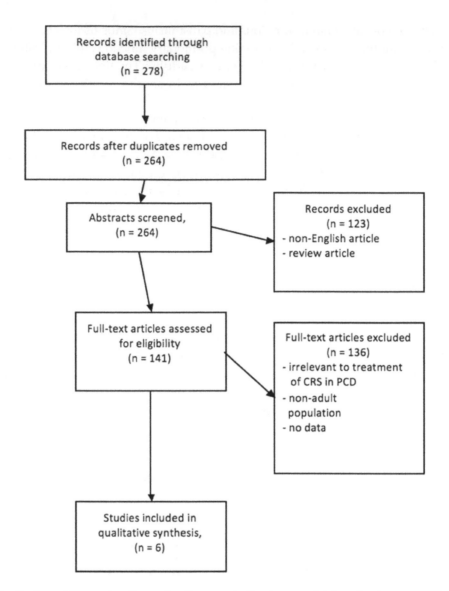

Figure 1. Preferred Reporting Items for Systematic Reviews and Meta-Analyses (PRISMA) flow diagram literature selection process. CRS: chronic rhinosinusitis; PCD: primary ciliary dyskinesia.

3. Results

The initial database query identified 278 articles. After screening and removal of duplicates, 141 articles were included for full-text review. A total of 136 articles were then excluded for irrelevance to treatment of CRS in PCD, non-adult population, or insufficient data. Manual searching of reference lists of the full text articles yielded no additional eligible studies. One study was published after the original search date and subsequently included. Six studies were included for qualitative analysis.

The six studies with direct thematic relevance to CRS in adult are summarized in Table 2. These manuscripts included one prospective single-arm trial [13], one retrospective cohort study [14], one cross-sectional study [7], two case series [15,16], and one case report [17]. The number of people included in each study ranged from one to 44. Antibiotic therapy was addressed in four studies, with two studies describing on treatment with long-term macrolides. Four studies addressed surgical treatment and outcomes including endoscopic sinus surgery. Outcome measures utilized for assessment included lung infection status (1 study), precipitins against pseudomonas (2 studies), author-created questionnaire (1 study), chest computerized tomography (CT) findings and/or pulmonary function (3 studies), arterial blood gases (1 study), and physical symptoms (5 studies).

Table 2. Summary of studies meeting criteria for qualitative analysis. CT, computerized tomography. FEV1, forced expiratory volume in 1 s. PCD, primary ciliary dyskinesia. PE, pressure equalization. SNOT: sinonasal outcome test.

Study	N	Setting	Level of Evidence	Intervention	Outcome Assessment	Results	Limitations
Alanin et al., 2016	24	Denmark	3	Endoscopic Sinus Surgery	SNOT-22, spirometry, precipitins, BMI, infection status of upper and lower airways	Improvement in CRS-related symptoms, reduced lung infection	Small, lacks control group
Alanin et al., 2015	8	Denmark	3	Endoscopic sinus surgery	Number of precipitins against *Pseudomonas* pre- and post-operatively	Reduced precipitins in $\frac{3}{4}$ patients after surgery	Small number of adults, pre and post-operative testing not performed in all patients
Kido et al., 2012	2	Japan	4	Long-term macrolide therapy	Chest CT findings, FEV1, physical symptoms	Improvement of outcome assessments in one case, decline in the other	Small case series
Mygind et al., 1983	27	Denmark	4	Antibiotics, nasal saline, sinus surgery, PE tube insertion	Physical symptoms	Improvement of sinonasal symptoms with antibiotics, nasal saline, and sinus surgery (Caldwell-Luc)	Case series, subjective outcome measures
Sommer et al., 2010	44	Germany	3	Antibiotic treatment, sinus surgery, tympanostomy tube placement	Questionnaire of treatment history in adults with PCD	19% needed antibiotics up to 10 times, 24% up to 30 times and 32% more than 30 times. 69% of patients underwent sinus surgery	Lack of age-specific data, non-validated questionnaire
Yoshioka et al., 2010	1	Japan	5	Long-term clarithromycin	Physical symptoms, pulmonary function, arterial blood gases, chest CT findings	Improvement in all outcome assessments	Single case report, subjective outcome measures

4. Discussion

There is a paucity of literature related to treatment and outcomes of CRS in adults with PCD. A recent consensus statement by the PCD Foundation noted the lack of randomized, controlled, or long-term prospective studies on CRS in PCD [6]. Data on outcomes of medical and surgical therapy is limited [6,10]. Standardized therapy has yet to be described, although the PCD foundation is making a strong effort towards a multi-disciplinary approach to improve long-term outcomes [6].

Medical management of CRS in adults with PCD is ill defined, and no consensus currently exists. Treatment of cystic fibrosis (CF), another recessive genetic disease with impaired mucociliary clearance, has been more substantially studied [18–22]. Intranasal glucocorticoids have been demonstrated to decrease nasal obstruction and nasal polyp size in CF patients [19]. Nasally nebulized dornase alfa, culture directed oral or systemic antibiotics, and topical antibiotic irrigation have all demonstrated benefit in CF patients after sinus surgery [20–22]. Less data is available for PCD, but current guidelines for general treatment of include daily chest physiotherapy and cardiovascular exercise as routine therapy, with antibiotics reserved for acute exacerbations [6,23,24]. Additionally, vaccination schedules should be followed, including annual influenza and pneumococcal vaccines [25,26]. General therapies utilized on an individual basis include inhaled or oral long-term suppressive antibiotics, inhaled hyperosmolar agents, deoxyribonuclease, and inhaled bronchodilators [6]. Long-term macrolide therapy has demonstrated some benefit in CRS patients [15,17], but robust data is lacking. Nasal saline is recommended for patients with CRS, and may improve symptoms in patients with PCD, although no studies exist examining their direct benefit.

A high percentage of PCD patients suffer from CRS and nasal polyposis, which can significantly affect quality of life. A recent study developed a metric to assess health-related quality of life in adults with PCD [27], demonstrating the multi-dimensional effects of the disease, including treatment burden and its effects on social and emotion functioning. Endoscopic sinus surgery (ESS) has been shown to help improve quality of life, lung infections, and lung function in adults with PCD [13], and the performance of ESS demonstrated benefit to children with PCD in one study [28], but outcomes in both children and adults are poorly defined, with high variation from study to study. The rarity of the disease makes long-term prospective studies difficult to perform, highlighting the need for multicenter data sharing. It is possible that ESS may decrease the need for numerous courses of antibiotics and allow for improved drug delivery for better disease control. However, the lack of evidence-based literature makes it difficult to provide any treatment recommendations or clinical practice guidelines.

Limitations of this review include the relatively small number of studies meeting inclusion criteria and low level of evidence based on CEBM criteria. The total number of patients in the studies was small (106) and dominated by single-institution case series. The limited number of studies and small sample size eligible for systematic review highlight the lack of available literature and may help guide further study. The use of a non-validated questionnaire further dampens the validity of treatment assessment. Validated outcome measures in future studies in this population are necessary to assess preoperative disease burden, response to medical and surgical treatment, and long-term outcomes. BESTCILIA, a European Commission funded consortium dedicated to improving care of PCD, is currently conducting a prospective study investigating long-term macrolide therapy in PCD patients [29]. Similar prospective studies will be needed to provide evidence for formal treatment recommendations.

5. Conclusions

The findings of this systematic review demonstrate a lack of evidence-based literature documenting the treatment and outcomes of PCD in adults. There is currently only one long-term prospective study of treatment of this rare disease. Efforts should be made toward a database for prospective data collection, which would allow for long-term multicenter studies investigating the treatment and outcomes of CRS in adults with PCD.

Author Contributions: Jacob P. Brunner, study design, data collection, drafting, revision, final approval, accountability for all aspects of the work; Charles A. Riley, study design, data collection, drafting, final approval, accountability for all aspects of the work; Edward D. McCoul, study design, revision, final approval, accountability for all aspects of the work.

Conflicts of Interest: The authors declare no conflict of interest.

References

1. Afzelius, B.A. A human syndrome caused by immotile cilia. *Science* **1976**, *193*, 317–319. [CrossRef] [PubMed]
2. Knowles, M.R.; Daniels, L.A.; Davis, S.D.; Zariwala, M.A.; Leigh, M.W. Primary ciliary dyskinesia. Recent advances in diagnostics, genetics, and characterization of clinical disease. *Am. J. Respir. Crit. Care Med.* **2013**, *188*, 913–922. [CrossRef] [PubMed]
3. Kartagener, M. Zur pathogenese der bronkiectasien. Bronkiectasien bei situs viscerum inversus. *Beitr Klin Tuberk Spezif Tuberk.* **1933**, *83*, 489–501. [CrossRef]
4. Torgersen, J. Transposition of viscera, bronchiectasis and nasal polyps; a genetical analysis and a contribution to the problem of constitution. *Acta Radiol.* **1947**, *28*, 17–24. [CrossRef] [PubMed]
5. Katsuhara, K.; Kawamoto, S.; Wakabayashi, T.; Belsky, J.L. Situs inversus totalis and Kartagener's syndrome in a Japanese population. *Chest* **1972**, *61*, 56–61. [CrossRef] [PubMed]
6. Shapiro, A.J.; Zariwala, M.A.; Ferkol, T.; Davis, S.D.; Sagel, S.D.; Dell, S.D.; Rosenfeld, M.; Olivier, K.N.; Milla, C.; Daniel, S.J.; et al. Diagnosis, monitoring, and treatment of primary ciliary dyskinesia: PCD foundation consensus recommendations based on state of the art review. *Pediatr. Pulmonol.* **2016**, *51*, 115–132. [CrossRef] [PubMed]

7. Sommer, J.U.; Schafer, K.; Omran, H.; Olbrich, H.; Wallmeier, J.; Blum, A.; Hormann, K.; Stuck, B.A. ENT manifestations in patients with primary ciliary dyskinesia: Prevalence and significance of otorhinolaryngologic co-morbidities. *Eur. Arch. Otorhinolaryngol.* **2011**, *268*, 383–388. [CrossRef] [PubMed]

8. Campbell, R. Managing upper respiratory tract complications of primary ciliary dyskinesia in children. *Curr. Opin. Allergy Clin. Immunol.* **2012**, *12*, 32–38. [CrossRef] [PubMed]

9. Knowles, M.R.; Zariwala, M.; Leigh, M. Primary Ciliary Dyskinesia. *Clin. Chest Med.* **2016**, *37*, 449–461. [CrossRef] [PubMed]

10. Mener, D.J.; Lin, S.Y.; Ishman, S.L.; Boss, E.F. Treatment and outcomes of chronic rhinosinusitis in children with primary ciliary dyskinesia: Where is the evidence? A qualitative systematic review. *Int. Forum Allergy Rhinol.* **2013**, *3*, 986–991. [CrossRef] [PubMed]

11. Moher, D.; Liberati, A.; Tetzlaff, J.; Altman, D.G. Preferred reporting items for systematic reviews and meta-analyses: The PRISMA statement. *Int. J. Surg.* **2010**, *8*, 336–341. [CrossRef] [PubMed]

12. Howick, J.; Chalmers, I.; Glasziou, P.; Greenhalgh, T.; Heneghan, C.; Liberati, A.; Moschetti, I.; Phillips, B.; Thornton, H. *The Oxford Levels of Evidence. 2*; Oxford Centre for Evidence-Based Medicine: London, UK, 2015.

13. Alanin, M.C.; Aanaes, K.; Høiby, N.; Pressler, T.; Skov, M.; Nielsen, K.G.; Johansen, H.K.; von Buchwald, C. Sinus surgery can improve quality of life, lung infections, and lung function in patients with primary ciliary dyskinesia. *Int. Forum Allergy Rhinol.* **2016**, 1–8. [CrossRef] [PubMed]

14. Alanin, M.C.; Johansen, H.K.; Aanaes, K.; Høiby, N.; Pressler, T.; Skov, M.; Nielsen, K.G.; von Buchwald, C. Simultaneous sinus and lung infections in patients with primary ciliary dyskinesia. *Acta Oto-Laryngol.* **2015**, *135*, 58–63. [CrossRef] [PubMed]

15. Kido, T.; Yatera, K.; Yamasaki, K.; Nagata, S.; Choujin, Y.; Yamaga, C.; Hara, K.; Ishimoto, H.; Hisaoka, M.; Mukae, H. Two Cases of Primary Ciliary Dyskinesia with Different Responses to Macrolide Treatment. *Intern. Med.* **2012**, *51*, 1093–1098. [CrossRef] [PubMed]

16. Mygind, N.; Pedersen, M. Nose-, sinus- and ear-symptoms in 27 patients with primary ciliary dyskinesia. *Eur. J. Respir. Dis.* **1983**, *64*, 96–101.

17. Yoshioka, D.; Sakamoto, N.; Ishimatsu, Y.; Kakugawa, T.; Ishii, H.; Mukae, H.; Kadota, J.; Kohno, S. Primary Ciliary Dyskinesia that Responded to Long-Term, Low-Dose Clarithromycin. *Intern. Med.* **2010**, *49*, 1437–1440. [CrossRef] [PubMed]

18. Hamilos, D. Chronic rhinosinusitis in patients with cystic fibrosis. *J. Allergy Clin. Immunol.* **2016**, *4*, 605–612. [CrossRef] [PubMed]

19. Costantini, D.; di Cicco, M.; Giunta, A.; Amabile, G. Nasal polyposis in cystic fibrosis treated by beclomethasone dipropionate. *Acta Univ. Carol. Med.* **1990**, *36*, 220–221.

20. Cimmino, M.; Nardone, M.; Cavaliere, M.; Plantulli, A.; Sepe, A.; Esposito, V.; Mazzarella, G.; Raia, V. Dornase alfa as postoperative therapy in cystic fibrosis sinonasal disease. *Arch. Otolaryngol. Head Neck Surg.* **2005**, *131*, 1097–1101. [CrossRef] [PubMed]

21. Virgin, F.; Rowe, S.; Wade, M.; Gaggar, A.; Leon, K.J.; Young, K.R.; Woodworth, B.A. Extensive surgical and comprehensive postoperative medical management for cystic fibrosis chronic rhinosinusitis. *Am. J. Rhinol. Allergy* **2012**, *26*, 70–75. [CrossRef] [PubMed]

22. Moss, R.B.; King, V.V. Management of sinusitis in cystic fibrosis by endoscopic surgery and serial antimicrobial lavage: Reduction in recurrence requiring surgery. *Arch. Otolaryngol. Head Neck Surg.* **1995**, *121*, 566–572. [CrossRef] [PubMed]

23. Gremmo, M.L.; Guenza, M.C. Positive expiratory pressure in the physiotherapeutic management of primary ciliary dyskinesia in paediatric age. *Monaldi Arch. Chest Dis.* **1999**, *54*, 255–257. [PubMed]

24. Madsen, A.; Green, K.; Buchvald, F.; Hanel, B.; Nielsen, K.G. Aerobic fitness in children and young adults with primary ciliary dyskinesia. *PLoS ONE* **2013**, *8*, e71409. [CrossRef] [PubMed]

25. Chang, C.C.; Morris, P.S.; Chang, A.B. Influenza vaccine for children and adults with bronchiectasis. *Cochrane Database Syst. Rev.* **2007**, *3*, CD006218.

26. Chang, C.C.; Singleton, R.J.; Morris, P.S.; Chang, A.B. Pneumococcal vaccines for children and adults with bronchiectasis. *Cochrane Database Syst. Rev.* **2009**, *2*, CD006316.

27. Lucas, J.S.; Behan, L.; Dunn Galvin, A.; Alpern, A.; Morris, A.M.; Carroll, M.P.; Knowles, M.R.; Leigh, M.W.; Quittner, A.L. A quality-of-life measure for adults with primary ciliary dyskinesia: QOL-PCD. *Eur. Respir. J.* **2015**, *46*, 375–383. [CrossRef] [PubMed]

28. Parsons, D.S.; Greene, B.A. A treatment for primary ciliary dyskinesia: Efficacy of functional endoscopic sinus surgery. *Laryngoscope* **1993**, *103*, 1269–1272. [CrossRef] [PubMed]

29. BESTCILIA. Available online: http://bestcilia.eu (accessed on 16 January 2017).

6

Rhabdomyosarcoma of the Paranasal Sinuses Initially Diagnosed as Acute Sinusitis

Amanda E. Dilger [1,*], Alexander L. Schneider [1], John Cramer [1] and Stephanie Shintani Smith [1,2]

[1] Department of Otolaryngology-Head and Neck Surgery, Northwestern University Feinberg School of Medicine, Chicago, IL 60611, USA; alexander.schneider@northwestern.edu (A.L.S.); john.cramer@northwestern.edu (J.C.); sshintani@gmail.com (S.S.S.)

[2] Center for Healthcare Studies, Northwestern University Feinberg School of Medicine, Chicago, IL 60611, USA

[*] Correspondence: amanda.dilger@northwestern.edu

Academic Editor: César Picado

Abstract: Rhabdomyosarcoma (RMS) is an uncommon soft tissue malignancy that is typically found in the pediatric population. Here we describe a rare case of widely metastatic alveolar RMS of the right paranasal sinuses in an adult woman who presented with several months of unilateral sinus symptoms that was initially misdiagnosed as acute sinusitis. A middle-aged female presented with two months of right sinus pressure and unilateral epistaxis. She had previously been diagnosed with acute sinusitis and was treated with antibiotics without improvement. Nasal endoscopy demonstrated a fungating right nasal cavity mass. On computed tomography scan (CT), she was found to have metastatic disease in the mediastinum, lungs, bones, pancreas, and right ovary. Pathology of the nasal cavity mass was consistent with alveolar RMS. The patient initially responded well to chemotherapy, but subsequently developed brain and leptomeningeal metastases. This case of sinonasal rhabdomyosarcoma is unique in the extent of metastatic disease at the time of diagnosis and the initial misdiagnosis despite concerning unilateral symptoms and imaging. This thus highlights the importance of maintaining a high index of suspicion for malignancy in patients with unilateral sinus symptoms.

Keywords: unilateral; sinusitis; rhabdomyosarcoma

1. Introduction

Soft tissue sarcomas are rarely occurring heterogeneous tumors derived from embryonic mesoderm [1]. They are primarily pediatric malignancies, having been shown to comprise up to 12% of pediatric malignancies, but as little as 1% of all adult malignancies [2]. Sarcomas account for only 1% to 2% of all head and neck malignancy [3–5]. The rhabdomyosarcoma (RMS) subtype is even more rare in adults, representing less than 1% of all malignant solid tumors in adults. When it does occur, one of the most common RMS subsites is the head and neck region [6].

Within the head and neck, RMS is further sub-divided into three main sub-types: orbital, nonorbital parameningeal (including the sinonasal region), and nonorbital nonparameningeal. RMS of the head and neck often produces non-specific symptoms secondary to local mass effect, including headache, nasal congestion, and otorrhea, all of which mimic benign disease. Thus, it is often diagnosed late in its course. Parameningeal sites confer a significant risk of central nervous system dissemination, and unfortunately are often unresectable by the time of diagnosis [7]. It is thus not surprising that parameningeal RMS are associated with a poor prognosis, and are at high risk of early recurrence [8].

Here, we describe a rare case of widely metastatic alveolar rhabdomyosarcoma of the paranasal sinus in an adult woman who presented with several months of unilateral sinus and ophthalmologic symptoms.

2. Case Report

A previously healthy middle-aged woman initially presented to an outside hospital Emergency Room with the complaint of headache and right sided sinus/facial pressure. Computed tomography scan (CT) brain at that time showed complete opacification of the right maxillary, ethmoid, and sphenoid sinuses (Figure 1). She was presumptively diagnosed with acute on chronic sinusitis and prescribed a course of oral antibiotics, oral steroids, and intra-nasal steroids. Approximately two weeks after this presentation, she had a breast biopsy for a newly noted mass, the pathology of which was consistent with poorly differentiated malignant neoplasm.

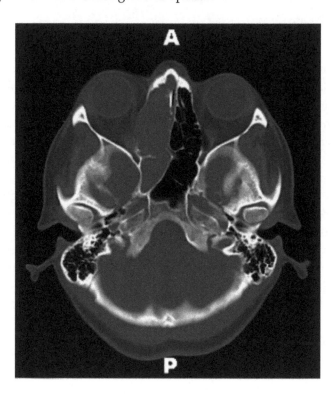

Figure 1. Prehospitalization computed tomography scan (CT) Brain without Contrast, axial view. Initial CT obtained by primary care physician, which demonstrates complete opacification of the right ethmoid and sphenoid sinuses. Abbreviations: A = anterior; P = posterior.

Three months after her initial presentation, she re-presented to the Emergency Department with right-sided epistaxis, hemoptysis, shortness of breath, and worsening right sinus pressure. Physical exam was notable for right-sided exophthalmos and epiphora with diplopia on far lateral gaze. Cranial nerve exam demonstrated paresthesias in the right V2 distribution. An otolaryngologist was consulted and nasal endoscopy revealed a fungating, bleeding mass that appeared to be originating from the head of the inferior turbinate and obstructing the entire right nasal cavity. The left nasal cavity appeared normal. Routine laboratory tests were notable for thrombocytopenia with platelets of 49,000.

CT Neck/Sinus demonstrated a large, enhancing mass in the right nasal cavity measuring 5.9 cm × 3.7 cm × 5.3 cm, which involved the entire right ethmoid sinuses and right maxillary sinus with post-obstructive opacification of the right frontal and sphenoid sinuses (Figure 2). There was also extension into the right orbit, with mass effect on the medial rectus and optic nerve as well extension into the right anterior cranial fossa. Multiple enlarged retropharyngeal, supraclavicular, and mediastinal lymph nodes were also identified (Figure 3). Magnetic resonance imaging (MRI) of the brain was significant for mass extension 4 mm into the right anterior cranial fossa. CT Chest, Abdomen, and Pelvis were notable for a large right breast mass as well as metastatic disease in the hilum, chest wall, lungs, liver, pancreas, peritoneal cavity, and right ovary.

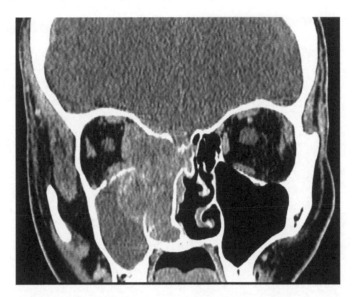

Figure 2. CT Sinus with Contrast on presentation to our hospital, coronal view. Large, heterogeneously enhancing mass of the right nasal cavity with post-obstructive opacificaiton of the right maxillary sinus. Bony destruction of the right lamina paprycea and cribiform plate.

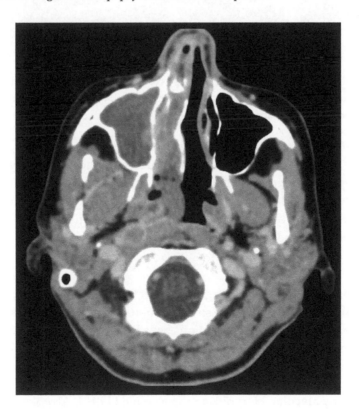

Figure 3. CT Sinus with Contrast on presentation to our hospital, axial view. Multiple enlarged pathologic-appearing lymph nodes seen in the right retropharyngeal space.

The decision was made to proceed to the operating room for endoscopic biopsy of the right nasal cavity mass and control of epistaxis. The right nasal cavity was notable for a friable mass that occupied the entire nasal cavity beyond the head of the inferior turbinate. Frozen sections were consistent with small blue cell neuroendocrine tumor, with similar morphology to the previously taken breast mass biopsy. A diagnosis of alveolar rhabdomyosarcoma was confirmed by pathology, which demonstrated the presence of a PAX3/7-FOXO1 fusion transcript (Figure 4).

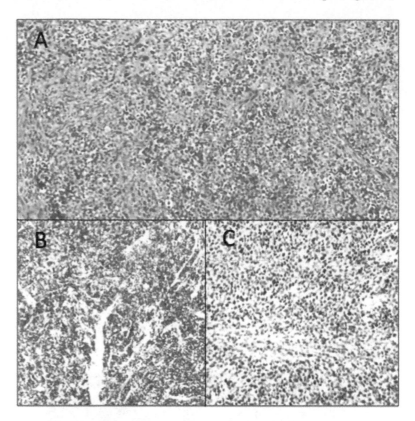

Figure 4. Pathology from nasal mass biopsy consistent with alveolar rhabdomyosarcoma. (**A**) Hematoxylin and eosin (H&E) stain demonstrating a small round blue cell tumor. (**B,C**) Positive stain for desmin and myogen, respectively. Markers of skeletal muscle differentiation.

Final pathological review and tumor board discussion concluded that the patient's findings were consistent with widely metastatic alveolar rhabdomyosarcoma of the nasal cavity. She elected to pursue palliative chemotherapy, consisting of Vincristine/Dactinomycin/Cyclophosphomide. She initially responded well, but developed leptomeningeal metastases after cycle five. She completed palliative whole brain and sinus-directed radiation. Her neurologic symptoms progressed, and approximately six months after her biopsies, she transitioned to comfort care only.

3. Discussion

Rhabdomyosarcoma (RMS) is a rare, aggressive soft tissue malignancy that commonly occurs in the head and neck, albeit significantly more so in children and adolescents than in adults. Given the relative rarity of this malignancy, many institutions have limited experience in treating RMS. As such, although the relative survival of standard risk RMS patients has improved over the last 30 years, the prognosis for patients with relapsed and/or metastatic disease remains poor [8].

Among both adults and children, the most commonly encountered histopathological RMS subtype is embryonal, followed by alveolar, botryoid, and unclassified [9,10]. Alveolar RMS has been found to be the most unfavorable subtype in terms of both recurrence rate and overall survival [8,10]. Many large retrospective studies have found that pediatric patients with head and neck RMS have significantly better outcomes than adults, and this may be in part to the higher predominance of embryonal subtype in the pediatric population.

Head and neck rhabdomyosarcoma can be further sub-classified by primary site: orbital, parameningeal, and non-orbital non-parameningeal. Parameningeal sites account for 41%–51.2% of head and neck RMS, and include the nasopharynx/nasal cavity, middle ear, paranasal sinuses, and the infratemporal fossa/pterygopalatine space [8,11]. Parameningeal RMS have been identified as unfavorable due to the fact that the lesions often invade critical anatomic structures, precluding complete resection [12]. Survival outcomes are significantly worse for parameningeal subsites; furthermore, there is a higher rate of direct meningeal extension, which is typically not found in patients with RMS of other sub-sites [13].

The development of distant metastases in patients with head and neck RMS is associated with significantly worse outcomes, specifically a 16% disease-specific survival at 5 years [9]. Although the specific locations and extent of distant disease is not quantified in the larger retrospective studies, prior case reports on adult head and neck RMS have only described metastatic disease to the lungs, bone, and liver. Here, we describe a patient with extensive distant metastases, including the breast, hilum, chest wall, lungs, liver, pancreas, peritoneal cavity, and right ovary. Of note, the finding of breast metastases in our patient is concordant with prior studies that have found RMS breast metastases only in female patients with alveolar subtype [14–16]. The extent of metastatic disease at the time of diagnosis raises the question of how impactful the month-long delay in diagnosis in terms of disease progression and overall likelihood of survival.

Although alveolar rhabdomyosarcoma is a rare cause of unilateral sinus opacification in adults, neoplasm in general should be considered in the setting of unilateral symptoms or radiologic findings. This is particularly true in cases of unilateral disease, where an anatomical etiology—such as a deviated septum, bony spur, or polyp—or odontogenic source is not identified on imaging or exam. Furthermore, neoplasm should be suspected in the setting of progressive disease that does not respond to traditional medical management. One retrospective study of 63 patients with unilateral sinus symptoms plus unilateral disease on CT, who underwent sinus surgery, identified neoplasm as the cause of opacification in 15.4% of cases, with malignancy representing a smaller but still significant proportion of cases. Additionally, unilateral epistaxis—as was seen in our patient—was more frequently associated with neoplastic disease than benign causes such as chronic rhinosinusitis and nasal polyposis in that particular study population [17]. The existing literature on unilateral sinusitis and its association with underlying malignancy is limited and primarily focused on inverted papilloma, which has a rate of malignant degeneration to squamous cell carcinoma of between 3.4% [18] and 9.7% [19]. The majority of other studies in this area focus specifically on unilateral maxillary sinusitis secondary to odontogenic sources. Nevertheless, given the potential for underlying malignancy in patients with unilateral sinus opacification on imaging, a comprehensive evaluation by an otolaryngologist including nasal endoscopy and consideration of imaging and biopsy should be considered. This is particularly true for patients like the one described here, with concerning signs or symptoms such as lack of anatomical cause for unilateral disease, progression of symptoms despite antibiotic management, and epistaxis.

4. Conclusions

Rhabdomyosarcoma of the paranasal sinuses is a rare malignancy, particularly in adults. Given the significantly worse outcomes in adults than children and the implications of distant metastases on survival, early diagnosis is of utmost importance. A high degree of clinical suspicion for neoplasm, including RMS, should be maintained when evaluating a patient with unilateral sinus disease.

Acknowledgments: No sources of funding were used in this study.

Author Contributions: Amanda E. Dilger, Alexander L. Schneider and Stephanie Shintani Smith were involved in the initial consultation, management and surgical procedure for the patient described in this case report. Amanda E. Dilger and John Cramer conceived the themes for this paper. Amanda E. Dilger, Alexander L. Schneider and John Cramer conducted the literature review and wrote this manuscript.

Conflicts of Interest: The authors declare no conflict of interest.

References

1. Gonzalez-Gonzalez, R.; Bologna-Molina, R.; Molina-Frechero, N.; Domínguez-Malagon, H.R. Prognostic factors and treatment strategies for adult head and neck soft tissue sarcoma. *Int. J. Oral Maxillofac. Surg.* **2012**, *41*, 569–575. [CrossRef] [PubMed]

2. Chang, A.E.; Chai, X.; Pollack, S.M.; Loggers, E.; Rodler, E.; Dillon, J.; Parvathaneni, U.; Moe, K.S.; Futran, N.; Jones, R.L. Analysis of clinical prognostic factors for adult patients with head and neck sarcomas. *Otolaryngol. Head Neck Surg.* **2014**, *151*, 976–983. [CrossRef] [PubMed]

3. Tajudeen, B.A.; Fuller, J.; Lai, C.; Grogan, T.; Elashoff, D.; Abemayor, E.; John, M.S. Head and neck sarcomas: The UCLA experience. *Am. J. Otolaryngol.* **2014**, *35*, 476–481. [CrossRef] [PubMed]

4. Lindford, A.; McIntyre, B.; Marsh, R.; MacKinnon, C.A.; Davis, C.; Tan, S.T. Outcomes of the treatment of head and neck sarcomas in a tertiary referral center. *Front. Surg.* **2015**, *2*, 19. [CrossRef] [PubMed]

5. Peng, K.A.; Grogan, T.; Wang, M.B. Head and neck sarcomas: Analysis of the SEER database. *Otolaryngol. Head Neck Surg.* **2014**, *151*, 627–633. [CrossRef] [PubMed]

6. Ruiz-Mesa, C.; Goldberg, J.M.; Munoz, A.J.C.; Dumont, S.N.; Trent, J.C. Rhabdomyosarcoma in adults: New perspectives on therapy. *Curr. Treat. Options Oncol.* **2015**, *16*, 27. [CrossRef] [PubMed]

7. Ahmed, A.A.; Tsokos, M. Sinonasal rhabdomyosarcoma in children and young adults. *Int. J. Surg. Pathol.* **2007**, *15*, 160–165. [CrossRef] [PubMed]

8. Turner, J.H.; Richmon, J.D. Head and neck rhabdomyosarcoma: A critical analysis of population-based incidence and survival data. *Otolaryngol. Head Neck Surg.* **2011**, *145*, 967–973. [CrossRef] [PubMed]

9. Callender, T.A.; Weber, R.S.; Janjan, N.; Benjamin, R.; Zaher, M.; Wolf, P.; El-Naggar, A. Rhabdomyosarcoma of the nose and paranasal sinuses in adults and children. *Otolaryngol. Head Neck Surg.* **1995**, *112*, 252–257. [CrossRef]

10. Thompson, C.F.; Kim, B.J.; Lai, C.; Grogan, T.; Elashoff, D.; St John, M.A.; Wang, M.B. Sinonasal rhabdomyosarcoma: Prognostic factors and treatment outcomes. *Int. Forum Allergy Rhinol.* **2013**, *3*, 678–683. [CrossRef] [PubMed]

11. Wharam, M.D., Jr. Rhabdomyosarcoma of Parameningeal Sites. *Semin. Radiat. Oncol.* **1997**, *7*, 212–216. [CrossRef]

12. Douglas, J.G.; Arndt, C.A.; Hawkins, D.S. Delayed radiotherapy following dose intensive chemotherapy for parameningeal rhabdomyosarcoma (PM-RMS) of childhood. *Eur. J. Cancer* **2007**, *43*, 1045–1050. [CrossRef] [PubMed]

13. Tefft, M.; Fernandez, C.; Donaldson, M.; Newton, W.; Moon, T.E. Incidence of meningeal involvement by rhabdomyosarcoma of the head and neck in children: A report of the Intergroup Rhabdomyosarcoma Study (IRS). *Cancer* **1978**, *42*, 253–258. [CrossRef]

14. Persic, M.; Roberts, J.T. Alveolar rhabdomyosarcoma metastatic to the breast: Long-term survivor. *Clin. Oncol.* **1999**, *11*, 417–418. [CrossRef]

15. Audino, A.N.; Setty, B.A.; Yeager, N.D. Rhabdomyosarcoma of the breast in adolescent and young adult (AYA) women. *J. Pediatr. Hematol. Oncol.* **2017**, *39*, 62–66. [CrossRef] [PubMed]

16. Kebudi, R.; Koc, B.S.; Gorgun, O.; Celik, A.; Kebudi, A.; Darendeliler, E. Breast metastases in children and adolescents with rhabdomyosarcoma: A large single-institution experience and literature review. *J. Peadiatr. Hematol. Oncol.* **2017**, *39*, 67–71. [CrossRef] [PubMed]

17. Habesoglu, T.E.; Habesoglu, M.; Surmeli, M.; Uresin, T.; Egeli, E. Unilateral sinonasal symptoms. *J. Craniofac. Surg.* **2010**, *21*, 2019–2022. [CrossRef] [PubMed]

18. Pasquini, E.; Sciarretta, V.; Farneti, G.; Modugno, G.C.; Ceroni, A.R. Inverted papilloma: Report of 89 cases. *Am. J. Otolaryngol.* **2004**, *25*, 178–185. [CrossRef] [PubMed]

19. Yoskovitch, A.; Braverman, I.; Nachtigal, D.; Frenkiel, S. Sinonasal schneiderian papilloma. *J. Otolaryngol.* **1998**, *27*, 122–126. [PubMed]

7

Eosinophilia and Quality of Life in Patients Receiving a Bioabsorbable Steroid-Eluting Implant during Endoscopic Sinus Surgery

Jason D. Pou [1], Charles A. Riley [1], Kiranya E. Tipirneni [2], Anna K. Bareiss [1] and Edward D. McCoul [1,2,3,*]

[1] Department of Otolaryngology, Head and Neck Surgery, Tulane University School of Medicine, New Orleans, LA 70121, USA; jpou@tulane.edu (J.D.P.); criley2@tulane.edu (C.A.R.); abareiss@tulane.edu (A.K.B.)

[2] Ochsner Clinic School, University of Queensland, New Orleans, LA 70121, USA; kiranya.tipirneni@gmail.com

[3] Department of Otorhinolaryngology, Ochsner Clinic Foundation, New Orleans, LA 70121, USA

* Correspondence: emccoul@gmail.com

Academic Editor: César Picado

Abstract: Introduction: Bioabsorbable steroid-eluting implants are available as an adjunct for endoscopic sinus surgery (ESS) in the treatment of chronic rhinosinusitis (CRS). It is unclear which patients are most likely to benefit from this technology. We sought to determine if the severity of preoperative sinonasal inflammation influences the postoperative changes in patient-reported quality of life (QOL) and endoscopic appearance following ESS with implant placement; Methods: Consecutive adult patients undergoing ESS for CRS with ethmoidectomy and placement of a steroid-eluting implant over an 18-month period were prospectively included for study. Pre-operative sinus computed tomography (CT) opacification was evaluated using the Lund-Mackay score (LMS). Sinonasal Outcome Test (SNOT-22) scores and Lund-Kennedy endoscopic scores (LKES) for each patient were collected preoperatively and at three- and six-month intervals postoperatively. Serum eosinophilia (>6.0% on peripheral smear) and sinus tissue eosinophilia were recorded; Results: One hundred and thirty-six patients were included for analysis. Of these, 36.7% had polyposis, 15.4% had serum eosinophilia and 64.0% had tissue eosinophilia. The mean (standard deviation) SNOT-22 score was 45.5 (19.4) preoperatively, which improved postoperatively to 18.8 (14.1) at three months ($p < 0.001$) and 16.5 (14.0) at six months ($p < 0.001$). Similar results were found when stratified by the presence of polyposis, serum eosinophilia, tissue eosinophilia or high-grade CT findings (LMS > 6). Higher baseline LKES was observed for patients with eosinophilia or high-grade LMS, but these differences normalized at six months postoperatively; Conclusions: Patient-reported QOL and endoscopic appearance show improvement six months after placement of a steroid-eluting implant during ESS, irrespective of the presence of polyposis or eosinophilia.

Keywords: steroid-eluting implant; endoscopic sinus surgery; quality of life; eosinophil; chronic rhinosinusitis

1. Introduction

Chronic rhinosinusitis (CRS) is estimated to affect over 12% of adults in the United States [1]. The clinical manifestations of CRS are variable, though in nearly all cases quality of life (QOL) is diminished [2], with associations with impaired productivity, lost workdays, more healthcare visits, and increased spending on treatment. Validated metrics such as the 22-item Sinonasal Outcomes Test

(SNOT-22) have been created to determine the severity of disease, to monitor progression, and to demonstrate the response to medical and surgical treatment [3].

Endoscopic sinus surgery (ESS) has a role in the management of CRS to improve sinus ventilation and mucociliary clearance as well as to facilitate the topical administration of medication [4]. Adjunct, long-term medical therapy is necessary for the effective treatment and maintenance of CRS [5]. The beneficial effect of steroids is well-known in CRS; however, the side effects of long-term systemic steroid use are not desirable and can lead to serious complications [6]. Topical intranasal steroids can minimize systemic effects and are an integral component in treatment; however, penetration into the middle meatus and sinus cavities can be limited by postoperative edema and crusting [7]. Current efforts are focused on improving steroid delivery to the diseased sinuses while limiting their systemic effects [8].

Bioabsorbable steroid-eluting implants are a relatively new technology that may be utilized within the ethmoid sinus lumen following ESS [9,10]. Only one such implant is currently available, marketed under the trade name Propel (Intersect ENT, Menlo Park, CA, USA), which combines the release of 370 μg of mometasone furoate with a spring-like spacer activity that is designed for gradual release over 30 days [11]. This offers the potential benefits of decreasing postoperative inflammation and mucosal edema, reducing polyposis and adhesions, securing the middle turbinate in a medialized position, and separating raw mucosal edges [8,10].

Previous studies examining the utility of adjuvant use of a bioabsorbable steroid-eluting implant in ESS have demonstrated its safety and clinical effectiveness in CRS patients in general [6–8,12]. However, it is unclear which patient groups are most likely to benefit from this technology. Study of patient-reported QOL outcomes with use of this device has been limited, and the differential effect of this device upon phenotypes of CRS has not been fully studied. The aim of the present study was to determine if changes in patient-reported QOL after ESS with implant placement are related to the severity of baseline sinonasal inflammation. Objective measures of tissue eosinophilia, serum eosinophilia, polyposis and degree of radiographic sinus opacification were used as indicators of inflammation severity. A secondary aim was to determine if surgeon-reported endoscopic appearance showed similar postoperative improvements in patients with mild versus severe baseline inflammation.

2. Methods

A single-cohort before-after study design was utilized to evaluate outcomes of ESS for CRS performed by a single surgeon (EDM) from October 2014 to March 2016. During this time period, 151 consecutive adult patients undergoing ethmoidectomy for CRS had placement of a Propel implant. This implant is composed of a bioabsorbable polymer, poly-(LL-lactide-co-glycolide), woven into a scaffold and impregnated with 370 μg of mometasone furoate, and is deployed into the sinus cavity using an specialized catheter. ESS cases performed for other indications besides CRS did not receive an implant and were not included in the study. Patients were excluded who received postoperative systemic corticosteroids (nine cases), who had a diagnosis of cystic fibrosis (five cases), or who received an implant but were found incidentally to have a sinonasal neoplasm (one case). All included participants underwent unilateral or bilateral total (anterior and posterior) ethmoidectomy, and each operated ethmoid cavity received an implant. Treatment of other paranasal sinuses was permitted, as was concurrent septoplasty or inferior turbinate reduction. In addition to ethmoidectomy, 96.3% (131/136) underwent concurrent maxillary antrostomy, 83.8% (114/136) underwent frontal sinus exploration, and 56.6% (77/136) underwent sphenoidotomy.

CRS was defined as symptomatic mucosal inflammation of the paranasal sinuses of at least 12 consecutive weeks duration. Pre-operative sinus computerized tomography (CT) within three months of the procedure was reviewed. Opacification was evaluated for each patient using the Lund-Mackay score (LMS) on all preoperative CT scans, with LMS = 6 considered the median score in this cohort. Pre-operative Lund-Kennedy Endoscopic score (LKES) was determined on all patients with in-office nasal endoscopy performed by the senior author. The presence of preoperative serum eosinophilia (>6.0% on peripheral smear) and presence of polyps were recorded. The presence of tissue eosinophilia (>10 cells/hpf) was documented on histopathologic examination of ethmoid tissue specimens. Relevant comorbidities were obtained from the medical history provided by the patient or recorded in the medical record.

Patients were seen approximately seven days and 28 days postoperatively for nasal endoscopy and debridement. If stent fragments were present on post-operative day 28, they were removed during the office visit. At 28 days all patients were then started on a daily application of an intranasal topical steroid. LKES was reported during nasal endoscopy at the three- and six-month post-operative visits. Patient-reported SNOT-22 scores were gathered preoperatively and at three and six months postoperatively, and were grouped for analysis relative to the median score of 45. The study was approved by the institutional review board of the senior author's primary institution.

Sample size calculation was based on the expected mean (SD) postoperative change score, previously reported in a large cohort as 16.2 (20.0) [13]. Assuming an alpha level of 0.05 and a power of 0.8, the calculated sample size was 48. A larger cohort was sampled to account for dropouts. Pre- and post-operative continuous variables were compared using two-tailed paired t-tests. Nonparametric variables were compared using Fisher's exact test. p-values less than 0.05 were considered significant. Statistical analysis was completed using SAS software (version 9.3, SAS Institute Inc., Cary, NC, USA).

3. Results

One hundred and thirty-six patients met inclusion criteria. Of these, 50 (36.8%) had polyposis, 21 (15.4%) had serum eosinophilia and 87 (64.0%) had tissue eosinophilia. None of these cases received systemic steroids during the study period. Baseline characteristics of eosinophilic (serum eosinophilia >6.0% on peripheral smear) and non-eosinophilic (serum eosinophilia $\leq$ 6.0%) groups were comparable, although more males presented with high-grade LMS and lower preoperative SNOT-22 scores (Table 1). Comorbid conditions that could affect QOL were equally distributed. Patients with serum eosinophilia had a mean LMS of 11.9 versus 7.4 in patients without eosinophilia (p = 0.003), whereas those with and without tissue eosinophilia had LMS scores of 9.11 and 6.96, respectively (p = 0.211). Tissue eosinophilia and serum eosinophilia were weakly correlated (Spearman rho = 0.265). Two patients (1.5%) required revision ESS during the study period.

The mean (standard deviation) SNOT-22 score for all patients was 45.5 (19.4) preoperatively, which improved postoperatively to 18.8 (14.1) at three months (p < 0.001), and to 16.5 (14.0) at six months (p < 0.001). Similar results were found in the subgroup analysis of tissue eosinophilia, serum eosinophilia, the presence of polyps, and high-grade presentation of disease on CT (LMS > 6) (Figure 1A–D, Table 2). Three and six-month SNOT-22 scores were significantly lower than the preoperative SNOT-22 scores in all subgroups (Figure 1A–D). The presence or absence of serum eosinophilia and the grade of disease on CT did not significantly affect postoperative SNOT-22 scores (Figure 1A,D, Table 2). Three-month postoperative SNOT-22 scores were significantly higher in patients with tissue eosinophilia and polyps compared to those without; however, at six months, there was no significant difference (Figure 1B,C, Table 2).

Table 1. Baseline characteristics.

Basline Characteristic	Total Subjects, n (%)	Serum Eosinophilia Present, n (%)	p-Value [1]	LMS $\geq$ 6, n (%)	p-Value [2]	Preoperative SNOT-22 Score $\geq$ 45, n (%)	p-Value [3]
Sex							
Male	55/136 (40.4)	12/55 (21.8)	0.089	42/55 (76.4)	0.027	14/55 (25.5)	0.008
Female	81/136 (59.6)	9/81 (11.1)	-	47/81 (58.0)	-	49/81 (60.5)	-
Prior surgery							
Yes	47/136 (34.6)	10/47 (21.3)	0.171	34/47 (72.3)	0.219	25/47 (53.2)	0.242
No	89/136 (65.4)	11/89 (12.4)	-	55/89 (61.8)	-	38/89 (42.7)	-

Table 1. *Cont.*

Baseline Characteristic	Total Subjects, n (%)	Serum Eosinophilia Present, n (%)	p-Value [1]	LMS ≥ 6, n (%)	p-Value [2]	Preoperative SNOT-22 Score ≥ 45, n (%)	p-Value [3]
Age							
>50 years	70/136 (51.5)	12/70 (17.1)	0.569	46/70 (65.7)	0.944	31/70 (44.3)	0.263
≤50 years	66/136 (48.5)	9/66 (13.6)	-	43/66 (65.2)	-	32/66 (48.5)	-
Asthma							
Present	21/136 (15.4)	4/21 (19.0)	0.617	17/21 (81.0)	0.103	12/21 (57.1)	0.280
Absent	115/136 (84.5)	17/115 (14.8)	-	72/115 (62.6)	-	51/115 (44.4)	-
AR							
Present	63/136 (46.3)	15/63 (23.8)	0.012	42/63 (66.7)	0.779	30/63 (47.6)	0.779
Absent	73/136 (53.7)	6/73 (8.2)	-	47/73 (74.6)	-	33/73 (45.2)	-
Anxiety							
Present	25/136 (18.3)	6/25 (24.0)	0.190	14/25 (56.0)	0.271	13/25 (52.0)	0.529
Absent	111/136 (81.6)	15/111 (10.8)	-	75/111 (67.5)	-	50/111 (45.0)	-
Depression							
Present	15/136 (11.0)	4/15 (26.7)	0.200	10/15 (66.7)	0.912	9/15 (60.0)	0.258
Absent	121/136 (89.0)	17/121 (14.0)	-	79/121 (65.3)	-	54/121 (44.3)	-
Migraine							
Present	19/136 (14.0)	1/19 (5.3)	0.187	9/19 (47.4)	0.073	12/19 (63.2)	0.112
Absent	117/136 (86.0)	20/117 (17.1)	-	80/117 (68.4)	-	51/117 (43.6)	-

LMS, Lund-Mackay Score; SNOT-22, Sinonasal Outcome Test; AR, Allergic Rhinitis; [1] *p*-value represents comparison of percentages of patients with serum eosinophilia; [2] *p*-value represents comparison of percentages of patients with LMS ≥ 6; [3] *p*-value represents comparison of percentages of patients with preoperative SNOT-22 ≥ 45.

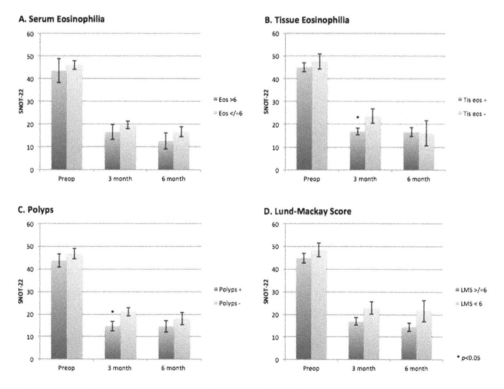

Figure 1. Comparisons of preoperative, three-month postoperative, and six-month postoperative SNOT-22 scores. (**A**) Presence versus absence of serum eosinophilia; (**B**) Presence versus absence of tissue eosinophilia; (**C**) Presence versus absence of polyposis; (**D**) High-grade versus low-grade Lund-Mackay score of CT opacification. * *p* < 0.05 for between-group comparisons. SNOT-22: Sinonasal Outcome Test; CT: computed tomography; LMS: Lund-Mackay Score.

The baseline LKES scores were significantly higher for patients with serum and tissue eosinophilia, polyps and high-grade CT disease (Figure 2A–D; Table 3). The three- and six-month LKES scores were significantly lower for patients with and without serum eosinophilia, with no significant difference between the groups (Figure 2A, Table 3). Patients with tissue eosinophilia and high-grade CT disease had significantly higher three-month postoperative LKES scores ($p = 0.017$ and $p = 0.006$, respectively); however, this difference was not seen at six months postoperatively ($p = 0.189$ and $p = 0.144$, respectively) (Figure 2B,D; Table 3).

Table 2. Between-group comparisons of Sinonasal Outcome Test (SNOT-22) scores before and after endoscopic sinus surgery.

Disease Characteristic	Preop	p-Value [1]	3 Month Postop	p-Value [2]	6 Month Postop	p-Value [3]
Serum eosinophilia						
Present	43.44	0.609	16.5	0.461	12.57	0.474
Absent	46.01	-	19.6	-	16.61	-
Tissue eosinophilia						
Present	45.01	0.512	18.86	0.034	16.55	0.924
Absent	47.57	-	23.54	-	16.09	-
Polyps						
Present	43.74	0.419	14.71	0.032	14.63	0.362
Absent	46.67	-	21.08	-	17.97	-
Lund-Mackay score						
LMS ≥ 6	44.77	0.350	16.84	0.050	14.42	0.093
LMS < 6	48.33	-	22.82	-	21.6	-

LMS, Lund-Mackay score. [1] p-value represents comparison of preoperative SNOT-22 scores; [2] p-value represents comparison of three-month postoperative SNOT-22 scores; [3] p-value represents comparison of six-month postoperative SNOT-22 scores.

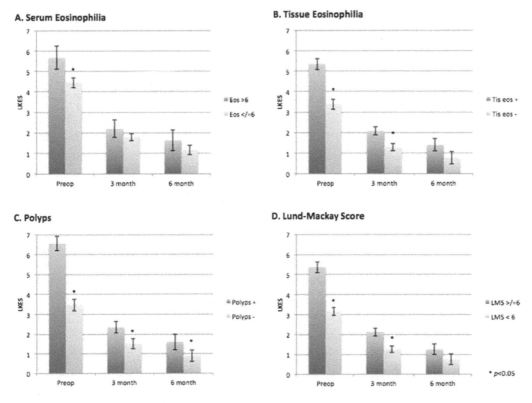

Figure 2. Comparisons of preoperative, three-month postoperative, and six-month postoperative Lund-Kennedy Endoscopic scores. (**A**) Presence versus absence of serum eosinophilia. (**B**) Presence versus absence of tissue eosinophilia. (**C**) Presence versus absence of polyposis. (**D**) High-grade versus low-grade Lund-Mackay score of CT opacification. * $p < 0.05$ for between-group comparisons.

Table 3. Between-group comparisons of Lund-Kennedy endoscopic score (LKES) before and after endoscopic sinus surgery.

Disease Characteristic	Preop	p-Value [1]	3 Month Postop	p-Value [2]	6 Month Postop	p-Value [3]
Serum eosinophilia						
Present	5.67	0.036	2.2	0.349	1.63	0.420
Absent	4.45	-	1.79	-	1.16	-
Tissue eosinophilia						
Present	5.35	<0.001	2.08	0.017	1.4	0.189
Absent	3.39	-	1.29	-	0.77	-
Polyps						
Present	6.56	<0.001	2.34	0.006	1.72	0.032
Absent	3.48	-	1.51	-	0.87	-
Lund-Mackay score						
LMS $\geq$ 6	5.37	<0.001	2.13	0.006	1.36	0.144
LMS < 6	3.17	-	1.26	-	0.73	-

LMS, Lund-Mackay score. [1] p-value represents comparison of preoperative LKES; [2] p-value represents comparison of three-month postoperative LKES; [3] p-value represents comparison of six-month postoperative LKES.

4. Discussion

CRS is a heterogeneous disease consisting of multiple variants with different underlying pathophysiologies [14]. In the United States and Europe, patients with CRS are classified into two phenotypes: CRS with nasal polyps (CRSwNP) and CRS without nasal polyps [15]. CRSwNP patients that have recurrence of nasal polyps after surgery are more likely to have pronounced eosinophilic infiltration of the nasal mucosa [15,16]. Eosinophilic CRS is a subtype of CRS that predicts less post-operative improvement in patient-reported QOL and disease-specific measures [17,18]. Peripheral blood eosinophilia and tissue eosinophilia are associated with more severe CRSwNP, higher recurrence rates of nasal polyps after surgery [14,15], and higher revision surgery rates [19].

The availability of bioabsorbable steroid-eluting implants in the treatment of CRS offers the potential for decreased inflammation, adhesions, recurrent polyposis, and improved sinus ostia patency in the postoperative period after ESS [10,20]. However, few studies have focused on patient-reported QOL outcomes with the use of this device, and the relative efficacy in the treatment of different phenotypes of CRS has not been analyzed in previous studies [6–8,12]. The goal of this study was to determine if a bioabsorbable steroid-eluting implant would have a differential effect on patient-reported QOL relative to the status of baseline eosinophilia. We found that QOL scores showed comparable improvement among patients with eosinophilic CRS and those without. Similar results were found when comparing low- versus high-grade sinus CT opacification, as well as patients with CRSwP versus those without polyps. These findings suggest that the benefit from these implants may not be limited to one particular CRS phenotype, and could be beneficial to a wider range of patients undergoing ESS.

In addition to patient-reported outcomes, the clinician assessment of endoscopic appearance may be a useful outcome to assess disease control. Patients with eosinophilic CRS are often noted to have persistent postoperative edema and polypoid changes on endoscopy during the postoperative period. As expected, our data showed higher preoperative LKES for patients with polyposis, eosinophilia or higher-grade CT opacification. Moreover, subsequent improvement in postoperative LKES was observed for patients with both low- and high-grade disease. At six months postoperatively, patients with preoperative eosinophilia or high-grade CT opacification were found to have an endoscopic appearance comparable to those without eosinophilia or with low-grade CT opacification. Though future controlled studies are necessary to better examine this effect, our data suggest that the steroid-eluting implant in conjunction with ESS might assist with suppression of inflammation that persists for several months after implant degradation. Further studies are required to determine whether these effects are significantly better than surgery performed without placement of a bioabsorbable steroid-eluting implant.

Revision ESS rates as reported in the literature are variable. Patients with serum and tissue eosinophilia often require systemic steroids and have significantly higher recurrence and revision rates [15,21–23]. In a previous study of the steroid-eluting implant, revision ESS was indicated in 2.2% (2/90) of cases with use of the Propel stent, which is consistent with the revision rate (1.5%) in the present study [6]. Of this, only one patient of 21 (4.8%) with serum and tissue eosinophilia required revision surgery after one year, which is significantly less than revision rates reported in the literature, though long-term follow up is necessary.

Several notable limitations are relevant in the present study. As a single-armed study without a comparison treatment group, conclusions about causation and comparative effectiveness are not possible. Additionally, although approximately 80% of patients continued to follow up six months from the time of surgery, there is a risk of follow-up bias, as postoperative outcomes could have influenced both follow-up and completion of the forms. Finally, some patients in this study also received a septoplasty and/or inferior turbinate reduction, which may be a confounding variable that overestimates the improvement in QOL measures.

Although the present study indicates that improvements occur regardless of the severity of preoperative inflammation, it remains unclear how these effects would compare to cases in which an implant was not utilized. Future studies with controlled trials of patient-reported QOL following ESS with bioabsorbable steroid-eluting implants are needed, which may utilize postoperative objective markers of inflammation to supplement the effects on patient-reported QOL. Investigation of the effect of simultaneous additional symptom scores or QOL measures may help elucidate the confounding potential of septoplasty and inferior turbinate reduction in conjunction with ESS. Lastly, examination into specific items of the SNOT-22 score that are most affected by implant placement may result in better preoperative counseling and patient selection.

5. Conclusions

Irrespective of the presence of polyposis or eosinophilia, patient-reported QOL scores are improved up to six months after placement of a steroid-eluting implant during ESS for patients with CRS. Endoscopic appearance shows comparable normalization over time regardless of the extent of preoperative inflammation. Controlled studies are necessary to determine the comparative effectiveness of the steroid-eluting implant.

Author Contributions: Edward D. McCoul conceived and designed the study; Jason D. Pou, Charles A. Riley, Anna K. Bareiss, Kiranya E. Tipirneni and Edward D. McCoul collected the data; Jason D. Pou, Charles A. Riley and Edward D. McCoul analyzed the data; Jason D. Pou, Charles A. Riley and Edward D. McCoul wrote and revised the paper; all authors approved the final manuscript.

Conflicts of Interest: There was no financial or material support for the research of this work. Edward D. McCoul is a consultant for Acclarent, which is unrelated to the current study. The other authors have no financial affiliations to disclose. The authors declare no conflict of interest.

References

1. Pleis, J.R.; Ward, B.W.; Lucas, J.W. Summary health statistics for U.S. adults: National health interview survey, 2009. *Vital Health Stat.* **2010**, *10*, 1–207.

2. Schlosser, R.J.; Gage, S.E.; Kohli, P.; Soler, Z.M. Burden of illness: A systematic review of depression in chronic rhinosinusitis. *Am. J. Rhinol. Allergy* **2016**, *30*, 250–256. [CrossRef] [PubMed]

3. Hopkins, C.; Gillett, S.; Slack, R.; Lund, V.J.; Browne, J.P. Psychometric validity of the 22-item sinonasal outcome test. *Clin. Otolaryngol.* **2009**, *34*, 447–454. [CrossRef] [PubMed]

4. Valentine, R.; Wormald, P.J. Are routine dissolvable nasal dressings necessary following endoscopic sinus surgery? *Laryngoscope* **2010**, *120*, 1920–1921. [CrossRef] [PubMed]

5. Wei, C.C.; Kennedy, D.W. Mometasone implant for chronic rhinosinusitis. *Med. Devices* **2012**, *5*, 75–80.

6.   Forwith, K.D.; Chandra, R.K.; Yun, P.T.; Miller, S.K.; Jampel, H.D. ADVANCE: A multisite trial of bioabsorbable steroid-eluting sinus implants. *Laryngoscope* **2011**, *121*, 2473–2480. [CrossRef] [PubMed]

7.   Marple, B.F.; Smith, T.L.; Han, J.K.; Gould, A.R.; Jampel, H.D.; Stambaugh, J.W.; Mugglin, A.S. Advance II: A prospective, randomized study assessing safety and efficacy of bioabsorbable steroid-releasing sinus implants. *Otolaryngol. Head Neck Surg.* **2012**, *146*, 1004–1011. [CrossRef] [PubMed]

8.   Murr, A.H.; Smith, T.L.; Hwang, P.H.; Bhattacharyya, N.; Lanier, B.J.; Stambaugh, J.W.; Mugglin, A.S. Safety and efficacy of a novel bioabsorbable, steroid-eluting sinus stent. *Int. Forum Allergy Rhinol.* **2011**, *1*, 23–32. [CrossRef] [PubMed]

9.   Campbell, R.G.; Kennedy, D.W. What is new and promising with drug-eluting stents in sinus surgery? *Curr. Opin. Otolaryngol. Head Neck Surg.* **2014**, *22*, 2–7. [CrossRef] [PubMed]

10.   Bednarski, K.A.; Kuhn, F.A. Stents and drug-eluting stents. *Otolaryngol. Clin. N. Am.* **2009**, *42*, 857–866. [CrossRef] [PubMed]

11.   Intersect ENT Inc. Propel Mometasone Implant. Available online: http://propelopens.com/the-propel-advantage/how-it-works (accessed on 10 September 2016).

12.   Forwith, K.D.; Han, J.K.; Stolovitzky, J.P.; Yen, D.M.; Chandra, R.K.; Karanfilov, B.; Matheny, K.E.; Stambaugh, J.W.; Gawlicka, A.K. RESOLVE: Bioabsorbable steroid-eluting sinus implants for in-office treatment of recurrent sinonasal polyposis after sinus surgery: 6-month outcomes from a randomized, controlled, blinded study. *Int. Forum Allergy Rhinol.* **2016**, *6*, 573–581. [CrossRef] [PubMed]

13.   Hopkins, C.; Rudmik, L.; Lund, V.J. The predictive value of the preoperative sinonasal outcome test-22 score in patients undergoing endoscopic sinus surgery for chronic rhinosinusitis. *Laryngoscope* **2015**, *125*, 1779–1784. [CrossRef] [PubMed]

14.   Kim, J.H.; Choi, G.E.; Lee, B.J.; Kwon, S.W.; Lee, S.H.; Kim, H.S.; Jang, Y.J. Natural killer cells regulate eosinophilic inflammation in chronic rhinosinusitis. *Sci. Rep.* **2016**, *6*, 27615. [CrossRef] [PubMed]

15.   Akdis, C.A.; Bachert, C.; Cingi, C.; Dykewicz, M.S.; Hellings, P.W.; Naclerio, R.M.; Schleimer, R.P.; Ledford, D. Endotypes and phenotypes of chronic rhinosinusitis: A PRACTALL document of the European academy of allergy and clinical immunology and the American academy of allergy, asthma & immunology. *J. Allergy Clin. Immunol.* **2013**, *131*, 1479–1490. [PubMed]

16.   Shah, S.A.; Ishinaga, H.; Takeuchi, K. Pathogenesis of eosinophilic chronic rhinosinusitis. *J. Inflamm.* **2016**, *13*, 11. [CrossRef] [PubMed]

17.   Ferguson, B.J. Eosinophilic mucin rhinosinusitis: A distinct clinicopathological entity. *Laryngoscope* **2000**, *110*, 799–813. [CrossRef] [PubMed]

18.   Soler, Z.M.; Sauer, D.; Mace, J.; Smith, T.L. Impact of mucosal eosinophilia and nasal polyposis on quality-of-life outcomes after sinus surgery. *Otolaryngol. Head Neck Surg.* **2010**, *142*, 64–71. [CrossRef] [PubMed]

19.   Vlaminck, S.; Vauterin, T.; Hellings, P.W.; Jorissen, M.; Acke, F.; Van-Cauwenberge, P.; Bachert, C.; Gevaert, P. The importance of local eosinophilia in the surgical outcome of chronic rhinosinusitis: A 3-year prospective observational study. *Am. J. Rhinol. Allergy* **2014**, *28*, 260–264. [CrossRef] [PubMed]

20.   Janisiewicz, A.; Lee, J.T. In-office use of a steroid-eluting implant for maintenance of frontal ostial patency after revision sinus surgery. *Allergy Rhinol* **2015**, *6*, 68–75. [CrossRef] [PubMed]

21.   Tansavatdi, K.P.; McGill, L.; Riggs, S.; Orlandi, R.R. Development of an animal model for wound healing in chronic rhinosinusitis. *Arch. Otolaryngol. Head Neck Surg.* **2010**, *136*, 807–812. [CrossRef] [PubMed]

22.   Jakobsen, J.; Svendstrup, F. Functional endoscopic sinus surgery in chronic sinusitis—A series of 237 consecutively operated patients. *Acta Otolaryngol. Suppl.* **2000**, *543*, 158–161. [CrossRef] [PubMed]

23.   Lee, S.H.; Kim, H.J.; Lee, J.W.; Yoon, Y.H.; Kim, Y.M.; Rha, K.S. Categorization and clinicopathological features of chronic rhinosinusitis with eosinophilic mucin in a Korean population. *Clin. Exp. Otorhinolaryngol.* **2015**, *8*, 39–45. [CrossRef] [PubMed]

8

The Impact of Endonasal Endoscopic Sinus Surgery on Patients with Chronic Pulmonary Diseases

Basel Al Kadah [1],*, Gudrun Helmus [1], Quoc Thai Dinh [2] and Bernhard Schick [1]

[1] Department of Otorhinolaryngology, University Medical Center Homburg/Saar, D-66424 Homburg, Germany; gudrunhelmus@gmx.de (G.H.); bernhard.schick@uks.eu (B.S.)

[2] Department of Pneumology and Experimental Pneumology, University Medical Center Homburg/Saar, D-66424 Homburg, Germany; thai.dinh@uks.eu

* Correspondence: basel.al-kadah@uks.eu

Academic Editor: César Picado

Abstract: Introduction: The impact of endoscopic sinus surgery on bronchial asthma has been studied by several groups. According to the latest studies, patients with chronic obstructive pulmonary disease (COPD) seem to have frequent symptoms of chronic rhinosinusitis. Our study compares the impact of endoscopic sinus surgery on both the upper and lower airways of patients with bronchial asthma as well as those with COPD. Methods: This study includes 43 patients (bronchial asthma, $n = 32$, COPD, $n = 11$) undergoing surgical treatment for chronic rhinosinusitis at the ENT-Department, University of Homburg (Homburg, Germany). To assess the effect of sinus surgery, the Sino-Nasal Outcome Test 20 German Adapted Version (SNOT-20 GAV) and St. George's Respiratory Questionnaire (SGRQ) were used both pre- and postoperatively. Results: Both SNOT-20 ($p < 0.001$) and SGRQ ($p = 0.021$) scores improved significantly after sinus surgery. The postoperative improvement in bronchial asthma and COPD was similar in both groups, indicating no difference of the diseases in regards to postoperative symptom improvement. There was no difference indicated in SNOT-20 GAV or SGRQ when grouping patients by polyps, aspirin (ASS) intolerance, allergies, eosinophilia or previous surgery. Conclusions: The treatment of chronic rhinosinusitis by sinus surgery may help to improve the therapy outcome of patients with bronchial asthma as well as patients with COPD.

Keywords: endoscopic sinus surgery; COPD; asthma; SGRQ; SNOT-20 GAV

1. Introduction

Several research groups have studied the impact of sinus surgery on bronchial asthma and have often noticed the term sinubronchial syndrome [1,2]. However, there is no exact definition for this term. A current chronic rhinosinusitis guideline prefers collaboration with pneumologists [3], and a current study by Ehnhage et al. shows the impact of sinus surgery on the symptoms and lung function parameters in patients with bronchial asthma [4].

Hurst et al. (2006) reported investigations of chronic obstructive pulmonary diseases (COPD) patients showing an inflammatory marker in the sputum and nasal lavage with the finding that the entire respiratory system was affected by the inflammatory reaction [5]. Considering the aspect of inflammatory reactions along the entire respiratory system, recent studies focused on the incidence of rhinosinusitis in patients with chronic bronchitis and COPD. Hens et al. (2008) and Piotrowska et al. (2010) found higher endoscopic rhinosinusitis symptom scores in patients with COPD than in the healthy population [6,7]. In 90 patients with COPD in different disease stages, Kelemence et al. detected clinical criteria for rhinosinusitis in 53% of the patients [8]. In a review,

Kim and Rubin (2007) reported that 75% of all patients with COPD collectively complained of nasal symptoms [9].

There have been multiple studies of bronchial asthma which have examined the influence and impact of sinus surgery on pulmonary disease, however, the influence of sinus surgery on chronic bronchitis has yet to be investigated. The aim of this study is to investigate any changes after performing sinus surgery, in the patients' quality of life and any symptom changes in patients with chronic sinusitis in combination with COPD or with bronchial asthma.

2. Materials and Methods

This study includes 43 patients (22 male, 21 female) within a period ranging from January 2010 until April 2011. The median age was 50.8 years with a standard deviation of 16 years. The 43 patients (bronchial asthma: $n = 32$, COPD: $n = 11$) underwent surgical treatment for chronic rhinosinusitis in the ENT-Department at Saarland University Medical Center Homburg (Homburg Germany). The patients were examined by pneumologists before being included in the study, and the pneumologists had outlined the definition of a diagnosis of asthma or COPD. All patients gave their informed consent. All procedures performed in studies involving human participants were in accordance with the ethical standards of the institutional research committee and with the 1964 Helsinki declaration and its later amendments or comparable ethical standards.

Of a possible 57 patients, 43 patients were included in the study, which resulted in a 75% recirculation rate. There were 14 patients who were excluded due to an incomplete data source. Patient data was anonymized. An endonasal endoscopic sinus surgery according to the concepts of functional endoscopic sinus surgery developed by Heerman, Messerklinger, Draf, Wigand and Stammberger [10] was performed in intubation anesthesia after informed consent. Patient file evaluations were retrospective. A medical history and CT-Score according to Lund-Mackay was available for every patient. To assess the effect of functional endoscopic surgery, the Sino-Nasal Outcome Test 20 German Adapted Version (SNOT-20 GAV) and St. George's Respiratory Questionnaire (SGRQ) were used one week preoperatively and for a minimum of three months postoperatively. In addition, the patients' medical treatment for bronchial asthma and COPD was evaluated.

The SGRQ has been developed by Jones et al. [11]. The SGRQ covers the quality of life of patients with COPD, bronchial asthma and bronchiectasis in three sub-scales (symptom, activity and strain) and has been validated for a three month time frame [11]. The SNOT-20 is a validated questionnaire reported by Piccirillo et al. [12], and the SNOT-20 GAV is validated by Baumann et al. [13].

Statistical analysis was tested by using a cross table and Chi-Square-Test. When the requirements for Chi-Square-Test had not been reached, we used the Fisher-Exact-Test. The postoperative run was tested with the Wilcoxon-Test. The Kruskal-Wallis-Test was used to compare more than two groups. We calculated the grade of correlation coefficient according to Spearman. Level $\alpha = 0.05$ was defined as a significant level. The statistical data base was analyzed and processed under the application SPSS "Statistical Package for the Social Sciences" (SPSS®, IBM Corporation, New York, NY, USA), Version 19 for Windows, as well as Microsoft Office Excel 2007 for Windows (Microsoft Corporation, Redmond, WA, USA).

3. Results

There were 43 cases with at least a one-year follow-up that were analyzed after functional endoscopic sinus surgery: There were 32 patients (74.4%) with bronchial asthma and 11 patients (25.6%) with COPD. There were 29 patients (67.4%) who had nasal polyps, 12 patients (27.9%) who had aspirin intolerance, and 11 patients (25.6%) who had Samter-syndrome. (Figure 1).

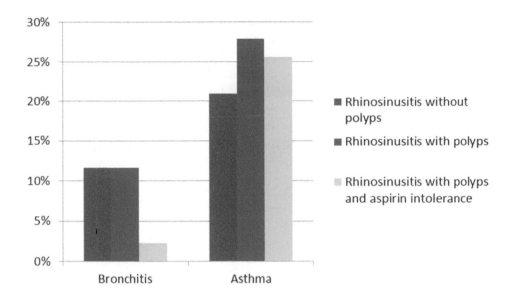

Figure 1. Incidence of Aspirin-Intolerance and nasal polyp.

Eosinophily was found in the histopathological nasal mucosa analysis of 30 patients (73.2%). Seasonal allergies were reported in 11 patients (25.6%), and 22 patients (51.2%) reported perennial allergies.

The median CT-score according to Lund-Mackay resulted in a preoperative CT-score of 13.5 with no difference between asthma patients and COPD patients ($p = 0.277$). Most patients were on their first or second sinus operation. A third operation was performed in six patients, a fourth operation was performed in two patients and a seventh operation was performed in one patient. The questionnaires were completed in an average postoperative rate of 4.3 ± 2.2 month. Figure 2 shows the medication level pre- and post- operative. The medication intake, before and after the sinus surgery, was insignificantly different in both groups according to the result of the Wilcoxon-Test ($p = 0.429$).

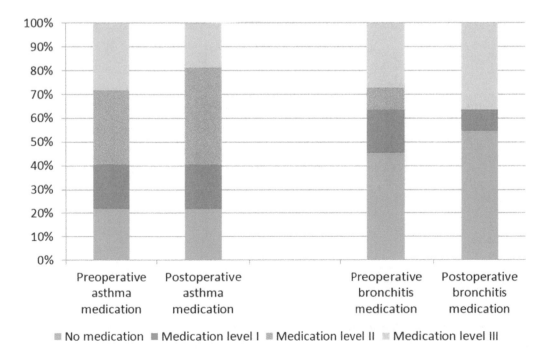

Figure 2. Medication level pre- and postoperative.

The total score of the SGRQ in all patients shows a preoperative median value of 36.3% and a postoperative median value of 24.8% (Figure 3a). Additionally, the average improvement of the SGRQ score, 8.3 points in asthma patients and 7.9 points in COPD patients, was statistically significant after sinus surgery compared to the preoperative value (Figure 3b, Wilcoxon-Test: $p = 0.021$). The preoperative median symptom score was 50.2% and the postoperative score was 44.6% (Figures 4 and 5). The preoperative median activity score was 42.7% and the postoperative score was 36.5%. The preoperative median impact score was 26.9% and the postoperative score was 14.4%. The activity score ($p = 0.001$) and the impact score ($p = 0.003$) were statistically significant, while the symptom score was insignificant with $p = 0.132$ (Figure 6).

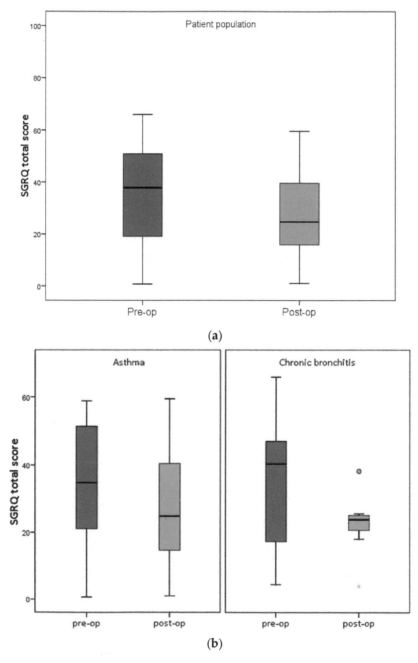

Figure 3. (a) St. George's Respiratory Questionnaire (SGRQ) total score; (b) SGRQ total score pre-op and post-op in asthma and chronic bronchitis group. pre-op: preoperative; post-op: postoperative. Green asterisk and circle are outliers.

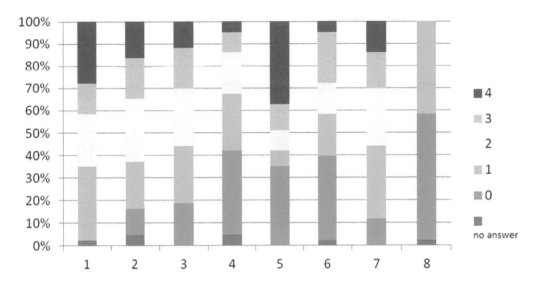

Figure 4. SGRQ subscale symptoms pre-op (0 = no symptom, 1 = light symptom, 2 = mild symptom, 3 = intense symptom, 4 = heavy symptom, 0% no impairment to 100% heavy impairment).

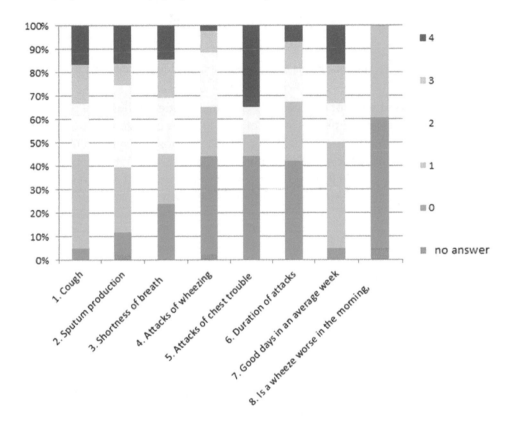

Figure 5. SGRQ subscale symptoms post-op (0 = no symptom, 1 = light symptom, 2 = mild symptom, 3 = intense symptom, 4 = heavy symptom, 0% no impairment to 100% heavy impairment).

No statistically significant difference was found when comparing the average improvement of the SGRQ in asthma patients and in COPD patient groups both preoperatively and postoperatively, using the Fisher-Exact-Test ($p = 0.695$), (Figure 4). Dividing the groups into patients with polyps, patients without polyps, patients with allergies, patients without allergies, patients with ASS-intolerance, and patients without ASS-intolerance, the Fisher-Exact-Test showed no statistical significance between the different sub-groups preoperatively nor postoperatively. All sub-groups had better results after having sinus surgery.

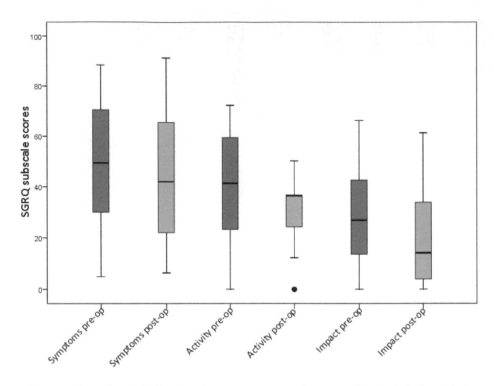

Figure 6. Box plots SGRQ subscale scores pre-op and post-op (black circle is outlier).

(Figures 7–10). The total score of the SNOT-20 GAV in all patients showed a preoperative median value of 44% and a postoperative median value of 22% and the change was significant before and after sinus surgery (Wilcoxon-Test: $p < 0.001$, Figure 11). Almost all symptoms in SNOT-20 GAV questionnaires were significantly better postoperatively in both groups (Table 1). Dividing the patients into an asthma group and a COPD group did not result in a significant difference between groups, ($p = 0.089$) both groups saw significant changes after sinus surgery.

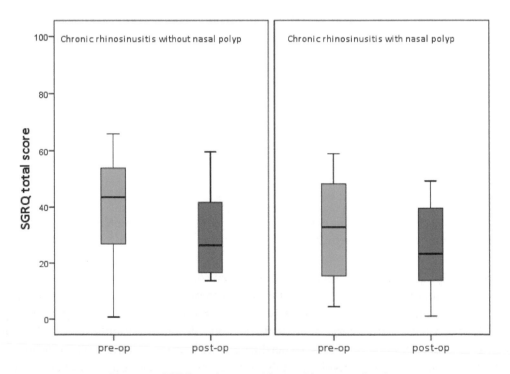

Figure 7. SGRQ total score with or without nasal polyp.

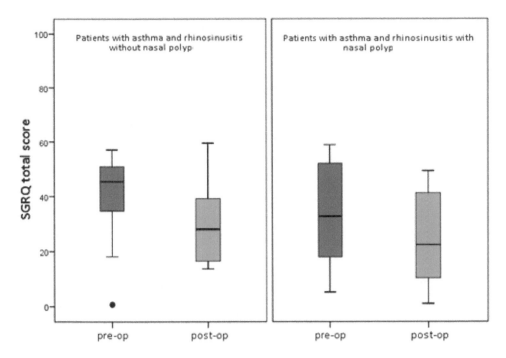

Figure 8. SGRQ total score in asthma patient with or without nasal polyp (black circle is outlier).

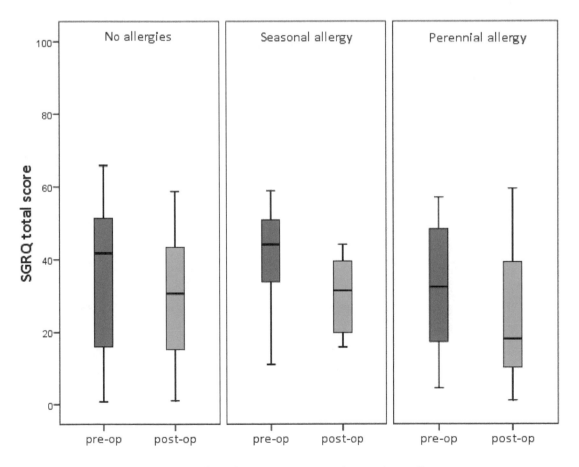

Figure 9. SGRQ total score in patient with or without allergy.

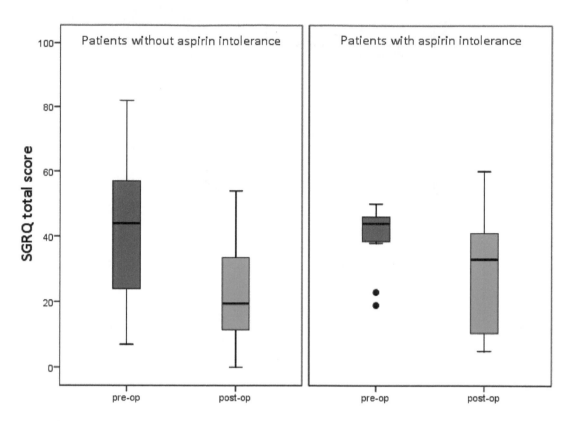

Figure 10. SGRQ total score with or without aspirin intolerance (black circles are outliers).

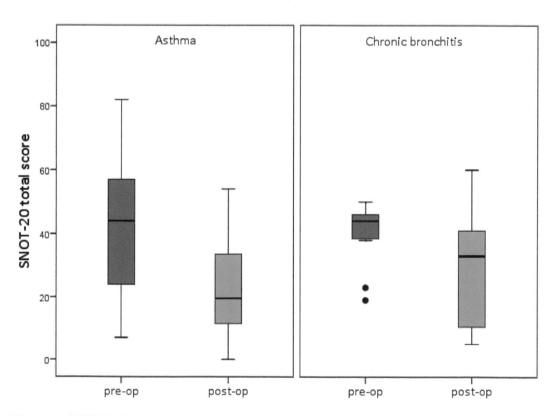

Figure 11. SNOT-20 GAV total score pre-op and post-op in asthma and chronic bronchitis group (black circles are outliers).

Table 1. Sino-Nasal Outcome Test 20 German Adapted Version (SNOT-20 GAV) symptom score pre-op and post-op.

Symptom	Pre-op (Ø)	Post-op (Ø)	p-value
Need to blow nose	2.51 ± 1.4	1.44 ± 1.2	<0.001
Sneezing	2.00 ± 1.5	0.93 ± 0.9	<0.001
Runny nose	2.21 ± 1.6	1.00 ± 1.1	<0.001
Cough	2.23 ± 1.6	1.67 ± 1.5	0.010
Postnasal discharge	2.72 ± 1.7	1.67 ± 1.4	0.001
Thick nasal discharge	2.67 ± 1.6	1.49 ± 1.4	<0.001
Ear fullness	1.91 ± 1.5	0.81 ± 1.2	<0.001
Dizziness	1.16 ± 1.4	0.67 ± 1.1	0.005
Ear pain	0.93 ± 1.1	0.51 ± 0.8	0.033
Facial pain/pressure	2.37 ± 1.8	1.12 ± 1.2	<0.001
Difficulty falling asleep	1.88 ± 1.7	1.26 ± 1.5	0.003
Wake up at night	2.60 ± 1.3	1.74 ± 1.4	<0.001
Lack of a good night's sleep	2.81 ± 1.6	1.53 ± 1.5	<0.001
Wake up tired	2.49 ± 1.6	1.65 ± 1.5	0.001
Fatigue	2.70 ± 1.6	1.70 ± 1.2	<0.001
Reduced productivity	2.47 ± 1.6	1.60 ± 1.4	0.001
Reduced concentration	2.14 ± 1.5	1.21 ± 1.2	<0.001
Frustrated/restless/irritable	2.14 ± 1.5	1.09 ± 1.2	<0.001
Sad	1.65 ± 1.6	0.84 ± 1.1	0.001
Embarrassed	1.02 ± 1.4	0.42 ± 0.8	<0.001

4. Discussion

This study focuses on possible improvements in the quality of life of COPD patients after sinus surgery.

The study found SGRQ improvements in patients with asthma to be 8.3 points and in patients with COPD to be 7.9 points. 69.0% of the asthma patients and 62.5% of the COPD patients showed postoperative improvements in a minimum of four points. In 2002, a differentiation of four points in SGRQ was identified by Jones as being clinically relevant [14]. Therefore, this study proves for the first time that in both groups there was a relevant improvement in the quality of life after sinus surgery.

Additionally, this study demonstrates the impact of upper airway on the lower airway independent of the pathology in patients with COPD. The impact of sinus surgery on the lower airway has previously been demonstrated in patients with bronchial asthma and bronchial hyperreagibility. A significant improvement of lung function in patients with bronchial asthma was found in different studies [4,15]. Stahl et al. [16] reported on the relation between severity of the COPD, GOLD (Global Initiative for Chronic Obstructive Lung Disease) classification and SGRQ-score in patients with a medial SGRQ score of 32.9%. An improvement of the peak flow in 75% was reported in Dejima et al. Study [17]. Improvements of the subjective feeling of the patients with asthma of 70% have been noted by Uri et al. 2002 [18].

The quality of life for patients in our study was improved after sinus surgery independent of an additional disease pattern such as nasal polyps or ASS intolerance. Similar results have been reported by Batra et al. (2003), which analysed 17 patients with nasal polyps and bronchial asthma as well as nine patients with ASS-intolerance and bronchial asthma, showing the improvement of bronchial asthma independent of ASS intolerance [19].

Comparing the results of SNOT-20 GAV and SGRQ, patients with a high preoperative SNOT-20 GAV score obviously experienced greater improvements in their postoperative quality of life. The correlation coefficient between preoperative SGRQ and the improvement of the postoperative run, as well as for SNOT and SGRQ, found an adequate rank level in both.

In this study, the second data acquisition was taken at a minimum of three months after sinus surgery. Usually the oedema phase takes approximately 30 days, and after three months the healing process is complete [20]. Baumann et al. [21] and Hopkins et al. [22] determined there was no difference or significant outcome of SNOT-20 GAV between the three month and the one year data collection results and the five year results. Not all patients in this study had preoperative medication for bronchial asthma or COPD. This was found to be a limitation when questioning medication changes post sinus surgery. A high percentage of the study patients (22%) needed no medication therapy pre- or postoperatively. In a European study conducted by Patridge et al. 2011, 50% of asthma patients and 23% of COPD patients needed no medication when first questioned [23].

In this study, 28% of the patients had ASS-intolerance with a quarter of those having nasal polyps. Based on previous studies, the prevalence of ASS-intolerance ranges from 0.6% to 2.5%, whilst the prevalence increases to 20% in patients with asthma [3,24]. In our study group, the eosinophily in the histopathological examination of the nasal mucosa was 72% in patients with asthma, and 64% in the COPD patients. An allergy was known to be present in 80% of the asthma patients. Various authors have reported the correlation of eosinophily in nasal mucosa and bronchial asthma [25,26]. Various studies have also shown a strong correlation, up to 80%, between patients with an allergy and patients with bronchial asthma [27,28].

In our study, the Lund-MacKay Score was 13.5 points. A score of five points was determined to be nonpathological [29]. Patients with chronic sinusitis were found to have a score ranging from 10 to 13.4 points [30,31]. A higher score was detected [32,33] in patients with bronchial asthma

In this study, 58% of the patients had sinus surgery as a revision surgery. In previous studies, note that the revision surgery rate ranges from 19% to 63% [34–36]. Risk factors for revision surgery include: ASS-intolerance [37], bronchial asthma [38], allergy [39] and nasal polyps [40]. Our study clearly demonstrates the improvement of the SNOT-20 GAV results with a preoperative median score of 44 points and a postoperative score of 22 points. The improvement was high and statistically significant ($p < 0.001$). This improvement in the SNOT-20 GAV score was independent of pulmonary disease, ASS-intolerant, nasal polyp, allergy, CT-Score and revision surgery. Numerous studies have confirmed the success of the operation for patients with chronic sinusitis based on a SNOT-20 score [30,31,33,41,42].

5. Conclusions

This study shows the positive impact of sinus surgery for patients with bronchial asthma as well as for patients with COPD. The postoperative improvement was independent of pulmonary disease, nasal polyp, allergy, eosinophily, ASS-intolerance, CT-score or revision surgery. Sinus surgery for chronic rhinosinusitis may help to improve the therapy outcome of patients with bronchial asthma and COPD.

Acknowledgments: The authors would like to acknowledge the valuable contribution of Mei Fang Ong from the institute for Medical Biometry, University Medical Center Homburg/Saar, Germany in performing the statistical analysis. The authors would also like to acknowledge the valuable contribution made by native English speaker Jane C. Crofts in proof-reading this manuscript.

Author Contributions: Basel Al Kadah, study design, data collection, statistical analysis, drafting, final approval, accountability for all aspects of the work, correspondence; Gudrun Helmus, study design, data collection, statistical analysis, drafting, final approval; Quoc Thai Dinh and Bernhard Schick, revision, drafting, final approval, accountability for all aspects of the work.

Conflicts of Interest: The authors declare no conflict of interest.

References

1. Huzly, A. Sinobronchial Syndrome. *Beitr. Klin. Tuberk.* **1969**, *139*, 265–282. [CrossRef]
2. Singleton, M.A. The sinobronchial syndrome: An old fashioned, modern-day entity. *South Med. J.* **1971**, *64*, 754–756. [CrossRef] [PubMed]
3. Stuck, B.A.; Bachert, C.; Federspil, P.; Hosemann, W.; Klimek, L.; Mösges, R.; Pfaar, O.; Rudack, C.; Sitter, H.; Wagenmann, M.; et al. German Society of Otorhinolaryngology, Head and Neck Surgery. Rhinosinusitis guidelines—unabridged version: S2 guidelines from the German Society of Otorhinolaryngology, Head and Neck Surgery. *HNO* **2012**, *60*, 141–162. [CrossRef] [PubMed]

4.   Ehnhage, A.; Olsson, P.; Kolbeck, K.G.; Skedinger, M.; Stjärne, P. One year after endoscopic sinus surgery in polyposis: Asthma, olfaction, and quality-of-life outcomes. *Otolaryngol. Head Neck Surg.* **2012**, *146*, 834–841. [CrossRef] [PubMed]

5.   Hurst, J.R.; Perera, W.R.; Wilkinson, T.M.; Donaldson, G.C.; Wedzicha, J.A. Systemic and upper and lower airway inflammation at exacerbation of chronic obstructive pulmonary disease. *Am. J. Respir. Crit. Care Med.* **2006**, *173*, 71–78. [CrossRef] [PubMed]

6.   Hens, G.; Vanaudenaerde, B.M.; Bullens, D.M.A.; Piessens, M.; Decramer, M.; Dupont, L.J.; Hellings, P.W. Sinonasal pathology in nonallergic asthma and COPD: "United airway disease" beyond the scope of allergy. *Allergy* **2008**, *63*, 261–267. [CrossRef] [PubMed]

7.   Piotrowska, V.M.; Piotrowski, W.J.; Kurmanowska, Z.; Marczak, J.; Górski, P.; Antczak, A. Rhinosinusitis in COPD: Symptoms, mucosal changes, nasal lavage cells and eicosanoids. *Int. J. Chronic Obstr. Pulm. Dis.* **2010**, *5*, 107–117.

8.   Kelemence, A.; Abadoglu, O.; Gumus, C.; Berk, S.; Epozturk, K.; Akkurt, I. The Frequency of Chronic Rhinosinusitis/Nasal Polyp in COPD and Its Effect on the Severity of COPD. *COPD J. Chronic Obstr. Pulm. Dis.* **2011**, *8*, 8–12. [CrossRef] [PubMed]

9.   Kim, J.S.; Rubin, B.K. Nasal and sinus inflammation in chronic obstructive pulmonary disease. *COPD* **2007**, *4*, 163–166. [CrossRef] [PubMed]

10.   Al Kadah, B.; Bumm, K.; Charalampaki, P.; Schick, B. First experience in endonasal surgery using a new 3D-Chipendoscope Laryngorhinootologie. *Laryngo-Rhino-Otol.* **2012**, *91*, 428–433.

11.   Jones, P.W. St. George's Respiratory Questionnaire: MCID. *COPD J. Chronic Obstr. Pulm. Dis.* **2005**, *2*, 75–79. [CrossRef]

12.   Piccirillo, J.F.; Merritt, M.G., Jr.; Richards, M.L. Psychometric and clinimetric validity of the 20-Item Sino-Nasal Outcome Test (SNOT-20). *Otolaryngol. Head Neck Surg.* **2002**, *126*, 41–47. [CrossRef] [PubMed]

13.   Baumann, I.; Blumenstock, G.; DeMaddalena, H.; Piccirillo, J.F.; Plinkert, P.K. Quality of life in patients with chronic rhinosinusitis Validation of the Sino-Nasal Outcome Test-20 German Adapted Version. *HNO* **2007**, *55*, 42–47. [CrossRef] [PubMed]

14.   Jones, P.W. Interpreting thresholds for a clinically significant change in health status in asthma and COPD. *Eur. Respir. J.* **2002**, *19*, 398–404. [CrossRef] [PubMed]

15.   Loehrl, T.A.; Ferre, R.M.; Toohill, R.J.; Smith, T.L. Long-term asthma outcomes after endoscopic sinus surgery in aspirin triad patients. *Am. J. Otolaryngol.* **2006**, *27*, 154–160. [CrossRef] [PubMed]

16.   Stahl, E.; Lindberg, A.; Jansson, S.-A.; Rönmark, E.; Svensson, K.; Andersson, F.; Lundbäck, B. Health-related quality of life is related to COPD disease severity. *Health Qual. Life Outcomes* **2005**, *3*, 56–64. [CrossRef] [PubMed]

17.   Dejima, K.; Hama, T.; Miyazaki, M.; Yasuda, S.; Fukushima, K.; Oshima, A.; Hisa, Y. A clinical study of endoscopic sinus surgery for sinusitis in patients with bronchial asthma. *Int. Arch. Allergy Immunol.* **2005**, *138*, 97–104. [CrossRef] [PubMed]

18.   Uri, N.; Cohen-Kerem, R.; Barzilai, G.; Greenberg, E.; Doweck, I.; Weiler-Ravell, D. Functional endoscopic sinus surgery in the treatment of massive polyposis in asthmatic patients. *J. Laryngol. Otol.* **2002**, *116*, 185–189. [CrossRef] [PubMed]

19.   Batra, P.S.; Kern, R.C.; Tripathi, A.; Conley, D.B.; Ditto, A.M.; Haines, G.K.; Grammar, L. Outcome analysis of endoscopic sinus surgery in patients with nasal polyps and asthma. *Laryngoscope* **2003**, *113*, 1703–1706. [CrossRef] [PubMed]

20.   Hosemann, W.; Wigand, M.E.; Gode, U.; Linger, F.; Dunker, I. Normal wound healing of the paranasal sinuses: Clinical and experimental investigations. *Eur. Arch. Otorhinolaryngol.* **1991**, *248*, 390–394. [CrossRef] [PubMed]

21.   Baumann, I.; Blumenstock, G.; Praetorius, M.; Sittel, C.; Piccirillo, J.F.; Plinkert, P.K. Patients with chronic rhinosinusitis: Disease-specific and general health-related quality of life. *HNO* **2006**, *54*, 544–549. [CrossRef] [PubMed]

22.   Hopkins, C.; Slack, R.; Lund, V.; Brown, P.; Copley, L.; Browne, J. Long-term outcomes from the English national comparative audit of surgery for nasal polyposis and chronic rhinosinusitis. *Laryngoscope* **2009**, *119*, 2459–2465. [CrossRef] [PubMed]

23.   Partridge, M.R.; Dal Negro, R.W.; Olivieri, D. Understanding patients with asthma and COPD: Insights from a European study. *Prim. Care Respir. J.* **2011**, *20*, 315–323. [CrossRef] [PubMed]

24. May, A.; Wagner, D.; Langenbeck, U.; Weber, A. Family study of patients with aspirin intolerance and rhinosinusitis. *HNO* **2000**, *9*, 650–655. [CrossRef]

25. Bourdin, A.; Gras, D.; Vachier, I.; Chanez, P. Upper airway 1: Allergic rhinitis and asthma: United disease through epithelial cells. *Thorax* **2009**, *64*, 999–1004. [CrossRef] [PubMed]

26. Ciprandi, G.; Cirillo, I.; Vizzaccaro, A.; Milanese, M.; Tosca, M.A. Airway function and nasal inflammation in seasonal allergic rhinitis and asthma. *Clin. Exp. Allergy* **2004**, *34*, 891–896. [CrossRef] [PubMed]

27. Awad, O.G.; Lee, J.H.; Fasano, M.B.; Graham, S.M. Sinonasal outcomes after endoscopic sinus surgery in asthmatic patients with nasal polyps: A difference between aspirin-tolerant and aspirin-induced asthma? *Laryngoscope* **2008**, *118*, 1282–1286. [CrossRef] [PubMed]

28. Vogelmeier, C.; Buhl, R.; Criee, C.P.; Gillissen, A.; Kardos, P.; Köhler, D.; Magnussen, H.; Morr, H.; Nowak, D.; Pfeiffer–Kascha, D.; et al. Leitlinie der Deutschen Atemwegsliga und der Deutschen Gesellschaft für Pneumologie und Beatmungsmedizin zur Diagnostik und Therapie von Patienten mit chronisch obstruktiver Bronchitis und Lungenemphysem (COPD). *Pneumologie* **2007**, *61*, e1–e40. (In German). [CrossRef] [PubMed]

29. Ashraf, N.; Bhattacharyya, N. Determination of the "incidental" Lund scores for the staging of chronic rhinosinusitis. *Otolaryngol. Head Neck Surg.* **2001**, *125*, 483–486. [CrossRef]

30. Baumann, I.; Blumenstock, G.; Zalaman, I.M.; Praetorius, M.; Klingmann, C.; Sittel, C.; Piccirillo, J.F. Impact of gender, age, and comorbidities on quality of life in patients with chronic rhinosinusitis. *Rhinology* **2007**, *45*, 268–272. [PubMed]

31. Bradley, D.T.; Kountakis, S.E. Correlation between computed tomography scores and symptomatic improvement after endoscopic sinus surgery. *Laryngoscope* **2005**, *115*, 466–469. [CrossRef] [PubMed]

32. Bonfils, P.; Tavernier, L.; Abdel Rahman, H.; Mimoun, M.; Malinvaud, D. Evaluation of combined medical and surgical treatment in nasal polyposis—III. Correlation between symptoms and CT scores before and after surgery for nasal polyposis. *Acta Otolaryngol.* **2008**, *128*, 318–323. [CrossRef] [PubMed]

33. Kountakis, S.E.; Bradley, D.T. Effect of asthma on sinus computed tomography grade and symptom scores in patients undergoing revision functional endoscopic sinus surgery. *Am. J. Rhinol.* **2003**, *17*, 215–219. [PubMed]

34. Lee, J.Y.; Lee, S.W.; Lee, J.D. Comparison of the surgical outcome between primary and revision endoscopic sinus surgery for chronic rhinosinusitis with nasal polyposis. *Am. J. Otolaryngol.* **2008**, *29*, 379–384. [CrossRef] [PubMed]

35. Seyring, C.; Bitter, T.; Boger, D.; Büntzel, J.; Esser, D.; Hoffmann, K.; Guntinas-Lichius, O. Health Services Research on Paranasal Sinus Surgery in Thuringia: Epidemiologic Key Data and Outcome. *Laryngorhinootologie* **2012**, *91*, 434–439. [PubMed]

36. Smith, T.L.; Mendolia-Loffredo, S.; Loehrl, T.A.; Sparapani, R.; Laud, P.W.; Nattinger, A.B. Predictive factors and outcomes in endoscopic sinus surgery for chronic rhinosinusitis. *Laryngoscope* **2005**, *115*, 2199–2205. [CrossRef] [PubMed]

37. Gosepath, J.; Pogodsky, T.; Mann, W.J. Characteristics of recurrent chronic rhinosinusitis after previous surgical therapy. *Acta Otolaryngol.* **2008**, *128*, 778–784. [CrossRef] [PubMed]

38. Seybt, M.W.; McMains, K.C.; Kountakis, S.E. The prevalence and effect of asthma on adults with chronic rhinosinusitis. *Ear Nose Throat J.* **2007**, *86*, 409–411. [PubMed]

39. Wilkinson, T.M.; Patel, I.S.; Wilks, M.; Donaldson, G.C.; Wedzicha, J.A. Airway bacterial load and FEV1 decline in patients with chronic obstructive pulmonary disease. *Am. J. Respir. Crit. Care Med.* **2003**, *167*, 1090–1095. [CrossRef] [PubMed]

40. Hosemann, W. Postoperative measures to prevent recurrence of chronic pansinusitis and polyposis nasi. *HNO* **2003**, *51*, 279–283. [CrossRef] [PubMed]

41. Bezerra, T.F.; Piccirillo, J.F.; Fornazieri, M.A.; Pilan, R.R.D.M.; Pinna, F.D.R.; Padua, F.G.D.M.; Voegels, R.L. Assessment of quality of life after endoscopic sinus surgery for chronic rhinosinusitis. *Braz. J. Otorhinolaryngol.* **2012**, *78*, 96–102. [CrossRef] [PubMed]

42. Ling, F.T.; Kountakis, S.E. Important clinical symptoms in patients undergoing functional endoscopic sinus surgery for chronic rhinosinusitis. *Laryngoscope* **2007**, *117*, 1090–1093. [CrossRef] [PubMed]

9

Multimodal Frequency Treatment for Facial Pain Caused by Chronic Rhinosinusitis

Michael Smith [1], Philippe G. Berenger [2], Peter Bonutti [3], Alisa P. Ramakrishnan [3], Justin Beyers [3] and Vivek Ramakrishnan [4],*

[1] Sarah Bush Lincoln Health Center, 1000 Health Center Dr., Mattoon, IL 61938, USA; msmith@sblhs.org
[2] Department of Pain Management, Cleveland Clinic Foundation, 9500 Euclid Avenue, Cleveland, OH 44195, USA; berengp@ccf.org
[3] Bonutti Technologies, 2600 S Raney St., Effingham, IL 62401, USA; peter@bonutti.net (P.B.); alisa@bonuttiresearch.com (A.P.R.); jbeyers@bonuttitechnologies.com (J.B.)
[4] AxioSonic, 2600 S Raney St., Effingham, IL 62401, USA
* Correspondence: vivek@axiosonic.com; Tel.: +1-217-342-3400

Abstract: Chronic rhinosinusitis (CRS) is a common disease that affects over 200 million patients worldwide. CRS often presents with facial pain, which is considered an important criterion for the diagnosis of CRS. A single-arm clinical study was designed to test the effect of simultaneous high (1 MHz) and low frequencies (70–80 Hz) on facial pain in 14 CRS patients at the Sarah Bush Lincoln Health Center, Mattoon, IL, USA. We used two quality of life (QOL) instruments to test the effect of multimodal frequencies on patients suffering from CRS: the Brief Pain Inventory Short Form (BPI-SF), and the Sino-Nasal Outcome Test (SNOT-22). Mean BPI-SF severity scores improved by 0.80 points (Wilcoxon rank sum test $p < 0.01$) in all 14 patients. In patients with baseline facial pain ($n = 9$), the scores improved by an average of 1.5 ($p < 0.01$) points in the pain severity domain and by 1.4 points in the pain interference domain. Additionally, the mean improvement in SNOT-22 scores was 14.11 ($p < 0.05$), which is above the minimal clinically-important difference (MCID) of nine points. Our pilot study indicates that multimodal vibration frequencies applied over the facial sinuses reduce pain, possibly through the reduction of the inflammatory response and modulation of the pain receptors. This study suggests the possibility that combining different frequencies could have an enhanced effect on reducing CRS-related facial pain.

Keywords: maxillary sinus; frontal sinus; chronic rhinosinusitis; facial pain; mechanical vibration; nociceptive modulation

1. Introduction

Chronic rhinosinusitis (CRS) is one of the most common conditions in North America, with almost 40 million patients [1]. Current research suggests that CRS is predominantly an inflammatory disease, with current therapies targeting inflammation within the sino-nasal cavity [2]. Symptoms of nasal congestion and facial pain significantly reduce the quality of life of CRS patients [3,4]. Many patients continue to experience pain after both medical and surgical management. Application of high frequency vibration to sinus regions in CRS patients has been shown to reduce pain and associated symptoms [5]. Chronic rhinosinusitis is characterized by the long-term presence of multiple symptoms including mucopurulent drainage and nasal congestion, and about 80% of CRS patients report facial pain/pressure [4,6,7]. Factors contributing to the pathophysiology of adult CRS include allergies, bacterial biofilms, asthma and exposure to various environmental pollutants [2,7–9]. Radiography or computed tomography (CT) scans are often used to identify mucosal thickening and to identify any comorbid factors such as anatomic abnormalities.

Treatment for CRS focuses on reducing inflammation and includes nasal irrigation, nasal corticosteroids [10], balloon sinuplasty and endoscopic sinus surgery [7,11]. Common pain relievers are also used [12]. Despite the best care, some patients will not respond to long-term medicinal therapy; these patients are recommended for endoscopic sinus surgery. Endoscopic sinus surgery carries some risks [13,14] and can be expensive [15]. Sinus surgery is also less effective for patients with mild symptoms [16], lower sinus microbial diversity [9], cystic fibrosis [17] or for eosinophilic CRS patients [18]. Chronic rhinosinusitis symptoms can continue for years [19], inflicting a significant financial burden [20] and a lower quality of life [4]. In one study, pain persisted for over two years after surgery in around 18% of patients [21]. Home-based, non-medicinal and non-intrusive treatment options are highly desirable both from a patient perspective and as a means to reduce burgeoning healthcare costs.

The causes of facial pain in CRS are unclear. Objective measures of disease severity do not correlate well with sinus pain [22,23]. One explanation is that stimulation in the sino-nasal cavity can cause referred pain, where pain is felt in a completely different location [24]. Another explanation is the observation that many patients complaining of sinus pain experience headaches or migraines [25,26]. Hypersensitization to pain from migraines could make innocuous stimuli more painful, which may contribute to the pain experienced by CRS patients [26,27]. Misuse of medication can also contribute to sinus pain [28].

Pain relief via cutaneous vibration has been demonstrated in chronic pain patients [29], osteoarthritis [30] and muscle pain [31]. Cutaneous vibration affects mechanoreceptors in the face [32,33], moderating pain by activating a pain gating pathway in the brainstem [34,35]. Though transcutaneous electrical stimulation can reduce headaches [36] and vibration has been used to reduce facial pain for injections [37], cutaneous vibration has not been tested on CRS patients.

Pain relief for CRS patients has been demonstrated using deep heating via application of 1-MHz frequency waves [38–40]. These high frequency waves raise deep tissue temperatures 1–5 °C [41], similar to the action of steam inhalation for nasal congestion [42]. High frequency waves may also reduce inflammation [43,44] and may also act on biofilms that have been hypothesized as a contributing factor in CRS [45]. A combination of cutaneous vibration and deep heat could more effectively alleviate facial pain associated with CRS, targeting both deep and surface mechano- and thermo-sensitive nerves.

CRS pain is usually reported as a single item in a larger suite of questions, affecting accurate interpretation of pain relief data [4]. Accurate measurements of pain are crucial to determining clinically-meaningful pain relief results [46,47]. The placebo effect is also strong in pain trials, increasing the need for accurate measurements [48]. The Brief Pain Inventory Short Form (BPI-SF) and the Short-Form McGill Pain Questionnaire are validated across many populations for use in pain studies, but have not been used to study the effect of vibration pain relief on CRS patients.

We combined cutaneous vibration at 70–80 Hz with deep heating at 1 MHz to test the effect of multimodal treatment on facial pain, quality of life and CRS symptoms in 14 patients with CRS. We hypothesized that cutaneous vibration would have an analgesic effect through stimulation of mechanosensors in the face, while deep heating would have effects similar to what has been observed in previous studies. Each patient was treated with a proprietary multimodal vibration therapy unit, designed by AxioSonic, with a specific transducer head that conforms to complex facial geometry. We used the BPI-SF to more accurately determine the extent of pain relief perceived by patients, while we used a similar measure used in a previous study (the Sino-Nasal Outcome Test, SNOT-22 instead of SNOT-20) for comparison and to quantify quality of life (QOL) changes due to CRS. Development of a cost-effective, non-medicinal and non-invasive therapy for CRS facial pain will be useful for both medical practitioners and patients.

2. Materials and Methods

2.1. Prospective Clinical Trial of Multimodal Frequencies for the Treatment of Chronic Rhinosinusitis Patients

This clinical trial was a prospective, single-arm study conducted at Sarah Bush Lincoln Health Center, Mattoon, IL, USA, from August–October 2016. Appropriate government and local reviews were obtained, including prior approval by the Medical Ethics and Institutional Review Board (IRB) committee at Sarah Bush Lincoln Health Center, Mattoon, IL, USA. All subjects gave written informed consent. Subjects who were included met the diagnostic criteria for CRS as defined by the American Academy of Otolaryngology–Head & Neck Surgery Foundation Clinical Practice Guidelines [7]. Patients were excluded who: had used immunosuppressive drugs for treatments besides CRS within 30 days of trial or who had a diagnosis of conditions that may interfere with the results of the study, such as: immotile cilia syndrome, cystic fibrosis, immune-deficiency, systemic autoimmune conditions with sinus involvement, had sino-nasal tumors or obstructive lesions, a history of facial trauma, uncontrolled diabetes, smoked or had cancer or brain tumor(s). Because the efficacy endpoints were related to pain and CRS symptoms, subjects were asked to make no changes to the pain or medications they were taking throughout the study.

Possible side effects of multimodal therapy on the face have not been reported in the literature, so our primary endpoint was safety, as measured by the proportion of patients with device-related serious adverse events. The secondary endpoints included facial pain as measured by the BPI-SF (pain severity and pain interference scores) and the Sino-Nasal Outcome Test-22 (SNOT-22) [16,49]. We used SNOT-22 scores to investigate changes in disease-related quality of life, because mechanical vibrations may improve CRS symptoms, as well as pain [43,50]. BPI-SF is a validated tool to measure clinical pain severity and interference and has become one of the most widely-used measurement tools for assessing clinical pain [51]. Questions are scored 0–10 [4,51], and averages are taken for six questions on severity of pain and for seven questions on interference with quality of life. The SNOT-22 questionnaire is a validated, widely-used 22-item tool used to assess CRS symptom severity [4]. Lower total scores (score range 0–110) indicate better overall symptom severity and quality of life [4]. Endoscopy was performed by Michael Smith before and after treatment to investigate possible changes in CRS symptom severity, and observations were noted.

Multimodal frequency treatments were administered using an AxioSonic therapeutic device (Figure 1) by trained clinical staff at the principal investigator's clinical site. The AxioSonic device is a hand-held portable device that can be administered either at home or at a clinic. The AxioSonic device operates at two simultaneous frequencies, one at 70–80 Hz and one at 1 MHz. The higher frequency wave has two settings for treatment: maxillary (1 W/cm^2, 5 min duration) and frontal (0.5 W/cm^2, 5-min duration). The device is coupled to the skin with the use of a gel. A proprietary cutaneous mechanical vibration treatment is activated when the applicator is adequately coupled to the skin. Each unit was independently calibrated to ensure acoustic intensity.

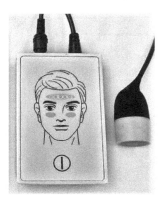

Figure 1. AxioSonic multimodal frequency treatment device.

The treatment regime consisted of three treatments per week for a total of six multimodal treatments over a two-week period (Figure 2). Each treatment session lasted a total of 15 min: 5 min on each maxillary sinus and 5 min on the frontal sinuses. Each unit was programmed to record total active usage time for each patient to ensure the units were functioning properly and to ensure treatment compliance. The study concluded for each participant 30 days after their last treatment with the AxioSonic device. All patients were treated with 3 treatments per week over the course of 2 weeks for a total of 6 treatments. All patients were followed for safety for 30 days after the last AxioSonic treatment session. Any adverse events were reported both with the number of patients experiencing events and the overall frequency of events. Adverse events were defined as any unfavorable and unintended diagnosis, symptom, sign, syndrome or disease occurring during the study, having been absent at baseline, or if present at baseline, appears to worsen. Because this was an initial assessment trial, no treatment control was included.

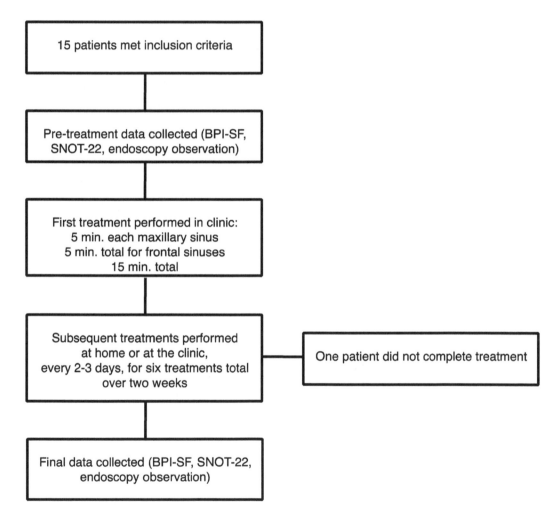

Figure 2. Clinical timeline. BPI-SF: Brief Pain Inventory Short Form; SNOT: Sino-Nasal Outcome Test.

Data analysis was performed using SAS Version 9.4 (SAS Institute, Cary, NC, USA) and R Version 3.2 (R Foundation for Statistical Computing, Vienna, Austria). We compared baseline to post-treatment scores with the Wilcoxon signed rank test to avoid violations of sphericity.

2.2. Analysis of Previously-Published Data

We were unable to find previous research that incorporated multiple analgesic frequencies to treat CRS pain. There are several studies that used 1-MHz frequencies to treat CRS symptoms, including pain [38–40,52–55], but only one was conducted in English with comparable data. We obtained raw data for this study; it had a total of 20 patients treated with a 1-MHz frequency (1 W/cm^2 and 0.5 W/cm^2) at a 10% duty cycle [40]. To evaluate the effect of their treatment, Young et al. [40] used the 20-question Sino-Nasal Outcome Test (SNOT-20), a list of questions where symptoms are rated 0–5. They also used a list of symptom-related questions, including pain, where each question was rated using a visual analog scale (1–7). We calculated standard statistical indices and estimated effect sizes using Cohen's d. Cohen's d is useful for quantifying the effectiveness of a particular intervention. It is a method of estimating the effectiveness of a treatment methodology, and is used to determine whether or not a significant difference in a study has a clinically-important outcome. It is calculated by dividing the difference in mean scores pre- and post-treatment by the standard deviation. Though other measures are also used, Cohen's d remains a useful tool in patient-reported outcome studies [56].

2.3. Ethical Standards

The authors assert that all procedures contributing to this work comply with the ethical standards of the relevant national and institutional guidelines on human experimentation as implemented by the Institutional Review Board for the Sarah Lincoln Bush Hospital (IRB00002130) and with the Helsinki Declaration of 1975, as revised in 2008.

3. Results

3.1. Clinical Trial Results

The average age of the 15 patients enrolled in this study was 60 years (34–83 years); six were male, and nine were female (Table 1). Subjects met inclusion and exclusion criteria. One patient was not considered in the final study because she did not continue treatment adequately after her device was damaged. Basic demographic data are presented in Table 1. Ten patients independently reported feelings of increased drainage and/or reduced pressure. Two patients specifically mentioned reduction in headache and pain. Most patients (13/14) felt that the treatment was helpful.

Table 1. Patient baseline demographic data. All patients maintained stable medication levels.

Patient Information	Value (SD*)
Patients enrolled	15
Patients completed study	14
Age (mean)	60 (12.64)
Male	6
Female	9
Diabetic (controlled)	3
Past sinus surgery	2
Hypertension	6
Patients reporting facial pain at the beginning of the study	9

* SD: standard deviation

Average post-treatment scores improved for both pain- and symptom-related domains (Tables 2 and 3). The treatment was more effective on patients with facial pain (Tables 2 and 3). Pain severity improved by one point on average for all patients and by 1.5 points for patients with facial pain (Figure 3). In the BPI-SF, there are seven questions relating to pain interference with daily life, called the interference domain. Patient mean scores in the interference domain improved from 2.0–0.89 for all patients (Table 4). Interestingly, the mean sleep domain scores of the BPI-SF interference assessment improved by 2.36 points in all subjects and by three points in subjects with pain at baseline.

Table 2. Changes in facial pain from Young et al. [40]. All 20 patients reported baseline facial pain. Mean scores, SD, mean change in scores, effect sizes (Cohen's *d*) and published *p*-values are included.

Item	Baseline	Post-Treatment	Change (SD)	Effect Size (Cohen's *d*)
Facial Pain (from SNOT-20)	2.20 (1.73)	1.45 (1.46)	0.75 (1.48)	0.51 *
Facial Pain Analog Scale	4 (2.12)	3 (1.67)	1 (1.65)	0.76
SNOT-20 total score	43.15 (24.75)	27.40 (21.18)	15.75 (17.41)	0.90 ***

*** $p < 0.001$, * $p < 0.05$.

Table 3. Treatment results for patients with baseline pain (*n* = 9). Mean scores, SD, mean change in scores, effect sizes (Cohen's *d*) and *p*-values are included.

Domain	Baseline	Post-Treatment	Change (SD)	Effect Size
BPI-SF Severity (Facial Pain)	2.78 (1.97)	1.28 (1.72)	1.50 (1.56)	0.96 **
BPI-SF Interference	2.65 (2.44)	1.25 (1.86)	1.40 (2.26)	0.62
SNOT-22 total score	47.11 (18.80)	33.00 (16.56)	14.11 (16.85)	0.84 *

** $p < 0.01$, * $p < 0.05$.

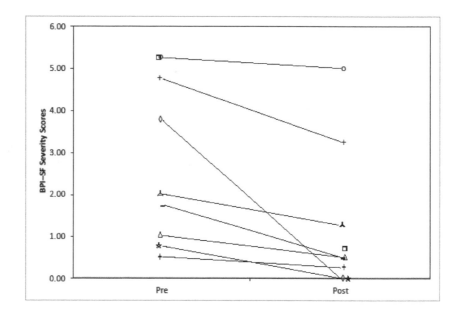

Figure 3. Improvement in BPI-SF severity domain pain scores for patients with baseline facial pain after six treatments.

Table 4. Treatment results for all patients (*n* = 14). Five patients reported no baseline facial pain. Mean scores, SD, effect sizes (Cohen's *d*) and *p*-values were calculated.

Domain	Baseline (SD)	Post-Treatment (SD)	Change (SD)	Effect Size
BPI-SF Severity (Facial Pain)	1.82 (2.00)	1.02 (1.62)	0.80 (1.52)	0.67 **
BPI-SF Interference	1.91 (2.11)	0.83 (1.51)	1.09 (1.78)	0.60 *
SNOT-22 total score	41.47 (17.56)	34.27 (15.73)	7.20 (19.18)	0.45

** $p < 0.01$, * $p < 0.05$.

Patient scores of overall symptom and quality of life as measured by SNOT-22 improved, with a medium effect size (Table 4 and Figure 4). The effect size of symptom improvement was larger (and statistically significant $p < 0.05$) for patients who reported pain at baseline (SNOT-22 *d* = 0.84, Table 3). Patients improved an average of 5.5 points in the symptoms domain of SNOT-22 (Questions 1–12) and an average of 3.14 points in the quality of life domain (Questions 13–22).

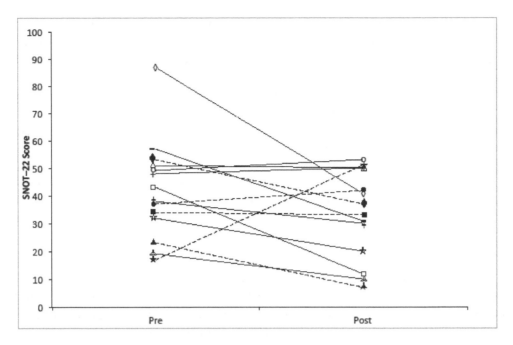

Figure 4. Change in SNOT-22 scores for all patients after six treatments. Patients with baseline facial pain are solid lines, and patients without baseline pain are dotted lines.

Total scores from BPI-SF and SNOT-22 were highly correlated (Figure 5), but there was one patient who reported a large decrease in quality of life using the SNOT-22 form that was not detected using the BPI-SF form. Similar questions are found in both forms, including quality of sleep, mood and productivity; it is unclear why the patient reported slight improvement on the BPI-SF form and a large decrease in quality of life on the SNOT-22 form.

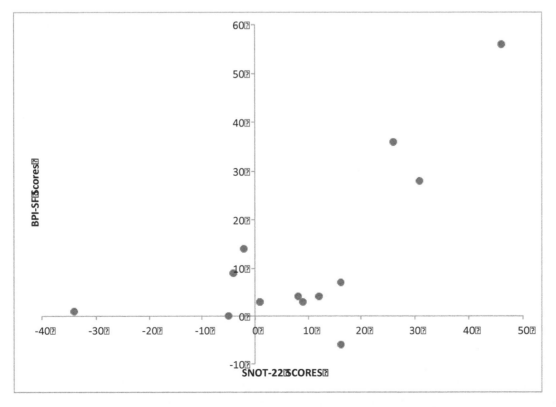

Figure 5. Correlation between SNOT-22 scores and BPI-SF scores ($R^2 = 0.51$).

Endoscopy results based on visual inspection by Michael Smith before and after treatment indicated reduced or completely resolved middle meatal edema in 13 out of 14 patients. Further studies with larger numbers of patients should include an objective scoring system, quantitative measures of edema and discharge, and based on our preliminary study, they should also focus on CRS patients that present with facial pain. No device-related adverse events were observed or reported for the 84 AxioSonic treatment sessions (six sessions for each of 14 patients), nor during the 30-day follow-up after the last AxioSonic treatment session. Overall, treatment of CRS pain with AxioSonic is safe, effective and has reduced side effects.

Effect sizes from Young et al. [40] were high and comparable to results from our paper for CRS symptoms (Table 2). All of these patients had pain of at least one on a scale of 0–7. When we compare results for patients that had facial pain, the AxioSonic multimodal treatment is more effective for treating pain.

4. Discussion

This study measured changes in CRS-related quality of life measurements including facial pain after treatment with multimodal frequency stimulation. Treatment with combined high frequency (1 MHz) and low frequency vibration (70–80 Hz) reduced both pain and quality of life measures. The effect size we observed for pain was larger than published results for a previous clinical trial that used only 1-MHz ultrasound frequency [40]. We also observed an improvement in the sleep subdomain of the SNOT-22, a crucial component of quality of life. There were no device-related adverse events. No research has yet reported effects of low frequency vibration (50–100 Hz) on CRS pain. Most of the published literature has focused on analgesia in the peripheral nervous system [30,31,57–60], though some research has reported success treating temporomandibular disorder pain [61,62]. Low frequency vibratory inhibition of nerves associated with the parasympathetic nervous system may be partly responsible for the beneficial effects of treatment [63,64]. The current study adds to previous research by testing the analgesic effects of vibrational neurostimulation for facial pain.

Several clinical trials have reported improvements in pain after treatment with 1-MHz ultrasound [40,52,54]. In a study by Ansari et al. [53], 95% of patients with facial pain at the beginning of the study reported significant improvement after the study. The facial pain effect size observed in our study ($d = 0.96$) was much higher than that estimated from Young et al.'s data ($d = 0.51$), likely due to the application of multimodal frequencies (70–80 Hz and 1 MHz) in the AxioSonic system. Our effect size for quality of life measures using the SNOT-22 questionnaire ($d = 0.45$) was lower than Young et al.'s paper [40] ($d = 0.9$). One possible reason for this discrepancy could be due to the fact most patients in Young et al.'s study [40] presented with facial pain, whereas in our study, five patients did not present with facial pain at the beginning of treatment. When we take patients presenting with facial pain into account, our symptom effect size ($d = 0.84$) is similar to Young et al. ($d = 0.90$) [40]. In addition, we used the pain-specific metric (BPI-SF) and the SNOT-22 questionnaires, had different treatment regimes, and our sample size was smaller, all of which can influence the end result. Chronic rhinosinusitis symptoms can have a negative impact on quality of life [47], especially in interference with sleep [65]. Lack of sleep is correlated with depression in CRS patients [3]. In our study, patients experienced better sleep after treatment and reported improvement in overall quality of life. In both questionnaires, the BPI-SF and the SNOT-22, patients reported increased ability for uninterrupted sleep. The observed effect size in questions related to sleep in the BPI-SF was $d = 0.64$ and $d = 0.61$ for SNOT-22 in all patients ($n = 14$). Treating CRS pain with vibrational stimulation could significantly decrease the burden of CRS on patients' quality of life.

Overall, the effect sizes we observed were largest for patients with facial pain, the main targeted symptom for AxioSonic multimodal treatment. Though this study only included nine patients with facial pain, the average change in SNOT-22 scores was 16.85 for those patients. This is larger than the minimal clinically-important difference (MCID) of 8.9 [66], indicating that patients with pain due to CRS could benefit significantly from this treatment. Further clinical studies should test the relative benefits of different wavelengths and include a placebo control to quantify the effects of various treatments.

Vibratory analgesia is based on the observation that stimulation of afferent nerves with mechanical vibration reduces perceived pain [67,68]. The analgesic effect of vibration is likely due to both afferent and cortical processes [64,67,69]. Combining vibratory stimulation with either electrical or thermal stimulation increases the analgesia effect, probably due to the activation and recruitment of multiple types of receptors [30,31,57]. Vibratory analgesia of 70–80 Hz has been successfully used to reduce pain in various procedures, including IV insertion [59], blood collection [58] and experimentally-induced pain [70]. In a study on patients with temporomandibular disorder, 20-Hz vibration on the cheek reduced pain, but not as much as 100-Hz vibration [62]. Dual-stimulation therapy with application of both heat and vibration could alleviate CRS pain, as we observed in this study.

The reduction in quality of life reported by CRS patients may be mediated in part by the sphenopalatine (pterygopalatine) ganglion (SPG), near the maxillary sinuses and accessible through the rear of the nasal cavity. The SPG is involved in tissue inflammation, lacrimation, mucus production and other parasympathetic processes [71–74]. Low frequency neurostimulation (20 Hz, much lower than ultrasound frequencies) of the SPG or the Vidian nerve leads to vasodilation and associated inflammation [75,76]. Stimulation of the SPG at higher frequencies (50 Hz) resolves nasal congestion and swelling due to cluster headaches [77] and may alleviate similar symptoms in CRS patients, as well. Electrical stimulation and mechanical stimulation of peripheral nerves target similar types of nerves [57], and both electrical [78,79] and vibratory stimulation [30,62,80] have analgesic effects [29]. Combining treatment modalities could lead to amplified analgesia [57].

Vibratory stimulation at 70–80 Hz could reduce facial pain in CRS patients through multiple pathways, specifically by modulating the parasympathetic response. Neuromodulation through vibratory stimulus can affect the activity of large diameter nerve fibers, subsequently exciting inhibitory cells and reducing perceived pain [81]. Nerves associated with the SPG may also be involved, and vibration could modulate the parasympathetic response [64,82]. These mechanisms of action could explain the reduction in facial pain observed in our study and also the observation that over half of the patients in our study reported that the AxioSonic device helped increase mucous discharge possibly due to the thinning of bacterial biofilms [40]. Visual inspection by endoscopy as part of patients' routine care showed improved edema and reduction or clearing of purulent discharge, suggesting a reduced inflammatory response [83]. The deep heating and thermal effects of the 1-MHz waves could also contribute to an additional reduced inflammatory response [40]. Our AxioSonic device is hypothesized to work by a combination of modulating nociceptive receptors, deep heating and reducing inflammation.

5. Conclusions

Chronic rhinosinusitis has a negative impact on the quality of life of at least 14% of the population in the United States [84]. The data from our prospective clinical study support previous studies showing improvement in facial pain and overall CRS symptom scores in patients treated with ultrasound at a 1-MHz frequency. In addition, our studies show that adding an additional low frequency vibration at 70–80 Hz could improve the pain response in patients suffering from CRS and suggests that multimodal vibration treatment would benefit patients, with few side effects and no risk of antibiotic overuse.

Acknowledgments: We are grateful to James Bartley for providing us with data from previous studies, Tonya Bierman for help designing the device and Patrick Balsmann for help with the clinical trial.

Author Contributions: P.B. and V.R. helped design the study. M.S. performed the clinical trial. A.P.R. helped with the statistics and data analysis. J.B. designed the device, programmed the software and helped with the study. P.B. gave input on the neurobiology of pain. The final manuscript was written by A.P.R. and V.R. with inputs from all authors. All authors approved the final manuscript.

Conflicts of Interest: The multimodal frequency clinical trial was funded by AxioSonic. M.S. was the principal investigator of the study and designed the study with the input of P.B. and V.R. Data were collected at each site using paper clinical report forms. All investigators had unrestricted access to the data.

References

1. Blackwell, D.L.; Lucas, J.W. Tables of Summary Health Statistics for U.S. Adults: 2014 National Health Interview Survey. 2015. Available online: http://www.cdc.gov/nchs/nhis/SHS/tables.htm (accessed on 13 July 2017).

2. Fokkens, W.J.; Lund, V.J.; Mullol, J.; Bachert, C.; Alobid, I.; Baroody, F.; Cohen, N.; Cervin, A.; Douglas, R.; Gevaert, P.; et al. European position paper on rhinosinusitis and nasal polyps 2012. *Rhinology* **2012**, *50*, 1–298. [PubMed]

3. Cox, D.R.; Asbhy, S.; Mace, J.C.; DelGaudio, J.M.; Smith, T.L.; Orlandi, R.R.; Alt, J.A. The pain-depression dyad and the association with sleep dysfunction in chronic rhinosinusitis. *Int. Forum Allergy Rhinol.* **2017**, *7*, 56–63. [CrossRef] [PubMed]

4. DeConde, A.M.; Made, J.C.; Ashby, S.; Smith, T.L.; Orlandi, R.R.; Alt, J.A. Characterization of facial pain associated wtih chronic rhinosinusitis using validated pain evaluation instruments. *Int. Forum Allergy Rhinol.* **2015**, *5*, 682–689. [CrossRef] [PubMed]

5. Bartley, J.; Ansari, N.N.; Naghdi, S. Therapeutic ultrasound as a treatment modality for chronic rhinosinusitis. *Curr. Infect. Dis. Rep.* **2014**, *16*, 398–404. [CrossRef] [PubMed]

6. Meltzer, E.O.; Hamilos, D.L. Rhinosinusitis diagnosis and management for the clinician: A synopsis of recent consensus guidelines. *Mayo Clin. Proc.* **2011**, *86*, 427–443. [CrossRef] [PubMed]

7. Rosenfeld, R.; Piccirillo, J.; Chandrasekhar, S.; Brook, I.; Kumar, K.; Kramper, M.; Orlandi, R.; Palmer, J.; Patel, Z.; Peters, A.; et al. Clinical practice guideline (update): Adult sinusitis. *Otolaryngol. Head Neck Surg.* **2015**, *152*, S1–S39. [CrossRef] [PubMed]

8. Lanza, D.C.; Kennedy, D.W. Adult rhinosinusitis defined. *Otolaryngol. Head Neck Surg.* **1997**, *117*, S1–S7. [CrossRef]

9. Ramakrishnan, V.R.; Hauser, L.J.; Feazel, L.M.; Ir, D.; Robertson, C.E.; Frank, D.N. Sinus microbiota varies among chronic rhinosinusitis phenotypes and predicts surgical outcome. *J. Allergy Clin. Immunol.* **2015**, *136*, 334–342. [CrossRef] [PubMed]

10. Schäcke, H.; Döcke, W.; Asdullah, K. Mechanisms involved in the side effects of glucocorticoids. *Pharmacol. Ther.* **2002**, *96*, 23–43. [CrossRef]

11. Patel, Z.M.; Thamboo, A.; Rudmik, L.; Nayak, J.V.; Smith, T.L.; Hwang, P.H. Surgical therapy vs continued medical therapy for medically refractory chronic rhinosinusitis: A systematic review and meta-analysis. *Int. Forum Allergy Rhinol.* **2017**, *7*, 119–127. [CrossRef] [PubMed]

12. Hinz, B.; Cheremina, O.; Brune, K. Acetaminophen (paracetamol) is a selective cyclooxygenase-2 inhibitor in man. *FASEB J.* **2008**, *22*, 383–390. [CrossRef] [PubMed]

13. Lund, V.J.; MacKay, I.S. Outcome assessment of endoscopic sinus surgery. *J. R. Soc. Med.* **1994**, *87*, 70–72. [PubMed]

14. Ragab, S.M.; Lund, V.J.; Scadding, G. Evaluation of the medical and surgical treatment of chronic rhinosinusitis: A prospective, randomised, controlled trial. *Laryngoscope* **2004**, *114*, 923–930. [CrossRef] [PubMed]

15. Friedman, M.; Schalch, P.; Lin, H.; Mazloom, N.; Neidich, M.; Joseph, N.J. Functional endoscopic dilatation of the sinuses: Patient satisfaction, postoperative pain, and cost. *Am. J. Rhinol.* **2008**, *22*, 204–209. [CrossRef] [PubMed]

16. Kennedy, J.L. Sino-nasal outcome test (SNOT-22): A predictor of postsurgical improvement in patients with chronic sinusitis. *Ann. Allergy Asthma Immunol.* **2013**, *111*, 246–251.e2. [CrossRef] [PubMed]

17. Chaaban, M.R.; Kejner, A.; Rowe, S.M.; Woodworth, B.A. Cystic fibrosis chronic rhinosinusitis: A comprehensive review. *Am. J. Rhinol. Allergy* **2013**, *27*, 387–395. [CrossRef] [PubMed]

18. Younis, R.T.; Ahmed, J. Predicting revision sinus surgery in allergic fungal and eosinophilic mucin chronic rhinosinusitis. *Laryngoscope* **2017**, *127*, 59–63. [CrossRef] [PubMed]

19. Benninger, M.S.; Ferguson, B.J.; Hadley, J.A.; Hamilos, D.L.; Jacobs, M.; Kennedy, D.W.; Lanza, D.C.; Marple, B.F.; Osguthorpe, J.D.; Stankiewicz, J.A.; et al. Adult chronic rhinosinusitis: Definitions, diagnosis, epidemiology, and pathophysiology. *Otolaryngol. Head Neck Surg.* **2003**, *129*, S1–S32. [CrossRef] [PubMed]

20. Bhattacharyya, N.; Orlandi, R.R.; Grebner, J.; Martinson, M. Cost burden of chronic rhinosinusitis: A claims-based study. *Otolaryngol. Head Neck Surg.* **2011**, *144*, 440–445. [CrossRef] [PubMed]

21. Jones, N.S.; Cooney, T.R. Facial pain and sinonasal surgery. *Rhinology* **2003**, *41*, 193–200. [PubMed]

22. Ryan, W.R.; Ramachandra, T.; Hwang, P.H. Correlations between symptoms, nasal endoscopy, and in-office computed tomography in post-surgical chronic rhinosinusitis patients. *Laryngoscope* **2011**, *121*, 674–678. [CrossRef] [PubMed]

23. Shields, G.; Seikaly, H.; LeBoeuf, M.; Guinto, F.; LeBoeuf, H.; Pincus, T.; Calhoun, K. Correlation between facial pain or headache and computed tomography in rhinosinusitis in Canadian and U.S. subjects. *Laryngoscope* **2003**, *113*, 943–945. [CrossRef] [PubMed]

24. Clerico, D.M. An experimental study of pain upon stimulation of the nasal and sinus cavities. *Am. J. Otolaryngol.* **2014**, *35*, 300–304. [CrossRef] [PubMed]

25. Mehle, M.E.; Schreiber, C.P. Sinus headache, migraine, and the otolaryngologist. *Otolaryngol. Head Neck Surg.* **2005**, *133*, 489–496. [CrossRef] [PubMed]

26. Jones, N.S. Sinus headaches: Avoiding over- and mis-diagnosis. *Expert Rev. Neurother.* **2009**, *9*, 439–444. [CrossRef] [PubMed]

27. Mehle, M.E.; Schreiber, C.P. What do we know about rhinogenic headache? *Otolaryngol. Clin. North Am.* **2014**, *47*, 255–268. [CrossRef] [PubMed]

28. Aaseth, K.; Grande, R.B.; Kværner, K.; Lundqvist, C.; Russell, M.B. Chronic rhinosinusitis gives a ninefold increased risk of chronic headache. *Cephalalgia* **2010**, *30*, 152–160. [CrossRef] [PubMed]

29. Lundeberg, T. The pain suppressive effect of vibratory stimulation and transcutaneous electrical nerve stimulation (TENS) as compared to aspirin. *Brain Res.* **1984**, *294*, 201–209. [CrossRef]

30. Kitay, G.S.; Koren, M.J.; Helfet, D.L.; Parides, M.K.; Markenson, J.A. Efficacy of combined local mechanical vibrations, continuous passive motion and thermotherapy in the management of osteoarthritis of the knee. *Osteoarthr. Cartil.* **2009**, *17*, 1269–1274. [CrossRef] [PubMed]

31. Gay, A.; Aimonetti, J.; Roll, J.; Ribot-Ciscar, E. Kinesthetic illusions attenuate experimental muscle pain, as do muscle and cutaneous stimulation. *Brain Res.* **2015**, *1615*, 148–156. [CrossRef] [PubMed]

32. Trulsson, M.; Essick, G.K. Sensations evoked by microstimulation of single mechanoreceptive afferents innervating the human face and mouth. *J. Neurophysiol.* **2010**, *103*, 1741–1747. [CrossRef] [PubMed]

33. Johansson, R.S.; Trulsson, M.; Olsson, K.Å.; Westbert, K.G. Mechanoreceptor activity from the human face and oral mucosa. *Exp. Brain Res.* **1988**, *72*, 204–208. [CrossRef] [PubMed]

34. Sessle, B.J. Acute and chronic craniofacial pain: Brainstem mechanisms of nociceptive transmission and neuroplasticity, and their clinical correlates. *Crit. Rev. Oral Biol. Med.* **2000**, *11*, 57–91. [CrossRef] [PubMed]

35. Woolf, C.J. Central sensitization: Implications for the diagnosis and treatment of pain. *Pain* **2011**, *152*, S2–S15. [CrossRef] [PubMed]

36. Miller, S.; Sinclair, A.J.; Davies, B.; Matharu, M. Neurostimulation in the treatment of primary headaches. *Pract. Neurol.* **2015**, *16*, 362–375. [CrossRef] [PubMed]

37. Nanitsos, E.; Vartuli, R.; Forte, A.; Dennison, P.J.; Peck, C.C. The effect of vibration on pain during local anaesthesia injections. *Aust. Dent. J.* **2009**, *52*, 94–100. [CrossRef] [PubMed]

38. Ansari, N.N.; Soofia, N.; Farhadi, M.; Jalaie, S. A preliminary study into the effect of low-intensity pulsed ultrasound on chronic maxillary and frontal sinusitis. *Physiother. Theory Pract.* **2007**, *23*, 211–218. [CrossRef] [PubMed]

39. Naghdi, S.; Ansari, N.N.; Farhadi, M. A clinical trial on the treatment of chronic rhinosinusitis with continuous ultrasound. *J. Phys. Ther. Sci.* **2008**, *20*, 233–238. [CrossRef]

40. Young, D.; Morton, R.; Bartley, J. Therapeutic ultrasound as treatment for chronic rhinosinusitis: Preliminary observations. *J. Laryngol. Otol.* **2010**, *124*, 495–499. [CrossRef] [PubMed]

41. Baker, K.G.; Robertson, V.J.; Duck, F.A. A review of therapeutic ultrasound: Biophysical effects. *Phys. Ther.* **2001**, *81*, 1351–1358. [CrossRef] [PubMed]

42. Tyrell, D.; Barrow, I.; Arthur, J. Local hyperthermia benefits natural and experimental common colds. *Br. Med. J.* **1989**, *298*, 1280–1283. [CrossRef]

43. Bartley, J.; Young, D. Ultrasound as a treatment for chronic rhinosinusitis. *Med. Hypotheses* **2009**, *73*, 15–17. [CrossRef] [PubMed]

44. Chung, J.-I.; Barua, S.; Choi, B.H.; Min, B.-H.; Han, H.C.; Baik, E.J. Anti-inflammatory effect of low intensity ultrasound (LIUS) on complete Freund's adjuvant-induced arthritis synovium. *Osteoarthr. Cartil.* **2012**, *20*, 314–322. [CrossRef] [PubMed]

45. Tan, N.C.; Foreman, A.; Jardeleza, C.; Douglas, R.; Tran, H.; Wormald, P.J. The multiplicity of *Staphylococcus aureus* in chronic rhinosinusitis: Correlating surface biofilm and intracellular residence. *Laryngoscope* **2012**, *122*, 1655–1660. [CrossRef] [PubMed]

46. Dworkin, R.H.; Turk, D.C.; Wyrwich, K.W.; Beaton, D.; Cleeland, C.S.; Farrar, J.T.; Haythornthwaite, J.A.; Jensen, M.P.; Kerns, R.D.; Ader, D.N.; et al. Interpreting the clinical importance of treatment outcomes in chronic pain clinical trials: IMMPACT recommendations. *J. Pain* **2007**, *9*, 105–121. [CrossRef] [PubMed]

47. Tarasidis, G.S.; DeConde, A.M.; Mace, J.C.; Ashby, S.; Smith, T.L.; Orlandi, R.R.; Alt, J.A. Cognitive dysfunction associated to pain and quality of life in chronic rhinosinusitis. *Int. Forum Allergy Rhinol.* **2015**, *5*, 1004–1009. [CrossRef] [PubMed]

48. Schedlowski, M.; Enck, P.; Rief, W.; Bingel, U. Neuro-bio-behavioral mechanisms of placebo and nocebo responses: Implications for clinical trials and clinical practice. *Pharmacol. Rev.* **2015**, *67*, 697–730. [CrossRef] [PubMed]

49. DeConde, A.S.; Mace, J.C.; Bodner, T.; Hwang, P.H.; Rudmik, L.; Soler, Z.M.; Smith, T.L. SNOT-22 quality of life domains differentially predict treatment modality selection in chronic rhinosinusitis. *Int. Forum Allergy Rhinol.* **2014**, *4*, 972–979. [CrossRef] [PubMed]

50. Sanderson, M.J.; Dirksen, E.R. Mechanosensitivity of cultured ciliated cells from the mammalian respiratory tract: Implications for the regulation of mucociliary transport. *Proc. Natl. Acad. Sci. USA* **1986**, *83*, 7302–7306. [CrossRef] [PubMed]

51. Cleeland, C.S. Brief Pain Inventory User's Guide. 2009. Available online: https://www.mdanderson.org/documents/Departments-and-Divisions/Symptom-Research/BPI_UserGuide.pdf (accessed on 27 June 2017).

52. Ansari, N.N.; Fathali, M.; Naghdi, S.; Hasson, S.; Jalaie, S.; Rastak, M.S. A randomized, double-blind clinical trial comparing the effects of continuous and pulsed ultrasound in patients with chronic rhinosinusitis. *Physiother. Theory Pract.* **2012**, *28*, 85–94. [CrossRef] [PubMed]

53. Ansari, N.N.; Naghdi, S.; Farhadi, M. Physiotherapy for chronic rhinosinusitis: The use of continuous ultrasound. *Int. J. Ther. Rehabil.* **2007**, *14*, 306–310. [CrossRef]

54. Ansari, N.N.; Naghdi, S.; Fathali, M.; Bartley, J.; Rastak, M.S. A randomized clinical trial comparing pulsed ultrasound and erythromycin phonophoresis in the treatment of patients with chronic rhinosinusitis. *Physiother. Theory Pract.* **2015**, *32*, 166–172. [CrossRef] [PubMed]

55. Høsøien, E.; Lund, A.B.; Vasseljen, O. Similar effect of therapeutic ultrasound and antibiotics for acute bacterial rhinosinusitis: a randomized trial. *J. Physiother.* **2010**, *56*, 27–32. [CrossRef]

56. Cohen, J. *Statistical Power Analysis for the Behavioral Sciences*, 2nd ed.; Lawrence Earlbaum Associates: Hillsdale, NH, USA, 1988.

57. Guieu, R.; Tardy-Gervet, M.; Roll, J. Analgesic effects of vibration and transcutaneous electrical nerve stimulation applied separately and simultaneously to patients with chronic pain. *Can. J. Neurol. Sci.* **1991**, *18*, 113–119. [CrossRef] [PubMed]

58. İnal, S.; Kelleci, M. Relief of pain during blood specimen collection in pediatric patients. *MCN* **2012**, *37*, 339–345. [CrossRef]

59. Moadad, N.; Kozman, K.; Shahine, R.; Ohanian, S.; Badr, L.K. Distraction using the BUZZY for children during an IV insertion. *J. Pediatr. Nurs.* **2016**, *31*, 64–72. [CrossRef] [PubMed]

60. Taddio, A.; Shah, V.; McMurtry, C.M.; MacDonald, N.E.; Ipp, M.; Riddell, R.P.; Noel, M.; Chambers, C.T. Procedural and physical interventions for vaccine injections. *Clin. J. Pain* **2015**, *31*, S20–S37. [CrossRef] [PubMed]

61. Hara, E.S.; Witzel, A.L.; De Luca, C.E.P.; Ballester, R.Y.; Kuboki, T.; Bolzan, M.C. A novel vibratory stimulation-based occlusal splint for alleviation of TMD painful symptoms: a pilot study. *J. Oral Rehabil.* **2013**, *40*, 179–184. [CrossRef] [PubMed]

62. Roy, E.A.; Hollins, M.; Maixner, W. Reduction of TMD pain by high-frequency vibration: A spatial and temporal analysis. *Pain* **2003**, *101*, 267–274. [CrossRef]

63. Rocha, W.A.; Rodrigues, K.M.; Pereira, R.R.; Nogueira, B.V.; Gonçalves, W.L. Acute effects of therapeutic 1-MHz ultrasound on nasal unblocking of subjects with chronic rhinosinusitis. *Braz. J. Otorhinolaryngol.* **2011**, *77*, 7–12. [CrossRef] [PubMed]

64. West, S.J.; Bannister, K.; Dickenson, A.H.; Bennett, D.L. Circuitry and plasticity of the dorsal horn—Toward a better understanding of neuropathic pain. *Neuroscience* **2015**, *300*, 254–275. [CrossRef] [PubMed]

65. Craig, T.J.; Ferguson, B.J.; Krouse, J.H. Sleep impairment in allergic rhinitis, rhinosinusitis, and nasal polyposis. *Am. J. Otolaryngol.* **2008**, *29*, 209–217. [CrossRef] [PubMed]

66. Hopkins, C.; Gillett, S.; Slack, R.; Lund, V.J.; Browne, J.P. Psychometric validity of the 22-item Sinonasal Outcome Test. *Clin. Otolaryngol.* **2009**, *34*, 447–454. [CrossRef] [PubMed]

67. Duan, B.; Cheng, L.; Bourane, S.; Britz, O.; Padilla, C.; Garcia-Campmany, L.; Krashes, M.; Knowlton, W.; Velasquez, T.; Ren, X.; et al. Identification of spinal circuits transmitting and gating mechanical pain. *Cell* **2014**, *159*, 1417–1432. [CrossRef] [PubMed]

68. Melzack, R.; Wall, P.D. Pain mechanisms: A new theory. *Science* **1965**, *150*, 971–979. [CrossRef] [PubMed]

69. Vierck, C.J.; Whitsel, B.L.; Favorov, O.V.; Brown, A.W.; Tommerdahl, M. Role of primary somatosensory cortex in the coding of pain. *Pain* **2013**, *154*, 334–344. [CrossRef] [PubMed]

70. Hollins, M.; McDermott, K.; Harper, D. How does vibration reduce pain? *Perception* **2014**, *43*, 70–84. [CrossRef] [PubMed]

71. Day, M. Sympathetic blocks: The evidence. *Pain Practice* **2008**, *8*, 98–109. [CrossRef] [PubMed]

72. Felisati, G.; Arnone, F.; Lozza, P.; Leone, M.; Curone, M.; Bussone, G. Sphenopalatine endoscopic ganglion block: A revision of a traditional technique for cluster headache. *Laryngoscope* **2006**, *16*, 1447–1450. [CrossRef] [PubMed]

73. Khan, S.; Schoenen, J.; Ashina, M. Sphenopalatine ganglion neuromodulation in migraine: What is the rationale? *Cephalalgia* **2014**, *34*, 382–391. [CrossRef] [PubMed]

74. Robbins, M.S.; Robertson, C.E.; Kaplan, E.; Ailani, J.; Charleston, L.; Kuruvilla, D.; Blumenfeld, A.; Berliner, R.; Rosen, N.L.; Duarte, R.; et al. The sphenopalatine ganglion: Anatomy, pathophysiology, and therapeutic targeting in headache. *Headache* **2015**, *56*, 240–258. [CrossRef] [PubMed]

75. Talman, W.T.; Corr, J.; Dragon, D.N.; Wang, D. Parasympathetic stimulation elicits cerebral vasodilatation in rat. *Auton. Neurosci.* **2007**, *133*, 153–157. [CrossRef] [PubMed]

76. Uddman, R.; Malm, L.; Fahrenkrug, J.; Sundler, F. Vip increases in nasal blood during stimulation of the Vidian nerve. *Acta Otolaryngol.* **1981**, *91*, 135–138. [CrossRef]

77. Ansarinia, M.; Rezai, A.; Tepper, S.J.; Steiner, C.P.; Stump, J.; Stanton-Hicks, M.; Machado, A.; Narouze, S. Electrical stimulation of sphenopalatine ganglion for acute treatment of cluster headaches. *Headache* **2010**, *50*, 1164–1174. [CrossRef] [PubMed]

78. Bjordal, J.M.; Johnson, M.I.; Lopes-Martins, R.A.; Bogen, B.; Chow, R.; Ljunggren, A.E. Short-term efficacy of physical interventions in osteoarthritic knee pain. A systematic review and meta-analysis of randomised placebo-controlled trials. *BMC Musculoskelet. Disord.* **2006**, *8*, 51. [CrossRef] [PubMed]

79. Johnson, M.; Martinson, M. Efficacy of electrical nerve stimulation for chronic musculoskeletal pain: A meta-analysis of randomized controlled trials. *Pain* **2007**, *130*, 157–165. [CrossRef] [PubMed]

80. Lobre, W.D.; Callegari, B.J.; Gardner, G.; Marsh, C.M.; Bush, A.C.; Dunn, W.J. Pain control in orthodontics using a micropulse vibration device: A randomized clinical trial. *Angle Orthod.* **2015**, *86*, 625–630. [CrossRef] [PubMed]

81. Mücke, M.; Cuhls, H.; Radbruch, L.; Weigl, T.; Rolke, R. Evidence of heterosynaptic LTD in the human nociceptive system: Superficial skin neuromodulation using a matrix electrode reduces deep pain sensitivity. *PLoS ONE* **2014**, *9*, e107718. [CrossRef] [PubMed]

82. Peirs, C.; Seal, R.P. Neural circuits for pain: Recent advances and current views. *Science* **2017**, *354*, 578–584. [CrossRef] [PubMed]

83. Smith, M.; Sarah Bush Lincoln Health Center, Matoon, IL, USA. Personal Communication, 2016.

84. Van Cauwenberge, P.; Watelet, J.B. Epidemiology of chronic rhinosinusitis. *Thorax* **2000**, *55*, S20–S21. [CrossRef] [PubMed]

10

Pediatric Chronic Sinusitis: What Art Thou?

Russell J. Hopp [1,2]

[1] Division of Allergy and Immunology, Creighton University, Omaha, NE 68131, USA; rhopp@creighton.edu
[2] Children's Hospital and Medical Center, Omaha, NE 68131, USA

Academic Editor: César Picado

Abstract: Pediatric chronic sinusitis has been re-termed, pediatric chronic rhinosinusitis, largely following the adult nomenclature. However, other large areas of medical management of the process have remained largely uninvestigated. This opinion piece discusses the gaps in our current knowledge of pediatric rhinosinusitis pathophysiology and limitations of current management protocols.

Keywords: children; pediatric; chronic sinusitis; chronic rhinosinusitis

1. Clinical Scenario

In 1979, a 3rd year pediatric resident was doing a preceptorship with a local pediatrician. In those days, a resident's time was largely unsupervised. A 10 year old male was seen by the resident with weeks of nasal congestion. The resident noticed purulent intra-nasal and posterior pharyngeal drainage. The resident told the mother it was a "cold" and it would resolve. Two days later the preceptor pediatrician asked the resident to accompany him to radiology. A Waters sinus view of the same child showed opacified maxillary sinuses. The mother had returned to see the pediatrician and a sinus X-ray was obtained. The pediatrician told the resident "Doctor, the boy you saw has a chronic sinusitis, and I took the X-ray to show you what it looks like".

Flash ahead to 2017. A 5 year old female is referred to an allergist for chronic nasal congestion lasting more than 1 year. The adenoids had been removed 6 months previous. The examination showed thin, mucopurulent nasal secretions. Allergy skin tests were negative. The sinus X-ray reveals bilateral ethmoid and maxillary opacification and absent adenoids.

What has changed in the past 38 years? Largely nothing!

2. Pediatric Chronic Sinusitis: What Art Thou?

The term chronic sinusitis, well recognized by providers and the lay public, acquired a new name in the early 2000s, and by time the first pediatric chronic rhinosinusitis consensus statement in 2014 was published, the condition had been re-termed "pediatric chronic rhinosinusitis (PCRS)" [1]. The authors admit that "many aspects of PCRS remain ill-defined" [1].

The term PCRS, in large part, mimics the terminology used to define adult disease(s) [2]; but using this phrase may in fact detract from the simplistic background leading to its presence: a chronically altered microbiology. A more accurate description is pediatric infectious chronic rhinosinusitis. Other concepts of PCRS remain largely unexplored.

3. Diagnosis

A recent review discussed the vagaries of the radiological assessment of PCRS [3]. Plain sinus films have acquired a negative connotation; and in another recent opinion paper any radiological procedure was considered unnecessary unless surgery was contemplated [4].

With regard to using a radiological approach to PCRS, the consensus for a diagnosis for pediatric rhinosinusitis as a condition is that the "disease" has existed for a minimum of 12 weeks; therefore, it seems curious that only expensive standards (CT of the sinuses), or no standards at all, are advocated for supporting its existence.

4. Treatment

There exists only two PCRS studies in children using antibiotics without a surgical option. Publications from 1982 and 1995 provide minimal current guidance [4,4]. In fact, none of the antibiotics in the studies are currently recommended or currently used: amoxicillin (ampicillin), erythromycin, trimethoprim-sulfamethoxazole, clindamycin, cefaclor.

As summarized elsewhere, many reports recommended various antibiotics, although amoxicillin-clavulanate potassium has extensive support [3]. However, to date no regulatory approval has arrived or prospective studies done in the clinical application of Amoxicillin-clavulanate in PCRS.

Equally lacking, is any guidance for alternative antibiotics for penicillin-allergic children.

5. Natural History

What remains totally undefined is the natural history of PCRS. Assuming the underlying dysfunctional microbiological process has taken 12 or more weeks to develop, how long does it take for the accompanying inflammatory process to resolve, and if the value of sinus X-rays is questioned, how is resolution to be determined? Since there is no standard for assessing if total resolution of a chronic rhinosinusitis infection has occurred (after antibiotic therapy), it is likely (although never studied) that recurrent (or recalcitrant) chronic pediatric sinusitis is actually non-resolved chronic pediatric rhinosinusitis.

6. Microbiology

Acceptance that PCRS is an alternation of the normal bacterial flora has morphed into the concept that all CRS, in general, has an altered microbiome. This has exclusively been explored in adult forms of CRS, which may not have a PCRS corollary. A recent adult study suggests the immune response to the microbiome is altered as compared to controls, suggesting a broader anti-inflammatory approach to treatment may be required [7]. Investigation of the sinus microbiome and inflammatory response in children does not exist.

7. Ancillary Therapy

Under what conditions is antibiotic therapy for PCRS sufficient? What situations require anti-inflammatory co-therapy (corticosteroids), and how much and for how long? Are topical corticosteroids useful, or is systemic therapy required? Would an extended course of low dose corticosteroids provide the same resolution potential as antibiotics?

At the end of the therapy period, what determines resolution after primary (antibiotic), with/without ancillary therapy? Symptoms? Examination findings?

8. Surgical Options

The 2014 consensus statement [1], which included surgical options, and others summarized previously, e.g., [3], did not provide one unifying surgical approach to PCRS.

9. Summary

Although more descriptive, the term pediatric chronic rhinosinusitis has provided no additional window into the condition. Adult CRS (with or without polyps) may actually, based on new studies, provide little pediatric equivalency [8]. As expressed by the authors of the 2014 consensus, the condition in 2017 is still "ill-defined" [1]. Or alternatively, "a bear by any other name is still a bear".

Conflicts of Interest: The author declares no conflict of interest.

References

1. Brietzke, S.; Shin, J.; Choi, S.; Lee, J.T.; Parikh, S.R.; Pena, M.; Prager, J.D.; Ramadan, H.; Veling, M.; Corrigan, C.; et al. Clinical Consensus Statement: Pediatric Chronic Rhinosinusitis. *Otolaryngol. Head Neck Surg.* **2014**, *151*, 542–553. [CrossRef] [PubMed]
2. Orlandi, R.R.; Kingdom, T.T.; Hwang, P.H.; Smith, T.L.; Alt, J.A.; Baroody, F.M.; Batra, P.S.; Bernal-Sprekelsen, M.; Bhattacharyya, N.; Chandra, R.K.; et al. International Consensus Statement on Allergy and Rhinology: Rhinosinusitis. *Int. Forum Allergy Rhinol.* **2016**, *6*, S22–S209. [CrossRef] [PubMed]
3. Hopp, R.J.; Alison, J.; Brooks, D. Pediatric Chronic Rhinosinusitis. *Pediatr. Ann.* **2014**, *43*, e201–e209.
4. Fokkens, W.J.; Lund, V.J.; Mullol, J.; Bachert, C.; Alobid, I.; Baroody, F.; Cohen, N.; Cervin, A.; Douglas, R.; Gevaert, P.; et al. EPOS 2012: European position paper on rhinosinusitis and nasal polyps 2012. A summary for Otorhinolaryngologists. *Rhinology* **2012**, *50*, 1–12. [PubMed]
5. Rachelefsky, G.S.; Katz, R.M.; Siegel, S.C. Chronic sinusitis in children with respiratory allergy: the role of antimicrobials. *J. Allergy Clin. Immunol.* **1982**, *69*, 382–387. [CrossRef]
6. Brook, I.; Yocum, P. Antimicrobial management of chronic sinusitis in children. *J. Laryngol. Otol.* **1995**, *109*, 1159–1162. [CrossRef] [PubMed]
7. Aurora, R.; Chatterjee, D.; Hentzleman, J.; Prasad, G.; Sindwani, R.; Sanford, T. Contrasting the microbiomes from healthy volunteers and patients with chronic rhinosinusitis. *JAMA Otolaryngol. Head Neck Surg.* **2013**, *139*, 1328–1338. [CrossRef] [PubMed]
8. Cho, S.H.; Bachert, C.; Lockey, R.F. Chronic Rhinosinusitis Pheonotypes: An Approach to Better Medical Care for Chronic Rhinosinusitis. *J. Allergy Clin. Immunol. Pract.* **2016**, *4*, 639–642. [CrossRef] [PubMed]

11

Do Adult Forms of Chronic Rhinosinusitis Exist in Children and Adolescents?

Russell J. Hopp

Department of Pediatrics, Creighton University School of Medicine, 2500 California Plaza, Omaha, NE 68131, USA; rhopp@creighton.edu

Abstract: Pediatric chronic sinusitis is currently designated as pediatric chronic rhinosinusitis. In most pediatric cases, sinusitis is considered as infectious. In the adult literature, a wider repertoire of chronic rhinosinusitis conditions is recognized. In this review, the adult forms of chronic rhinosinusitis are used as a framework for identifying and defining the potential spectrum of pediatric chronic rhinosinusitis that exists beyond the most recognized condition, pediatric infectious chronic rhinosinusitis.

Keywords: pediatric; children; adolescent; chronic sinusitis; chronic rhinosinusitis; nasal polyps; eosinophilic mucin chronic rhinosinusitis; Samter's triad

1. Introduction

Chronic rhinosinusitis (CRS) in adults is not uncommon and is often classified as CRS with or without polyps [1]. A recent extensive International Consensus Statement [2] and a theme issue of the Clinical Commentary Reviews [3] have provided insight into the pathophysiology, clinical presentation, and treatment of adult CRS. However, little to no comment is made about any equivalent disease(s) in the pediatric population. This review outlines what is known about pediatric CRS and uses the framework of the more established adult CRS conditions as a basis for determining where adult–pediatric CRS equivalencies (might) occur.

1.1. Definitions of Adult Chronic Rhinosinusitis

Based on the International Consensus Statement on Rhinosinusitis [2] and the Clinical Commentary Reviews [3], adult CRS can be divided into these different categories:

A.   Chronic rhinosinusitis without nasal polyps
B.   Chronic rhinosinusitis with polyps
C.   (Infectious) Chronic rhinosinusitis
D.   Aspirin or nonsteroidal drug-exacerbated chronic rhinosinusitis (AERD)
E.   Eosinophilic mucin rhinosinusitis (EMRS)

Deliberately excluded in this review is fungal rhinosinusitis (AFRS), based on its rarity and its accepted presence in children. Also excluded is pediatric CRS associated with cystic fibrosis (CF), primary ciliary dyskinesia (PCD), and primary immunodeficiency disorders (PID), but each of these other circumstances is discussed in the Clinical Commentary Reviews [3]. The above-listed adult categories (A–E) have a greater frequency and are, by large, stand-alone conditions.

Information on pediatric CRS, extracted from the International Consensus Statement [2], suggests that CRS is considered exclusively as an infectious form, and is further defined below. A brief mention is made of the presence of nasal polyps in children, and a further discussion of pediatric CF, PCD, and immunodeficiency round out the International Consensus discussion [2].

The collection of individual articles in Clinical Commentary Reviews [3] provides only a marginal expansion of the potential pediatric expression of any of the adult phenotypes. Individual manuscripts on the theme issue include findings that the presence of polyps raises the specter of CF [4,5] but CRS without polyps raises no pediatric discussion [6]. The authors of the manuscripts about infectious CRS and AERD provided no pediatric perspective [7,8], but children are briefly mentioned in a section of other phenotypes [5].

The Clinical Commentary Review mentions the term "eosinophilic (mucin) CRS" in the context of allergic fungal rhinosinusitis [9]. The broad topic of eosinophilic mucin is almost always linked to allergic fungal sinusitis, although it appears to have some support as a separate entity [10]. The "eosinophilic mucin CRS" term is also used in the International Consensus Statement, all in the context of allergic fungal sinusitis [2]. Limited literature exists for a non-allergic fungal sinusitis (non-AFS) form of eosinophilic mucin rhinosinusitis [10].

In summary, the listed definitions of adult CRS in both the International Consensus Statement [2] and Clinical Commentary Reviews [3] have minimal pediatric comment other than it being a chronic infectious process.

Until recently, numerous publications on pediatric chronic sinus disease have focused almost solely on the infectious nature of the condition. Two contemporary articles have presented an integrative approach to the discussion of pediatric chronic rhinosinusitis [11,12]. These two articles have provided brief discussions on additional phenotypes of pediatric CRS beyond its infectious nature.

To further expand the perspective on pediatric CRS, this review uses a systematic approach to expand the classification of potential pediatric CRS entities, using the framework of the adult processes of CRS as a guide.

1.2. Potential Definitions of Pediatric Chronic Rhinosinusitis

A.   Pediatric (infectious) chronic rhinosinusitis
B.   Aspirin or nonsteroidal drug-exacerbated pediatric CRS
C.   Pediatric CRS with polyps
D.   Pediatric CRS without polyps
E.   Pediatric eosinophilic mucin CRS (EMRS)
F.   Other
G.   Recognized but not discussed

A.   Pediatric (infectious) chronic rhinosinusitis

Pediatric chronic sinusitis has morphed, descriptively, to the term chronic pediatric rhinosinusitis [13]. A more accurate term would actually be pediatric chronic infectious rhinosinusitis. This author has published an extensive updated review on pediatric (infectious) CRS [14]. A Clinical Consensus Statement on pediatric chronic rhinosinusitis by otolaryngologists was published in 2014 [13]. The pediatric infectious CRS summary in The International Consensus Statement [2] largely mirrors the Clinical Consensus Statement on pediatric CRS [13].

Chronic infectious rhinosinusitis in children has reasonably defined time periods and symptoms (acute, subacute, chronic), although the route from the normal sinus to chronic rhinosinusitis is not well understood. The topic of pediatric infectious CRS has been recently extensively reviewed [14]. In brief, there is a good consensus as to the standards for diagnosis, the selection of a first-round antibiotic, and length of treatment, but the therapy for refractory patients and determining the presence of refractoriness is not well defined [12]. Areas of future research include the microbiome of pediatric chronic rhinosinusitis, imaging specificity, alternative antibiotic selection, ancillary therapy, and optimal surgical therapy [11,12,14]. Recent detailed discussions on pediatric CRS was presented by Hamilos and included proposals for the potential route from acute sinusitis to the more chronic state [11,12].

B. Aspirin or nonsteroidal drug-exacerbated pediatric CRS (AERD)

Aspirin or nonsteroidal-drug exacerbated CRS was discussed in the Clinical Commentary Review. The specific manuscript on the topic makes no mention of the occurrence in pediatrics [8]. The definition of hypersensitivity responses to nonsteroidal anti-inflammatory drugs was provided in a position paper in 2013 [15]. No specificity to a pediatric expression of aspirin or nonsteroidal drug-exacerbated respiratory disease was provided in that publication [15].

The pediatric presentation of asthma, nasal polyps (with CRS), and aspirin (ASA) or nonsteroidal anti-inflammatory drug (NSAID) allergy (Samter's triad) is not common and has minimal literature reference. A case report from 2013 details one child [16]. An otolaryngology tertiary referral center reported in 2013 on 28 children with nasal polyps, of which three had aspirin sensitivity and two were reported as having had an aspirin desensitization [17]. Of the two case reports, one child did not have defined asthma and one had mild asthma. Both underwent functional endoscopic sinus surgery. Neither publication referenced previous pediatric literature on Samter's triad [16,17]. An up-to-date 2017 literature review simply stated that children and adolescents are rarely affected [18].

Two published reports on aspirin-exacerbated respiratory disease (aspirin-induced asthma) were reported in the United States at a single site [19], and in Europe in 16 clinical centers [20]. The single American site, at Scripps Clinic in San Diego, examined the natural history of 300 subjects, all of who had a positive aspirin challenge [19]. The age of onset was 34 ± 12 years, thus indicating pediatric age in a percent of subjects; the youngest studied subject was 17 years old. In the European study, of the 500 study subjects with positive aspirin challenges, the ages of onset of rhinitis, asthma, and polyps were 29.7 ± 12.5, 31.9 ± 13.5, and 35.2 ± 12.1, respectively [20], again showing a pediatric onset of Samter's triad clinical symptoms.

A recent clinical commentary in 2016 presented three children with AERD. Several other publications with limited pediatric AERD inclusion were referenced in this report [21].

Both NSAID-associated CRS and Samter's triad is exceedingly rare in children and adolescents, but do exist. No collections of exclusively pediatric cases from one or collaborative centers are available. Limited information suggests a similar presentation in children as in adults, and therapy is likely similar to adults.

C. Pediatric CRS with polyps (pediatric CRSwNP)

The 3rd edition of the textbook Pediatric Allergy mentions in the allergic rhinitis chapter that nasal polyps are frequent in cystic fibrosis but not in pediatric allergic rhinitis [22]. The chapter on sinusitis makes no mention of nasal polyps [23].

The previously mentioned otolaryngology referral center publication on Samter's triad actually mentioned a total of 28 children with nasal polyposis over a 6-year period [17]. The three children with aspirin sensitivity were discussed in detail. No further details on the other children with CRSwNP were presented.

A South Korean publication stratified their CRS with nasal polyposis subjects by age. Twenty pediatric subjects with CRS and polyps were discussed. The surgical procedure and outcome was the focus of the manuscript [24].

Another Korean otolaryngology group selected pediatric patients with protracted sinus infection [25]. Children with a multitude of complicating factors including CF, immunodeficiency, aspirin-allergy, and antrochoanal polyps were excluded. Any "suspicious" polypoid tissue at surgery was examined histologically. Overall, 64% of the children with CRS who went to surgery had sinonasal polyposis proven histologically.

An Israeli study covering pediatric endoscopic sinus surgery due to nasal polyps from 2000 to 2010 was published in 2012 [26]. Thirty-one subjects, 8–18 years, met their criteria. Thirteen had an antrochoanal polyp, 16 had chronic sinusitis with nasal polyposis, and 3 had a mucocele. One child had previously undiagnosed CF. They further stated that chronic sinusitis with polyps is predominately seen in adults, and they speculated on whether it is the same disease process in children. They suggest that literature on pediatric CRSwNP in otherwise healthy children is absent.

A French study in 1997 reported on 14 children with nasal polyposis alone and 5 children with asthma and polyposis [27]. Children with CF were discussed separately. No comment was made of accompanying CRS in the non-CF children, but the surgical description suggests that sinus pathology was present.

A German study on functional endoscopic sinus surgery in children and adolescents with chronic rhinosinusitis was published in 2009; the study population was from a referral center between 1995 and 2004 [28]. Of the 115 children, 59 subjects had CRS without polyps and 45 cases had CRS with polyps (including 6 with CF). No results were presented on histological changes in any of the subjects, and the report focused on the surgical aspects of the disease.

A quality of life outcome study was reported in children with chronic rhinosinusitis with nasal polyps undergoing functional endoscopic sinus surgery (FESS) [29]. Published in 2013, the authors stated that although FESS is relatively successful, children with CRSwNP should undergo maximum medical therapy prior to surgery, and that data on this population is scarce.

CRS with polyps in adults is a complex immunological process with a strong emphasis on type 2 immunity, including interleukin-5 (IL-5), interleukin-13 (IL-13), eotaxin-2, and eosinophilia [30]. Similar information is lacking in children. An older study on eosinophilia in sinus tissue of children with chronic sinusitis has been published [31]. Children with chronic sinusitis with asthma ($n = 13$), without asthma ($n = 11$), and with CF ($n = 10$) were reported. Sinus tissue was histologically examined and compared to sinus tissue from sphenoid sinuses in six controls. In general, all three disease groups had higher eosinophils in tissue compared to the sphenoid sinus tissue, and the non-asthma children had the lowest among the disease groups. The degree of allergy between the disease groups did not influence the eosinophilia in the diseased sinus mucosa.

An older study of pediatric nasal polyps reported on 120 cases: 24 children had unilateral and 22 children had bilateral polyps, and the other cases were from CF or with antrochoanal polyps only [32]. The tissue of the polyp was uniformly reported as normal respiratory mucosa. Cellular infiltrates within the polyp were acute and chronic inflammatory cells, but eosinophilia was rarely found. The presence of concomitant CRS appears to have been present in the non-CF, non-antrochoanal patients, but was not well defined.

Other reports on the prevalence of nasal polyps in pediatric sinus surgery have ranged from 7% to 18.8% [33–35]. Tissue from pediatric nasal polyps might mimic an adult eosinophilic state or, less commonly, neutrophilia.

In summary, CRSwNP is rare in children and adolescents, with some evidence for eosinophilia within the extracted sinus tissue. Its separate pediatric existence without allergy, without a bacterial infectious component, and without CF or ciliary dyskinesia co-morbidity is not well defined. Any future reports in children and adolescents with CRSwNP should examine the immunological constitutionality of the sinus tissue, the cellular composition of the polyp, and bacteriological presence, including the spectrum of the microbiome. Since surgery is potentially performed on these children/adolescents, studies of this type could be performed.

D. Pediatric chronic rhinosinusitis without polyps (pediatric CRSsNP)

A condition of adult CRS without polyps appears to exist [6]. However, its presence as a distinct pediatric entity is non-existent in the literature. Any population of pediatric CRS without polyps, if clinically viable, must exclude infectious CRS, allergic rhinitis, nasal polyps, aspirin-exacerbated respiratory disease (ARED), CF, immunodeficiency, AFRS, and eosinophilic mucin CRS.

Hamilos proposed a scenario where persistent pediatric CRS might evolve into a complex condition, reflecting a potential for a CRSsNP status; however, he further proposed a "maladaptive-eosinophilic" state in a minority of children [11,12].

It is possible to speculate that a pediatric infectious CRS situation could, after a long duration, morph into a microbiomically (microbiologically) altered, neutrophilic-driven CRS. If true, it is also possible that at some point antibiotics cannot resolve the condition. These children may, in effect, drive surgically managed pediatric infectious CRS (recalcitrant) [14].

The adult condition of CRSsNP gathers no clinical correlation in children in virtually all historical publications. The true potential form of a pediatric non-polyp CRS that correlates with either a purely neutrophilic end-stage or with an eventually or separate eosinophilic end-stage needs further investigation.

E.   Pediatric eosinophilic mucin CRS (EMRS)

Separate from an entity associated with allergic fungal sinusitis, literature evidence has been summarized for a pediatric eosinophilic mucin CRS condition; although all were adolescents and of limited number compared to adults [10]. Another publication termed this entity as "AFS-like syndrome" [36]. In that report, a pediatric patient was included [36].

Histological comparisons between adult and pediatric CRS

Another way to potentially divide pediatric and adult CRS forms, other than by definitional standards, is to examine the histopathology of surgical tissue. Two studies have approached the differentiation in this way, and one older study has examined mucosal histology in older children with chronic (rhino)sinusitis as compared to normal adults. The 1995 publication compared the sinus tissue from 24 non-CF children with 6 normal adult sphenoidal tissue samples [31]. The mean age was 7 (range 3–16 years). A publication in 2004 reported on 19 children with ages 1.4 to 8 years and adult CRS controls [37], which was further extended in the same children in 2009 using immunopathology [38]. A 2011 publication examined sinus mucosa from 16 CRS children with mean age 11.6 (range 7–16) and 29 adult CRS controls [33]. Table 1 attempts to compare and contrast the findings, although methodologies between the three studies are not comparable (per se). The re-analysis [38] of the children in the 2004 study [37] stands alone and shows that pediatric CRS is less eosinophilic than adult CRS controls and more skewed based on cellularity from excessive microbiological stimulation.

Table 1. Comparison of published histological studies of chronic rhinosinusitis (CRS) in children.

		Eosinophils	Lymphocytes	Suggested Phenotype in Children
1995 [31] *	Pediatric CRS no asthma	Present	ND	
	Pediatric CRS asthma	Present **	ND	
	Adult normal controls	0	ND	
2004 [37] *	Pediatric CRS	Low	High	Infectious CRS
	Adult CRS	High	Low	
2011 [33] *	Pediatric CRS	Low	Equal	Infectious CRS
	Adult CRS	High	Equal	

* The same articles were descriptively discussed in a report by Hamilos [11]. ** Present or elevated.

F.   Other minor classifications of chronic rhinosinusitis

Publications are available that define a condition termed eosinophilic chronic rhinosinusitis [39–41]. In essence, it is made up of a collection of other more recognized CRS conditions, including CRS with polyps, allergic fungal sinusitis, aspirin or non-steroidal drug-exacerbated chronic rhinosinusitis, and eosinophilic mucin CRS. Each of these has been previously and separately discussed for a pediatric presence.

G.   Other recognized—or not reviewed—pediatric CRS phenotypes

1.   CRS associated with adenoid hypertrophy [42]
2.   CRS with anatomical abnormalities [43]
3.   CRS with ciliary motility defects
4.   CRS with immunodeficiency
5.   CRS with cystic fibrosis

CRS with adenoid hypertrophy/adenoiditis may be a co-morbid factor of chronic infectious pediatric rhinosinusitis, but with an exaggerated adenoid dysfunction due to chronic nasal dysbiosis [42]. This was further discussed by Hamilos [11].

Anatomical abnormalities, although uncommon in children, may also allow for the development of pediatric infectious rhinosinusitis, although the role of anatomical contributions in CRS has been downplayed [43].

The entities of CRS with ciliary motility defects, CRS with immunodeficiency, and CRS with cystic fibrosis have been intentionally excluded from this review.

Surgical Approach to Pediatric CRS

Surgical therapy for pediatric CRS can include children with recalcitrant pediatric infectious CRS or for other forms of pediatric CRS. These could include aspirin or nonsteroidal drug-exacerbated pediatric CRS, pediatric CRS with polyps, and eosinophilic mucin CRS (an uncommonly used classification). The surgical approach for any of these separate etiologies may overlap. The Consensus Surgical Review does not differentiate between different surgical approaches, unless polyps are present [13].

2. Summary

Pediatric CRS is not an uncommon clinical diagnosis but it is vastly under-represented in the literature with any phenotypic subtypes. CRS in the vast majority of children, especially pre-school age, likely starts as viral rhinosinusitis that, without resolution, develops into pediatric infectious CRS [11,12,14]. The natural history of pediatric infectious CRS is unknown, and some small percentage will require surgical intervention. Polyp growth in infectious CRS is rare.

Older children and adolescents appear to have a bigger repertoire of beginnings of their CRS. Undoubtedly, ARED can start in later childhood, with or without asthma. True CRSwNP without aspirin or NSAID allergy rarely occurs. Whether this is type 2 cytokine-driven, as in adults, needs further investigation. CRSsNP has no pediatric correlates in the literature; however, pediatric infectious CRS could morph into this condition if left untreated for an extended period (speculative).

Recently, a sophisticated immunological cluster analysis of the adult rhinosinusitis phenotypes with polyps and CRS phenotypes without polyps has been published [44]. Defining the phenotypes of adult CRS obviously has important mechanistic implications, and only further highlights the divide between adult disease and the continued under-emphasis of pediatric CRS. Establishing clinical patterns of CRS in pediatrics could provide a pathway to define these conditions using similar complex methodologies.

To our knowledge, this is the first review to attempt to systematically categorize pediatric CRS into definable conditions based on the current literature. Using an adult-based system may prove, ultimately, to be incorrect; however, enough evidence exists to support a number of adult–pediatric CRS equivalencies. Using the general term pediatric CRS limits the background by which each child reaches the level of medical care and investigation. Unfortunately, the ability to investigate a group of like-presenting children using more invasive means may always be limited by ethical and regulatory constraints. Until a time when less invasive biomarkers become available to investigate pediatric CRS, literature using broad terminology will continue to provide only a limited picture of a chronic pediatric condition.

Author Contributions: The author thanks Ryan Sewell, Muhammad Pasha, and Hana Niebur for their review and editorial comments.

Conflicts of Interest: The author declares no conflict of interest.

References

1. Fokkens, W.J.; Lund, V.J.; Mullol, J.; Bachert, C.; Alobid, I.; Baroody, F.; Cohen, N.; Cervin, A.; Douglas, R.; Gevaert, P.; et al. EPOS 2012: European position paper on rhinosinusitis and nasal polyps 2012. *Rhinology* **2012**, *50*, 1–12. [PubMed]

2. Orlandi, R.R.; Kingdom, T.T.; Hwang, P.H.; Smith, T.L.; Alt, J.A.; Baroody, F.M.; Batra, P.S.; Bernal-Sprekelsen, M.; Bhattacharyya, N.; Chandra, R.K.; et al. International consensus statement on allergy and rhinology: Rhinosinusitis. *Int. Forum Allergy Rhinol.* **2015**, *6*, S22–S209. [CrossRef] [PubMed]

3. Cho, S.H.; Bachert, C.; Lockey, R.F. Chronic rhinosinusitis pheonotypes: An Approach to Better Medical Care for Chronic Rhinosinusitis. *J. Allergy Immunol. Pract.* **2016**, *4*, 565–642.

4. Stevens, W.W.; Schleimer, R.P.; Kern, R. Chronic rhinosinusitis with polyps. *J. Allergy Immunol. Pract.* **2016**, *4*, 565–572. [CrossRef] [PubMed]

5. Naclerio, R.M.; Baroody, F.M. Other phenotypes and treatment of chronic rhinosinusitis. *J. Allergy Immunol. Pract.* **2016**, *4*, 613–620. [CrossRef] [PubMed]

6. Cho, S.G.; Kim, D.W.; Gevaert, P. Chronic rhinosinusitis without nasal polyps. *J. Allergy Immunol. Pract.* **2016**, *4*, 575–582. [CrossRef] [PubMed]

7. Bose, S.; Grammer, L.C.; Peters, A.T. Infectious chronic rhinosinusitis. *J. Allergy Immunol. Pract.* **2016**, *4*, 584–589. [CrossRef] [PubMed]

8. Ledford, D.K.; Lockey, R.F. Aspirin or nonsteroidal anti-inflammatory drug-exacerbated chronic rhinosinusitis. *J. Allergy Immunol. Pract.* **2016**, *4*, 590–598. [CrossRef] [PubMed]

9. Hoyt, A.E.W.; Borsh, L.; Gurrla, J.; Payne, S. Allergic fungal rhinosinusitis. *J. Allergy Immunol. Pract.* **2016**, *4*, 599–604. [CrossRef] [PubMed]

10. Ferguson, B.J. Eosinophilic mucin rhinosinusitis: A distinct clinicopathological entity. *Laryngoscope* **2000**, *110*, 799–813. [CrossRef] [PubMed]

11. Hamilos, D.L. Pediatric chronic rhinosinusitis. *Am. J. Rhinol. Allergy* **2015**, *29*, 414–420. [CrossRef] [PubMed]

12. Hamilos, D.L. Problem-based learning discussion: Medical treatment of pediatric chronic rhinosinusitis. *Am. J. Rhinol. Allergy* **2016**, *30*, 113–121. [CrossRef] [PubMed]

13. Brietzke, S.; Shin, J.; Choi, S.; Lee, J.T.; Parikh, S.R.; Pena, M.; Prager, J.D.; Ramadan, H.; Veling, M.; Corrigan, C.; et al. Clinical Consensus Statement: Pediatric Chronic Rhinosinusitis. *Otolaryngol. Head Neck Surg.* **2014**, *151*, 542–553. [CrossRef] [PubMed]

14. Hopp, R.J.; Alison, J.; Brooks, D. Pediatric chronic rhinosinusitis. *Pediatr. Ann.* **2016**, *43*, e201–e209.

15. Kowalski, M.L.; Asero, R.; Bavbek, S.; Blanca, M.; Blanca-Lopez, M.; Bochenek, G.; Brockow, K.; Campo, P.; Celik, G.; Cernadas, J.; et al. Classification and practical approach to the diagnosis and management of hypersensitivity to nonsteroidal anti-inflammatory drugs. *Allergy* **2013**, *68*, 1219–1232. [CrossRef] [PubMed]

16. Ameratunga, R.; Randall, N.; Dalziel, A.; Anderson, B.J. Samter's triad in childhood: A warning for those prescribing NSAIDs. *Pediatr. Anesth.* **2013**, *23*, 757–759. [CrossRef] [PubMed]

17. Chen, B.S.; Virant, F.S.; Parikh, S.R.; Manning, S.C. Aspirin sensitivity syndrome (Samter's Triad): An underrecognized disorder in children with nasal polyposis. *Int. J. Pediatr. Otorrhinolaryngol.* **2013**, *77*, 281–283. [CrossRef] [PubMed]

18. Laidlaw, T.M.; Israel, E. *Aspirin-Exacerbated Respiratory Disease*; UpToDate: Waltham, MA, USA, 2016.

19. Berges-Gimeno, M.P.; Simon, R.A.; Stevenson, D.D. The natural history and clinical characteristics of aspirin-exacerbated respiratory disease. *Ann. Allergy Asthma Immunol.* **2002**, *89*, 474–478. [CrossRef]

20. Szczekilk, A.; Nizankowska, E.; Duplaga, M.; On Behalf of AIANE Investigators. Natural history of aspirin-induced asthma. *Eur. Resp. J.* **2000**, *16*, 432–436. [CrossRef]

21. Tuttle, K.L.; Schneider, T.R.; Henrickson, S.E.; Morris, D.; Abonia, J.P.; Spergel, J.M.; Laidlaw, T.M. Aspirin-exacerbated respiratory disease: Not always "adult-onset". *J. Allergy Clin. Immunol. Pract.* **2016**, *4*, 756–758. [CrossRef] [PubMed]

22. Gentile, D.A.; Pleskovic, N.; Bartholow, A.; Skoner, D.P. Allergic Rhinitis. In *Pediatric Allergy: Principles and Practice*, 3rd ed.; Leung, D.Y.M., Szefler, S.J., Bonilla, F.A., Akdis, C.A., Sampson, H.A., Eds.; Elsevier: Philadelphia, PA, USA, 2016; pp. 210–218.

23. Chan, K.H.; Azbug, M.J.; Liu, A.H. Sinusitis. In *Pediatric Allergy: Principles and Practice*, 3rd ed.; Leung, D.Y.M., Szefler, S.J., Bonilla, F.A., Akdis, C.A., Sampson, H.A., Eds.; Elsevier: Philadelphia, PA, USA, 2016; pp. 228–237.

24. Lee, J.Y.; Lee, S.W. Influence of age on the surgical outcome after endoscopic sinus surgery for chronic rhinosinusitis with nasal polyposis. *Laryngoscope* **2007**, *117*, 1084–1089. [CrossRef] [PubMed]

25. Lee, T.J.; Liang, C.W.; Chang, P.H.; Huang, C.C. Risk factors for protracted sinusitis in pediatrics after endoscopic sinus surgery. *Auria Nasus Larynx* **2009**, *36*, 655–660. [CrossRef] [PubMed]

26. Segal, N.; Gluk, O.; Puterman, M. Nsal polyps in the pediatric population. *B-ENT* **2012**, *8*, 265–267. [PubMed]

27. Triglia, J.M.; Nicollas, R. Nasal and sinus polyposis in children. *Laryngoscope* **1997**, *107*, 963–966. [CrossRef] [PubMed]

28. Siedek, V.; Stelter, K.; Betz, C.S.; Berghaus, A.; Leunig, A. Functional endoscopic sinus surgery-A retrospective analysis of 115 children and adolescents with chronic rhinosinusitis. *Int. J. Pediatr. Otorhinolaryngol.* **2009**, *73*, 741–745. [CrossRef] [PubMed]

29. Cornet, M.J.; Georgalas, C.; Reinartz, S.M.; Fokkens, W.J. Long-term results of functional endoscopic sinus surgery in children with chronic rhinosinusitis with nasal polyps. *Rhinology* **2013**, *51*, 326–334. [CrossRef]

30. Ocampo, C.J.; Berdnikovs, S.; Sakashita, M.; Mahdavinia, M.; Suh, L.; Takabayashi, T.; Norton, J.E.; Hulse, K.E.; Conley, D.B.; Chandra, R.K.; et al. Cytokines in Chronic Rhinosinusitis. Role in Eosinophilia and Aspirin-exacerbated Respiratory Disease. *Am. J. Respir. Crit. Care Med.* **2015**, *192*, 682–694.

31. Baroody, F.; Hughes, C.A.; McDowell, P.; Hruban, R.; Zinreich, S.J.; Naclerio, R.M. Eosinophilic in chronic childhood sinusitis. *Arch. Otolaryngol. Head Neck Surg.* **1995**, *121*, 1396–1402. [CrossRef] [PubMed]

32. Schramm, V.L.; Effron, M.Z. Nasal polyps in children. *Laryngoscope* **1980**, *90*, 1488–1495. [CrossRef] [PubMed]

33. Berger, G.; Kogan, T.; Paker, M.; Berger-Achituv, S.; Ebner, Y. Pediatric chronic rhinosinusitis histopathology: Differences and similarities with the adult form. *Otolaryngol. Head Neck Surg.* **2011**, *144*, 85–90. [CrossRef] [PubMed]

34. El Sharkawy, A.A.; Elmorsy, S.M.; Eladl, H.M. Functional endoscopic sinus surgery in children: Predictive factors of outcome. *Eur. Arch. Oto-Rhino-Laryngol.* **2012**, *169*, 107–111. [CrossRef] [PubMed]

35. Lazar, R.H.; Younis, R.T.; Gross, C.W. Pediatric functional endonasal sinus surgery. *Head Neck* **1992**, *14*, 92–98. [CrossRef] [PubMed]

36. Cody, D.T.; Neel, H.D.; Ferreiro, J.A.; Roberts, G.D. Allergic fungal sinusitis: The Mayo clinic experience. *Laryngoscope* **1994**, *104*, 1074–1079. [CrossRef] [PubMed]

37. Chan, K.H.; Abzug, M.J.; Coffinet, L.; Simoes, E.A.F.; Cool, C.; Liu, A.H. Chronic rhinosinusitis in young children differs from adults: A histopathological study. *J. Pediatr.* **2004**, *144*, 206–212. [CrossRef] [PubMed]

38. Coffinet, L.; Chan, K.H.; Abzug, M.J.; Somoes, E.A.F.; Cool, C.; Liu, A.H. Immunopathology of chronic rhinosinusitis in young children. *J. Pediatr.* **2009**, *154*, 754–758. [CrossRef] [PubMed]

39. Shah, S.A.; Ishinaga, H.; Takeuchi, K. Pathogenesis of eosinophilic chronic rhinosinusitis. *J. Inflamm.* **2016**, *13*, 11. [CrossRef] [PubMed]

40. Sok, J.C.; Ferguson, B.J. Differential diagnosis of eosinophilic chronic rhinosinusitis. *Curr. Allergy Asthma Rep.* **2006**, *6*, 203–214. [CrossRef] [PubMed]

41. Steinke, J.W.; Borish, L. Chronic rhinosinusitis phenotypes. *Ann. Allergy Asthma Immunol.* **2016**, *117*, 234–240. [CrossRef] [PubMed]

42. Brietzke, S.E.; Brigger, M.T. Adenoidectomy outcomes in pediatric rhinosinusitis: A meta-analysis. *Int. J. Pediatr. Otorhinolaryngol.* **2008**, *72*, 1541–1545. [CrossRef] [PubMed]

43. Sivasli, E.; Sirikçi, A.; Bayazýt, Y.A.; Gümüsburun, E.; Erbagci, H.; Bayram, M.; Kanlýkama, M. Anatomic variations of the paranasal sinus area in pediatric patients with chronic sinusitis. *Surg. Radiol. Anat.* **2003**, *24*, 400–405. [PubMed]

44. Tomassen, P.; Vandeplas, G.; Van Zele, T.; Cardell, L.O.; Arebro, J.; Olze, H.; Förster-Ruhrmann, U.; Kowalski, M.L.; Olszewska-Ziąber, A.; Holtappels, G.; et al. Inflammatory endotypes of chronic rhinosinusitis based on cluster analysis of biomarkers. *J. Allergy Clin. Immunol.* **2016**, *137*, 1449–1456. [CrossRef] [PubMed]

12

State-of-the-Art Adult Chronic Rhinosinusitis Microbiome: Perspective for Future Studies in Pediatrics

M. Asghar Pasha

Division of Allergy and Immunology, Albany Medical College, 176 Washington Avenue Extension, Suite 102, Albany, NY 12203, USA; pasham@amc.edu

Abstract: Chronic rhinosinusitis (CRS) is a prevalent disease that causes persistent mucosal inflammation and is associated with bacterial infection, which is thought to play a role in the inflammatory process. Microbiome analysis provides insight to host–microbial interactions. Disturbances in the host and commensal bacteria interaction may lead to CRS. Culture-based methods are useful to isolate some microorganisms but are unable to grow a majority of the bacteria. A review of the literature shows that several recent studies attempted to overcome this issue by using molecular techniques, such as microbial RNA sequencing, to describe the CRS microbiome. All of these studies were performed in adults, with no comparative studies reported in the pediatric population. Similar studies, utilizing molecular techniques, are needed to better understand the mechanism of CRS in children. Because valuable data from these adult studies may help to bridge the gap in our knowledge of the microbiome in pediatric CRS, we present an overview of the methodology and results behind the current microbiomic approach to adult CRS to set the stage for its use in the study of CRS in children.

Keywords: microbiome; pediatric chronic rhinosinusitis; molecular techniques

1. Introduction

The field of the microbiological study of chronic rhinosinusitis (CRS) in adults has taken a quantum leap forward in only a few years. Unfortunately, similar approaches to the study of CRS in children have been totally lacking in the literature. A Medline search was performed for articles reporting on the microbiome in patients with CRS. Search terms included: 16S ribosomal RNA (rRNA) gene sequencing in chronic rhinosinusitis, chronic rhinosinusitis and microbiome, chronic rhinosinusitis and pyrosequencing, non-cultured molecular techniques in chronic rhinosinusitis, microbiome and 16S ribosome RNA. The following is an overview of the reported methodology and results behind the current microbiomic approach to adult CRS with the goal to set the stage for its use in the future studies of pediatric CRS.

Bacterial rhinosinusitis is one of the most common problems presented to the primary care physician's office and results in over $5 billion in direct costs annually [1]. CRS symptoms lasting >12 weeks with or without exacerbations, affects more than 30 million Americans, which results in over $2.4 billion in annual health care expenditures [2]. CRS is considered an inflammatory disorder of the paranasal sinuses. Analysis of direct microbial cultures, sinus secretions, and tissue samples has demonstrated the presence of bacteria. It has been speculated that the bacterial colonization in CRS plays a role in pathophysiology of the disease [3,4]. Despite these findings, the role of microbial stimuli causing inflammation in CRS remains controversial [5].

The normal flora 'microbiome', also called commensal bacteria, in the gastrointestinal tract, nasal cavity and oropharynx provide useful functions. Microbiome analysis provides insight to host–microbial interactions. In recent years, this has been done using molecular techniques based on microbial RNA. Several published studies have shown that in the healthy state, sinuses are not completely sterile [6–10]. Disturbances in the host and commensal bacteria interaction may lead to disease, including upper airway disease such as CRS. The majority of the published studies used culture-based techniques as the mainstay of microbial diagnostics in CRS. The range of microbes detected by these techniques may not be representative of the actual diversity present, particularly in environmental samples [11]. Although culture-based methods are still useful to isolate and culture some microorganisms, it has been suggested that no more than 90% of bacteria can be cultured from most environments and that culture-positive results range from only 1 to 10% [12]. This has led to the development and use of molecular methodologies which include the following: phylogenetic oligonucleotide array, 16S ribosomal RNA gene clone libraries, analysis of functional gene arrays, next-generation sequencing technologies, sequencing by mass spectrometry, and random "shotgun" metagenomics [13,14]. These sophisticated methods help to identify both culturable and non-culturable organisms. For identification purposes, some techniques will selectively enhance or restrict growth of microorganisms. CRS has a polymicrobial community, and identification of every microorganism can be a monumental task [9]. Several recent studies attempted to overcome this issue by using molecular techniques to describe the CRS microbiome [5,7,9,10,15,16]. Here we review the available non-culture-based bacterial 16S rRNA gene sequencing data using pyrosequencing to describe bacterial diversity in patients with CRS and in healthy controls.

Abreu et al. report data regarding the healthy normal sinus microbiome in adults [7]. In this study, sinus brushing at the time of functional endoscopic sinus surgery (FESS) in patients with CRS was obtained and compared with that from a control group without CRS. A standardized phylogenetic microarray, the 16S rRNA PhyloChip, was used to analyze samples. This study showed significantly reduced bacterial diversity in patients with CRS compared with normal controls. Another finding in this study was that *Lactobacillus sakei* appeared to play a protective role in the normal sinus microbiome. The authors hypothesized that as the pathophysiology of CRS is multifactorial: it is co-dependent on a microbiome with increased relative abundance of *Corynebacterium tuberculostearicum* [7]. The study results could have been impacted by preoperative antibiotic use in some CRS subjects and by controls.

Ramakrishnan et al. analyzed sinus swabs collected during sinus surgery from a cohort of 56 patients with CRS and compared them with swabs from 20 controls using molecular phylogenetic analysis of 16S rDNA pyrosequences [17]. The authors attempted to determine whether a specific adult CRS phenotype shows an alteration in the sinus microbiome. The initial assessment of overall bacterial densities between groups showed the amount of total bacteria present was not statistically different between the groups. Bacteroidetes and Fusobacteria showed significant expansion with purulence in one half of the CRS study group. The isolation of anaerobes in CRS patients highlights the probable role and importance of these bacteria in the pathogenesis of CRS. The presence of nasal polyps was not independently associated with general bacterial community alterations. Baseline abundance of species of phylum Actinobacteria and genus *Corynebacterium* at the time of surgery were predictive of better surgical outcome in this study.

Feazel and colleagues compared conventional culture-based and culture-independent methodologies for the identification of microorganisms in CRS [10]. Middle meatus swab samples obtained during endoscopic sinus surgery from 15 CRS patients were compared with swabs from 5 controls. The samples were analyzed by using standard bacteriologic cultures and DNA pyrosequencing. Standard cultures were positive for all subjects, CRS patients as well as controls. The most common organisms isolated were coagulase-negative streptococci (75%), *Staphylococcus aureus* (50%), and *Corynebacterium acnes* (30%). The most prevalent species detected by pyrosequencing included coagulase-negative staphylococci (100%), *Corynebacterium* spp. (85.7%), *Propionibacterium acnes* (76.2%), and *S. aureus* (66.7%). Pyrosequencing was superior to standard culture technique for identifying significantly more diversity, particularly of anaerobes, in CRS patients relative to controls. The high prevalence of anaerobes in this study is an important finding, because earlier culture-based studies had reported a low prevalence, which could be due to methodological errors. This study also highlights the importance of *S. aureus* species, which was highly prevalent and abundant in CRS patients compared to controls.

Stephenson et al. reported similar results in a prospective study of 18 patients undergoing endoscopic sinus surgery for CRS and 9 control patients with pituitary adenomas [5]. They utilized molecular culture (bacterial tag-encoded FLX amplicon pyrosequencing (bTEFAP)) for identification of bacterial species present on sinonasal mucosa and compared them with those identified using conventional standard cultures. Standard cultures showed mainly *S. aureus* and coagulase-negative *Staphylococcus*. Molecular cultures identified up to 20 organisms per sample, and anaerobic species (*Diaphorobacter* and *Peptoniphilus*) predominated. *S. aureus* was detected in 50% of samples. The authors concluded that molecular cultures such as bTEFAP are sensitive tools for bacterial identification in CRS. This study suggests anaerobic involvement in patients with CRS undergoing sinus surgery. This is in agreement with Feazel et al. [10] regarding the high prevalence of anaerobes in the microbiome of CRS patients.

Aurora and colleagues used deep sequencing of the bacterial 16S and fungal 18S ribosomes genes, a culture-independent method, to analyze lavage of adult patients with CRS and adult controls [16]. In addition to microbiome analysis, immune response in the lavage was measured for the number of cytokines. Peripheral blood leukocyte immune response was measured by quantifying various cytokines. A group of 30 patients with refractory CRS and 12 controls were recruited. Middle meatus lavage was obtained prior to surgical intervention, after induction of general anesthesia. *Corynobacterium accolens* was the most abundant species, with a statistically significant increase in CRS patients compared to controls. These findings are in accord with those of Abrue et al., as previously described [7]. Fungal microbiome analysis showed *Cryptococcus neoformans* was much higher in CRS patients than in controls. Cytokine response in the lavage of all CRS patients relative to controls showed significantly elevated levels of interleukin (IL)-4, IL-5, and IL-13. Peripheral leukocytes from CRS patients produced IL-5 in response to control lavage samples (commensals), indicating hyperresponsiveness to the normal microbiome. This study highlights the importance of *C. neoformans*, a fungus, as a major constituent of sinus fungal microbiome in addition to *Corynobacterium*.

In a small cross-sectional study, Ramakrishnan and colleagues analyzed middle meatus swabs in healthy subjects without CRS, utilizing quantitative PCR and 16 rRNA pyrosequencing [6]. The most prevalent and abundant species isolated included *S. aureus*, *Staphylococcus epidermidis*, and *P. acnes*. The study has potential limitation with a small sample size and possible contamination of nasal microorganisms into specimens during surgery. Also, middle meatus microorganisms may not be representative of the sinus microbiome.

Choi and colleagues performed analysis of nasal lavage fluid from healthy controls and CRS patients with and without nasal polyposis [18]. Bacterial 16S ribosomal RNA pyrosequencing showed increased bacterial abundance and lower diversity from both bacterial and EV (bacteria-derived extracellular vesicles) fractions among CRS patients compared to controls. The authors found higher *S. aureus* composition from both bacterial and EV fractions in CRS patients with polyps compared to CRS patients without polyps. *Prevotella*, a genus of gram-negative bacteria and a genus of Bacteroidetes phylum, significantly decreased in CRS patients compared to controls, suggesting that the reduction in the bacteria may contribute to CRS pathogenesis. The results of this study highlight the importance of *S. aureus* in the pathogenesis of CRS, particularly CRS with polyps, as reported previously [5,9,10]. The most important finding in this study was bacteria-derived EV in the nasal fluids, and the authors argue that it may serve as another useful biomarker of CRS in the future. However, the EV analysis was done on nasal fluids as opposed to sinus fluids. The study was also limited by small sample.

Studies of CRS patients have shown a close association between bacterial and fungal biofilms [19–25]. In a prospective study, Cleland and colleagues examined the fungal microbiome in CRS patients undergoing endoscopic sinus surgery [26]. The control group consisted of patients undergoing endoscopic transsphenoidal resection of pituitary adenomas. Swabs were collected from the patients with CRS, intraoperatively and postoperatively, at 6 and 12 weeks. Fungal detection utilized 18S ribosomal DNA (rDNA) fungal tag-encoded FLX amplification pyrosequencing. The authors did not find major differences in the fungal microbiome between controls and CRS patients intraoperatively. Postoperatively, there was a decline in richness and presence of genera *Fusarium* and *Neocosmospora*. The authors hypothesized that the presence of *Malassezia* in patients with CRS could potentially have a disease-modifying effect. *Malassezia* is considered part of the normal cutaneous flora and is found in areas such as the trunk and head [27], and therefore its presence in the sinonasal cavity could represent seeding from these sites rather than permanent sinus colonization. Moreover, surgery itself affects the microbiome, and the findings postsurgery may have shown this confounding effect.

The results of these studies show that the most common/abundant bacteria in all subjects, both CRS patients and healthy controls included *Corynebacterium*, *Staphylococcus*, *Propionibacterium*, and Actinobacteria. The relative abundance of *C. tuberculostearicum* and *Corynebacterium accolens* was associated with CRS inflammation [7,16]. Increased relative abundance and diversity—particularly of *Propionibacterium*, *Burkholderia*, and *L. sakei*—was associated with healthy sinuses. The first two bacteria are also called "gatekeepers" and are thought to play an important role in maintaining a stable sinonasal community [28]. It is important to note that the studies that examined the microbiome in healthy subjects demonstrated the presence of *Staphylococcus*, *Streptococcus*, and *Pseudomonas*, bacteria known to cause respiratory disease [6,7,16]. These studies also indicated that significant microbiome dysbiosis is associated with CRS [7,10]. The presence of certain bacteria in CRS does not provide information regarding functional capabilities that differentiate healthy people from disease-associated communities. Moreover, some of the conflicting results in these studies could be due to interpersonal variation of the sinus microbiota caused by environmental exposures and biogeography, i.e., sampling of sinus vs. middle meatus. Variation in sampling techniques used to obtain specimens, e.g., brush vs. swab, also may have significant impact. Most of the studies did not consider the impact of other factors that might influence the sinus microbiome, such as lower respiratory tract disease (asthma), smoking, use of antibiotics, and/or use of steroids (oral and/or topical).

The pathophysiology of CRS is likely multifactorial and may be dependent on the paranasal sinus microbiome composition. Our knowledge of microbiota in CRS is still evolving. Key findings from the microbiome studies in adult CRS patients show less richness, evenness, and diversity than in control groups, although the total microbial burden appears to be similar. All culture-independent CRS microbiome studies in the literature have been done in adults, with no comparative studies reported in the pediatric population. Advancement in the understanding of pathophysiology of pediatric CRS, particularly with respect to the microbiome, is limited. Although multiple studies have been published, they are limited to standard culture techniques [29–42]. The standard culture-based techniques are outdated, antiquated, and limited. Data on CRS microbiome analyses performed with the use of non-cultured molecular techniques utilizing microbial RNA are more sensitive. There is a need for culture-independent research methods for the identification of microbiomes as has been employed in other studies [5,10,43]. Valuable data from adult studies may bridge the gap in our knowledge and understanding of the microbiome in pediatric CRS. For now, we can only extrapolate the findings of studies in adults to their application in the pediatric population.

Microbiome dysbiosis is associated with CRS. Culture-independent technologies help to describe microbial diversity, composition, and functional changes, as well as specific immune responses. Future studies should examine larger, more diverse populations, particularly children, of CRS to characterize the microbiome of different CRS phenotypes in comparison with controls. Additionally, longitudinal studies evaluating the effects of antimicrobials, sinus surgery, and topical nasal treatments on microbial diversity and abundance in CRS will be invaluable.

Acknowledgments: Author would like to acknowledge Russell Hopp, Qi Yang, Paul Feustel, and Marcia Lamb for their manuscript review and helpful suggestions.

Conflicts of Interest: The author declares no conflicts of interest.

References

1. Ray, N.F.; Baraniuk, J.N.; Thamer, M.; Rinehart, C.S.; Gergen, P.J.; Kaliner, M.; Josephs, S.; Pung, Y.H. Healthcare expenditures for sinusitis in 1996: Contributions of asthma, rhinitis, and other airway disorders. *J. Allergy Clin. Immunol.* **1999**, *103*, 408–414. [CrossRef]

2. Wallace, D.V.; Dykewicz, M.S.; Bernstein, D.I.; Blessing-Moore, J.; Cox, L.; Khan, D.A.; Lang, D.M.; Nicklas, R.A.; Oppenheimer, J.; Portnoy, J.M.; et al. The diagnosis and management of rhinitis: An updated practice parameter. *J. Allergy Clin. Immunol.* **2008**, *122*. [CrossRef] [PubMed]

3. Biel, M.A.; Brown, C.A.; Levinson, R.M.; Garvis, G.E.; Paisner, H.M.; Sigel, M.E.; Tedford, T.M. Evaluation of the microbiology of chronic maxillary sinusitis. *Ann. Otol. Rhinol. Laryngol.* **1998**, *107*, 942–945. [PubMed]

4. Brook, I.; Frazier, E.H.; Gher, M.E., Jr. Microbiology of periapical abscesses and associated maxillary sinusitis. *J. Periodontol.* **1996**, *67*, 608–610. [CrossRef] [PubMed]

5. Stephenson, M.F.; Mfuna, L.; Dowd, S.E.; Wolcott, R.D.; Barbeau, J.; Poisson, M.; James, G.; Desrosiers, M. Molecular characterization of the polymicrobial flora in chronic rhinosinusitis. *J. Otolaryngol. Head Neck Surg.* **2010**, *39*, 182–187. [PubMed]

6. Ramakrishnan, V.R.; Feazel, L.M.; Gitomer, S.A.; Ir, D.; Robertson, C.E.; Frank, D.N. The microbiome of the middle meatus in healthy adults. *PLoS ONE* **2013**, *8*, e85507. [CrossRef] [PubMed]

7. Abreu, N.A.; Nagalingam, N.A.; Song, Y.; Roediger, F.C.; Pletcher, S.D.; Goldberg, A.N.; Lynch, S.V. Sinus microbiome diversity depletion and *Corynebacterium tuberculostearicum* enrichment mediates rhinosinusitis. *Sci. Transl. Med.* **2012**, *4*, 151ra124. [CrossRef] [PubMed]

8. Yan, M.; Pamp, S.J.; Fukuyama, J.; Hwang, P.H.; Cho, D.Y.; Holmes, S.; Relman, D.A. Nasal microenvironments and interspecific interactions influence nasal microbiota complexity and *S. aureus* carriage. *Cell Host Microbe* **2013**, *14*, 631–640. [CrossRef] [PubMed]

9. Boase, S.; Foreman, A.; Cleland, E.; Tan, L.; Melton-Kreft, R.; Pant, H.; Hu, F.Z.; Ehrlich, G.D.; Wormald, P.J. The microbiome of chronic rhinosinusitis: Culture, molecular diagnostics and biofilm detection. *BMC Infect. Dis.* **2013**, *13*. [CrossRef] [PubMed]

10. Feazel, L.M.; Robertson, C.E.; Ramakrishnan, V.R.; Frank, D.N. Microbiome complexity and staphylococcus aureus in chronic rhinosinusitis. *Laryngoscope* **2012**, *122*, 467–472. [CrossRef] [PubMed]

11. Dunbar, J.; White, S.; Forney, L. Genetic diversity through the looking glass: Effect of enrichment bias. *Appl. Environ. Microbiol.* **1997**, *63*, 1326–1331. [PubMed]

12. Sun, Y.; Wolcott, R.D.; Dowd, S.E. Tag-encoded flx amplicon pyrosequencing for the elucidation of microbial and functional gene diversity in any environment. *Methods Mol. Biol.* **2011**, *733*, 129–141. [PubMed]

13. Wilson, M.T.; Hamilos, D.L. The nasal and sinus microbiome in health and disease. *Curr. Allergy Asthma Rep.* **2014**, *14*. [CrossRef] [PubMed]

14. Dowd, S.E.; Sun, Y.; Secor, P.R.; Rhoads, D.D.; Wolcott, B.M.; James, G.A.; Wolcott, R.D. Survey of bacterial diversity in chronic wounds using pyrosequencing, dgge, and full ribosome shotgun sequencing. *BMC Microbiol.* **2008**, *8*. [CrossRef] [PubMed]

15. Stressmann, F.A.; Rogers, G.B.; Chan, S.W.; Howarth, P.H.; Harries, P.G.; Bruce, K.D.; Salib, R.J. Characterization of bacterial community diversity in chronic rhinosinusitis infections using novel culture-independent techniques. *Am. J. Rhinol. Allergy* **2011**, *25*, e133–e140. [CrossRef] [PubMed]

16. Aurora, R.; Chatterjee, D.; Hentzleman, J.; Prasad, G.; Sindwani, R.; Sanford, T. Contrasting the microbiomes from healthy volunteers and patients with chronic rhinosinusitis. *JAMA Otolaryngol. Head Neck Surg.* **2013**, *139*, 1328–1338. [CrossRef] [PubMed]

17. Ramakrishnan, V.R.; Hauser, L.J.; Feazel, L.M.; Ir, D.; Robertson, C.E.; Frank, D.N. Sinus microbiota varies among chronic rhinosinusitis phenotypes and predicts surgical outcome. *J. Allergy Clin. Immunol.* **2015**, *136*, 334–342. [CrossRef] [PubMed]

18. Choi, E.B.; Hong, S.W.; Kim, D.K.; Jeon, S.G.; Kim, K.R.; Cho, S.H.; Gho, Y.S.; Jee, Y.K.; Kim, Y.K. Decreased diversity of nasal microbiota and their secreted extracellular vesicles in patients with chronic rhinosinusitis based on a metagenomic analysis. *Allergy* **2014**, *69*, 517–526. [CrossRef] [PubMed]

19. Gosepath, J.; Brieger, J.; Vlachtsis, K.; Mann, W.J. Fungal DNA is present in tissue specimens of patients with chronic rhinosinusitis. *Am. J. Rhinol.* **2004**, *18*, 9–13. [PubMed]

20. Shin, S.H.; Ponikau, J.U.; Sherris, D.A.; Congdon, D.; Frigas, E.; Homburger, H.A.; Swanson, M.C.; Gleich, G.J.; Kita, H. Chronic rhinosinusitis: An enhanced immune response to ubiquitous airborne fungi. *J. Allergy Clin. Immunol.* **2004**, *114*, 1369–1375. [CrossRef] [PubMed]

21. Inoue, Y.; Matsuwaki, Y.; Shin, S.H.; Ponikau, J.U.; Kita, H. Nonpathogenic, environmental fungi induce activation and degranulation of human eosinophils. *J. Immunol.* **2005**, *175*, 5439–5447. [CrossRef] [PubMed]

22. Ebbens, F.A.; Georgalas, C.; Fokkens, W.J. Fungus as the cause of chronic rhinosinusitis: The case remains unproven. *Curr. Opin. Otolaryngol. Head Neck Surg.* **2009**, *17*, 43–49. [CrossRef] [PubMed]

23. Ponikau, J.U.; Sherris, D.A.; Kern, E.B.; Homburger, H.A.; Frigas, E.; Gaffey, T.A.; Roberts, G.D. The diagnosis and incidence of allergic fungal sinusitis. *Mayo Clin. Proc.* **1999**, *74*, 877–884. [CrossRef] [PubMed]

24. Braun, H.; Buzina, W.; Freudenschuss, K.; Beham, A.; Stammberger, H. 'Eosinophilic fungal rhinosinusitis': A common disorder in Europe? *Laryngoscope* **2003**, *113*, 264–269. [CrossRef] [PubMed]

25. Tosun, F.; Hidir, Y.; Saracli, M.A.; Caliskaner, Z.; Sengul, A. Intranasal fungi and chronic rhinosinusitis: What is the relationship? *Ann. Otol. Rhinol. Laryngol.* **2007**, *116*, 425–429. [CrossRef] [PubMed]

26. Cleland, E.J.; Bassiouni, A.; Boase, S.; Dowd, S.; Vreugde, S.; Wormald, P.J. The fungal microbiome in chronic rhinosinusitis: Richness, diversity, postoperative changes and patient outcomes. *Int. Forum Allergy Rhinol.* **2014**, *4*, 259–265. [CrossRef] [PubMed]

27. Ashbee, H.R. Update on the genus *Malassezia*. *Med. Mycol.* **2007**, *45*, 287–303. [CrossRef] [PubMed]

28. Wagner Mackenzie, B.; Waite, D.W.; Hoggard, M.; Douglas, R.G.; Taylor, M.W.; Biswas, K. Bacterial community collapse: A meta-analysis of the sinonasal microbiota in chronic rhinosinusitis. *Environ. Microbiol.* **2017**, *19*, 381–392. [CrossRef] [PubMed]

29. Brook, I. Bacteriologic features of chronic sinusitis in children. *JAMA* **1981**, *246*, 967–969. [CrossRef] [PubMed]

30. Brook, I.; Yocum, P.; Shah, K. Aerobic and anaerobic bacteriology of concurrent chronic otitis media with effusion and chronic sinusitis in children. *Arch. Otolaryngol. Head Neck Surg.* **2000**, *126*, 174–176. [CrossRef] [PubMed]

31. Erkan, M.; Ozcan, M.; Arslan, S.; Soysal, V.; Bozdemir, K.; Haghighi, N. Bacteriology of antrum in children with chronic maxillary sinusitis. *Scand. J. Infect. Dis.* **1996**, *28*, 283–285. [CrossRef] [PubMed]

32. Hsin, C.H.; Su, M.C.; Tsao, C.H.; Chuang, C.Y.; Liu, C.M. Bacteriology and antimicrobial susceptibility of pediatric chronic rhinosinusitis: A 6-year result of maxillary sinus punctures. *Am. J. Otolaryngol.* **2010**, *31*, 145–149. [CrossRef] [PubMed]

33. Brook, I. Microbiology of sinusitis. *Proc. Am. Thorac. Soc.* **2011**, *8*, 90–100. [CrossRef] [PubMed]

34. Brook, I.; Yocum, P. Antimicrobial management of chronic sinusitis in children. *J. Laryngol. Otol.* **1995**, *109*, 1159–1162. [CrossRef] [PubMed]

35. Slack, C.L.; Dahn, K.A.; Abzug, M.J.; Chan, K.H. Antibiotic-resistant bacteria in pediatric chronic sinusitis. *Pediatr. Infect. Dis. J.* **2001**, *20*, 247–250. [CrossRef] [PubMed]

36. Don, D.M.; Yellon, R.F.; Casselbrant, M.L.; Bluestone, C.D. Efficacy of a stepwise protocol that includes intravenous antibiotic therapy for the management of chronic sinusitis in children and adolescents. *Arch. Otolaryngol. Head Neck Surg.* **2001**, *127*, 1093–1098. [CrossRef] [PubMed]

37. Goldenhersh, M.J.; Rachelefsky, G.S.; Dudley, J.; Brill, J.; Katz, R.M.; Rohr, A.S.; Spector, S.L.; Siegel, S.C.; Summanen, P.; Baron, E.J.; et al. The microbiology of chronic sinus disease in children with respiratory allergy. *J. Allergy Clin. Immunol.* **1990**, *85*, 1030–1039. [CrossRef]

38. Muntz, H.R.; Lusk, R.P. Bacteriology of the ethmoid bullae in children with chronic sinusitis. *Arch. Otolaryngol. Head Neck Surg.* **1991**, *117*, 179–181. [CrossRef] [PubMed]

39. Orobello, P.W., Jr.; Park, R.I.; Belcher, L.J.; Eggleston, P.; Lederman, H.M.; Banks, J.R.; Modlin, J.F.; Naclerio, R.M. Microbiology of chronic sinusitis in children. *Arch. Otolaryngol. Head Neck Surg.* **1991**, *117*, 980–983. [CrossRef] [PubMed]

40. Otten, F.W. Conservative treatment of chronic maxillary sinusitis in children. Long-term follow-up. *Acta Oto-Rhino-Laryngol. Belg.* **1997**, *51*, 173–175.

41. Otten, F.W.; Grote, J.J. Treatment of chronic maxillary sinusitis in children. *Int. J. Pediatr. Otorhinolaryngol.* **1988**, *15*, 269–278. [CrossRef]

42. Tinkelman, D.G.; Silk, H.J. Clinical and bacteriologic features of chronic sinusitis in children. *Am. J. Dis. Child.* **1989**, *143*, 938–941. [CrossRef] [PubMed]

43. Feazel, L.M.; Frank, D.N.; Ramakrishnan, V.R. Update on bacterial detection methods in chronic rhinosinusitis: Implications for clinicians and research scientists. *Int. Forum Allergy Rhinol.* **2011**, *1*, 451–459. [CrossRef] [PubMed]

13

Prevalence and Determinants of Sinus Problems in Farm and Non-Farm Populations of Rural Saskatchewan, Canada

Ayami Kajiwara-Morita [1,2], Chandima P. Karunanayake [3], James A. Dosman [3,4], Joshua A. Lawson [3,4], Shelley Kirychuk [3,4], Donna C. Rennie [3,5], Roland F. Dyck [3,4], Niels Koehncke [3,4], Ambikaipakan Senthilselvan [6], Punam Pahwa [3,7,*] and Saskatchewan Rural Health Study Research Team [3]

[1]   Division of Pharmacology and Therapeutics, Graduate School of Pharmaceutical Sciences, Kumamoto University, 5-1 Oe-honmachi, Chuo-ku, Kumamoto 862-0973, Japan; ayami.morita77@gmail.com
[2]   Jinnouchi Clinic, Diabetes Care Center, 6-2-3 Kuhonji, Chuo-ku, Kumamoto 862-0976, Japan
[3]   Canadian Centre for Health and Safety in Agriculture, University of Saskatchewan, 104 Clinic Place, Saskatoon, SK S7N 2Z4, Canada; cpk646@mail.usask.ca (C.P.K.); james.dosman@usask.ca (J.A.D.); josh.lawson@usask.ca (J.A.L.); shelley.kirychuk@usask.ca (S.K.); donna.rennie@usask.ca (D.C.R.); roland.dyck@usask.ca (R.F.D.); niels.koehncke@usask.ca (N.K.); saskatchewan.rural@usask.ca (S.R.H.S.R.T.)
[4]   Department of Medicine, University of Saskatchewan, Royal University Hospital, 103 Hospital Drive, Saskatoon, SK S7N 0W8, Canada
[5]   College of Nursing, University of Saskatchewan, 104 Clinic Place, Saskatoon, SK S7N 2Z4, Canada
[6]   School of Public Health, 3-276 Edmonton Clinic Health Academy, University of Alberta, 11405-87 Ave, Edmonton, AB T6G 1C9, Canada; sentil@ualberta.ca
[7]   Department of Community Health and Epidemiology, University of Saskatchewan, Health Science Building, 104, Clinic Place, Saskatoon, SK S7N 5E5, Canada
*   Correspondence: pup165@mail.usask.ca

Abstract: Although sinus problems have long been recognized as the most common respiratory symptoms associated with agricultural work, there is a scarcity of recent studies and/or reliable estimates as to the true prevalence or risk factors of sinus problems related to farming. The aim of this study was to determine the prevalence of sinus problems in farming and non-farming rural populations and further investigate the association of individual (for example life-style, occupational), contextual (e.g., environmental), and important covariates (e.g., age, sex) with sinus problems. A large-scale cross-sectional study was conducted in farm and non-farm residents of rural Saskatchewan, Canada. A logistic regression model based on a generalized estimating equations approach were fitted to investigate the risk factors of sinus problems. Sinus problems were reported by 2755 (34.0%) of the 8101 subjects. Farm residents were more likely to spend their first year of life on farm compared with non-farm residents, and indicated a significantly lower risk of sinus problems. Meanwhile, occupational exposure to solvent and mold were associated with an increased risk of sinus problems. Some health conditions such as allergy and stomach acidity/reflux, family history, and female sex were also related to a higher risk of sinus problems. Farm residents had a significantly lower risk of sinus problems than non-farm residents, likely due to the exposure to farm specific environments in their early life.

Keywords: rhinitis; occupational exposure; environmental exposure; farm; rural health; allergy; respiratory; birth weight; gastroesophageal reflux; sinusitis

1. Introduction

Sinus problems including rhinitis and sinusitis are among the most common medical conditions, which can significantly decrease quality of life, aggravate comorbid conditions such as asthma, and require significant direct medical expenditures [1–5]. They also create even greater indirect costs to society by causing lost work and schooldays and reduced workplace productivity and school learning [2,3]. Based on the National Population Health Survey data from 1998 to 1999, the prevalence of self-reported doctor diagnosed chronic rhinosinusitis was 5.2% with 95% confidence interval (4.8–5.7%) [6].

Sinus problems have long been recognized as common respiratory symptoms associated with agricultural work, however, there is a scarcity of recent studies and/or reliable estimates as to the true prevalence or risk factors of sinus problems related to farming [3,7,8]. It has been reported that breeding and handling of livestock, dairy production, swine barn exposures, and grain farming increased nasal inflammation and symptoms [3,7]. Exposure to pesticides has also been associated with many respiratory symptoms including sinus problems [3,9]. On the other hand, several studies have identified some of the exposures associated with a farming lifestyle that contributed to the reduced risk of rhinitis, asthma, and allergic diseases in farm children (i.e., contact with livestock; contact with animal feed such as hay, grain, straw, and silage; and the consumption of unprocessed cow's milk) [1,4,5,10–15]. The reduced risk in farm children has been attributed to higher endotoxin levels and more diverse exposures to microbial components in the farm environment [1,4,10–12,15]. This so-called "hygiene hypothesis" has a theoretical basis that the type and level of stimulation from the microbial environment may influence the postnatal differentiation of T-helper lymphocytes [1,4,5,10,11,13,14], and it supports the lifelong protective effect of farm exposures in early childhood against the development of allergies [11,15]. Some studies, however, failed to identify this protective effect [16] and the others reported that some farming and poor hygiene exposures were associated with an increase in the prevalence of rhinitis in schoolchildren [16,17]. There is no evidence which can fully explain this heterogeneity of the effects, although some possible backgrounds were suggested such as type or quantity of exposure, allergic/non-allergic, and early-onset/late-onset outcome [7,15–18]. There are many potential causative factors of sinus problems, and they sometimes modify the effects of each other. This may contribute to difficulty in reliably identifying risk factors of sinus problems in clinical settings.

The aim of this study was to determine the prevalence of sinus problems in farming and non-farming rural populations and further investigate the association of individual (for example life-style, occupational), contextual (e.g., environmental), and important covariates (e.g., age, sex) with sinus problems. The interactive effects between risk factors on sinus problems were investigated simultaneously to explain accurately the associations among these risk factors and sinus problems.

2. Materials and Methods

2.1. Baseline Survey

The Saskatchewan Rural Health Study (SRHS) design is a prospective cohort study being conducted in two phases: baseline and follow-up. Details of the baseline study are given elsewhere [19]. In brief, 39 rural municipalities (RMs) of the 298 RMs in Saskatchewan and 16 of the 145 towns (population ranging from 500 to 5000) in Saskatchewan were selected to participate in the study. These RMs and towns were selected at random from four quadrants of the province (southeast, southwest, northeast, and northwest). Councils of 32 out of 39 RMs (82.1%) and 15 out of 16 towns (93.8%) agreed to participate on behalf of their residents and supplied mailing addresses. Dillman's method was utilized to recruit study participants [20]. The study population comprised 8261 individuals (males and females, 18 years of age or older) from 4624 households living in 32 rural municipalities and 15 towns in the study area.

2.2. *Variables*

Information on the variables described below was collected by self-administered, mailed questionnaires based on the Population Health Framework [21,22]. Some measures of lifestyle factors, occupational exposures, and socio-economic status used in our questionnaire were adopted from previous research studies that had validated these measures [22–24]. The SRHS was conducted with the understanding and the voluntary consent of the participants upon return of the questionnaire. The study was approved by the Biomedical Research Ethics Board (Bio# 09-56) of the University of Saskatchewan, Canada.

2.2.1. Primary Outcome

The primary outcome of interest was sinus problems based on a "yes or no" answer to the question "Has a doctor ever said you had sinus trouble ever in your life: yes or no?".

In our survey, when we asked the question about sinus trouble, we captured the information either on sinusitis (including acute/chronic sinusitis) or rhinitis (including allergic or non-allergic rhinitis) or a combination of both. Sinusitis is an inflammation or swelling of the tissue lining the sinuses, while rhinitis is an inflammation of the nasal mucous membranes. Rhinosinusitis refers to inflammation of the nasal cavities and sinuses [25]. The symptoms of rhinitis and sinusitis overlap, and sinusitis rarely occurs in the absence of rhinitis [2].

2.2.2. Contextual Factors

The contextual factors associated with sinus problems of interest in this study were environmental factors including residence location, indoor/outdoor environment, and socioeconomic status. Designation of residence in a rural dwelling was further classified as living on farm or non-farm based on the question "Where is your home located?" with options: "farm, in town, acreage". A non-farm category was created by combining town and acreage. This categorization was necessary because farming exposures can be unique compared to non-farming exposures among rural residents. Indoor environment was assessed by response to questions about smoking inside the house, filtered heating systems, dampness, indoor mold, any pets in home, and pesticides applied inside the residence. The outdoor environment was assessed using information about indoor (barn) intensive livestock operation (building), feedlot or corrals, balestack or bales, grain bins, and sewage pond or manure lagoon located near the home. Main drinking water source was also investigated. Socioeconomic status was assessed using household income adequacy, which was a derived variable with four categories based on various combinations of total household income and the number of people living in the household according to the Statistics Canada definition [26].

2.2.3. Individual Factors

The individual factors considered to be associated with sinus problems were: (i) lifestyle or behavior-related factors with an expected impact on health including smoking and alcohol consumption; (ii) early life exposures; (iii) occupational history and its exposures; (iv) co-morbid conditions; and (v) family history of lung disease. Early life exposures were assessed by the response to the questions regarding ever having lived on a farm, lived on a farm during first year of life, mother smoking in pregnancy, breastfed as a child and its term (for ≥ 6 month or not), and birth weight (<2500 g, 2500–3999 g or ≥ 4000 g) according to the national reports [27,28]. Information about occupational history was collected (job title; business, industry or service; total number of years at job). Based on the most frequent responses (i.e., farmers, farm managers, farm supervisors, specialized livestock workers and general farm workers) to occupational history questions, a variable farm worker was derived. An association of farm worker was investigated as a possible risk factor of sinus problems. Information on the following occupational exposures was collected: grain dust, mine dust, asbestos dust, wood dust, other dust (specify), livestock, smoke from stubble burning, diesel fumes, welding fumes, solvent fumes, oil/gas-well fumes, herbicides (to kill plants), fungicides (to treat grain), insecticides (to kill insects), molds, radiation, other (specify). As the co-morbid conditions, allergic conditions, ear infection in the past year, stomach acidity or reflux in past year, usual cough, usual phlegm, ever wheeze, ever asthma, ever hay fever, and chronic diseases (diabetes, heart disease, heart attack, arteriosclerosis, hypertension, cystic fibrosis, tuberculosis, stroke, cancer, other (specify)) were included in the analyses. In the present study, the number of chronic diseases (categorized as: ≥ 2 diseases, 1 disease, or 0 (no disease)) and not each individual disease, seemed appropriate for the analyses because of a very low prevalence of some chronic conditions such as cystic fibrosis (0.1%) or tuberculosis (0.4%). Information about a family history of lung disease was based on biological family member (father, mother, brother/sister) ever having had lung trouble (asthma, emphysema and chronic bronchitis).

2.2.4. Covariates

Information was obtained on covariates of importance such as age, sex, body mass index, and educational attainment. Body mass index (BMI) was derived from self-reported weight and height of the respondent and used to determine normal ($<25 \text{ kg/m}^2$), overweight ($\geq 25 \text{ kg/m}^2$, $<30 \text{ kg/m}^2$), or obese ($\geq 30 \text{ kg/m}^2$).

2.3. Statistical Analysis

Statistical analysis was completed using SPSS version 24.0 statistical software (IBM SPSS 24.0 Statistics for Windows, IBM Corp., Armonk, NY, USA). Prevalence was presented as observed/total and percentage. Chi-square tests were used to determine the association of prevalence of sinus problems and location of residence. A logistic regression model using generalized estimating equations to account for the within-subject (household—considered as level 2) dependencies that occur in the analysis due to multiple individuals (considered as level 1) from the same household was used in the analysis. Based on bi-variable analysis, variables with $p < 0.20$ became candidates for a multivariable model. All variables that were statistically significant ($p < 0.05$), important contextual factors (i.e., location of home and region), sex, and age were retained in the final multivariable model. A parsimonious model was selected based on the Quasilikelihood function under the Independence model criteria goodness-of-fit statistic [29,30]. The strength of associations is presented by odds ratios and their 95% confidence intervals.

3. Results

Of the 8261 participants, 160 were excluded because of missing data for sinus problems and/or location of home, leaving 8101 (98.1%) subjects for the analysis. The mean age of population was 55.8 ± 15.7 years (range 18–101 years). There were approximately equal proportions of males (49.2%) and females (50.8%) in this study. Although there were fewer farm residents (42.1%) than non-farm residents (57.9%), the difference was accounted for in the multivariable analyses. Farm residents were more likely to spend their first year of life on a farm compared with non-farm residents (79.4% vs. 59.6%, $p < 0.001$). Sinus problems were reported by 2755 (34.0%) of the 8101 subjects (Table 1). The prevalence of sinus problems among farm residents was lower than that among non-farm residents (32.3% vs. 35.2%, $p = 0.006$), especially southwest (33.3% vs. 39.7%, $p = 0.015$) and northwest of Saskatchewan (30.5% vs. 35.3%, $p = 0.013$).

Table 1. Prevalence of sinus problems stratified by geographic location and farm/non-farm residence.

Quadrant of Saskatchewan	Farm Residents		Non-Farm Residents		Total	
	Sinus Problems		Sinus Problems		Sinus Problems	
	Yes/Total	(%)	Yes/Total	(%)	Yes/Total	(%)
Southwest	182/546	33.3	383/965	39.7 **	565/1511	37.4
Southeast	239/699	34.2	376/1057	35.6	615/1756	35.0
Northeast	379/1176	32.2	366/1174	31.2	745/2350	31.7
Northwest	301/987	30.5	527/1493	35.3 **	828/2480	33.4
Not Identified	0/0	-	2/4	50.0	2/4	50.0
Total	1101/3408	32.3	1654/4693	35.2 *	2755/8101	34.0

There was a significant difference (* $p < 0.01$, ** $p < 0.05$) in prevalence of sinus problems between farm and non-farm residents using the chi-squared test statistic.

The bi-variable relationships between the contextual factors, individual factors, or covariates and sinus problems are shown in Tables 2–4. Univariate logistic regression analyses, adjusted for repeated households, showed that the diagnosis of sinus problems was associated with the following contextual factors, individual factors, and covariates: household income adequacy; region of Saskatchewan (quadrant); location of home (farm/non-farm); dampness in past year; mold inside (mildew odor or musty smell); any pets in the past year; application of insecticides inside the house in the past year; sewage pond or manure lagoon located near home; water source; smoking; alcohol consumption; early life exposures (ever lived on a farm, lived on a farm during first year of life, mother smoking in pregnancy, birth weight, breastfed as a child, breastfed for 6 months or longer); occupational history in farm; adult farming exposure years; occupational exposures (grain dust, asbestos dust, welding fumes, solvents, insecticides, mold, or radiation); health conditions (house dust allergy, cat allergy, dog allergy, grass allergy, pollen allergy, mold allergy, ear infection in past year, stomach acidity, or reflux in past year, usual cough, usual phlegm, ever wheeze, ever asthma, ever hay fever, number of chronic diseases); family histories (father lung disease, mother lung disease, brother/sister lung disease); sex, age, body mass index (BMI) and education.

Table 2. Bivariable analysis of an association between contextual factors and sinus problems.

	Sinus Problems		Unadjusted OR * (95% CI)
	Yes/Total	(%)	
Contextual Factors			
Socioeconomic			
Household Income Adequacy			
Lowest income	98/211	31.7	0.87 (0.67, 1.14)
Lower middle income	370/1183	31.3	**0.85 (0.74, 0.99)**
Upper middle income	815/2273	35.9	1.05 (0.93, 1.18)
Highest income	1081/3106	34.8	1
Unknown	391/1230	31.8	0.87 (0.75, 1.01)
Environmental			
Quadrant (Region)			
Southwest	565/1511	37.4	**1.19 (1.04, 1.37)**
Southeast	615/1756	35.0	1.07 (0.94, 1.23)
Northeast	745/2350	31.7	0.93 (0.81, 1.05)
Northwest	828/2480	33.4	1

Table 2. *Cont.*

	Sinus Problems		Unadjusted OR * (95% CI)
	Yes/Total	(%)	
Contextual Factors			
Location of Home			
Farm	1101/2307	32.3	**0.87 (0.79, 0.97)**
Non-farm	1654/4693	35.2	1
Household Smoking			
Yes	392/1222	32.1	0.90 (0.78, 1.03)
No	2355/6843	34.4	1
Filter of Heating system			
Yes	2385/6916	34.5	1.13 (0.97, 1.32)
No	283/890	31.8	1
Dampness in Past Year			
Yes	603/1551	38.9	**1.29 (1.14, 1.46)**
No	2135/6495	32.9	1
Mildew Odor or Musty Smell			
Yes	519/1350	38.4	**1.27 (1.11, 1.44)**
No	2158/6527	33.1	1
Any Pets in Home in Past Year			
Yes	1350/3688	36.6	**1.24 (1.13, 1.37)**
No	1405/4413	31.8	1
Pesticides Applied Inside Residence in Past Year			
Yes	653/1694	38.5	**1.28 (1.14, 1.43)**
No	2073/6315	32.8	1
Livestock Operation Located near Home			
Yes	442/1325	33.4	0.98 (0.86, 1.11)
No	2261/6649	34.0	1
Feedlot or Corrals Located near Home			
Yes	917/2690	34.1	1.01 (0.91, 1.12)
No	1793/5298	33.8	1
Balestack or Bales Located near Home			
Yes	1034/3017	34.3	1.03 (0.93, 1.14)
No	1678/4974	33.7	1
Grain Bins Located near Home			
Yes	1389/4082	34.0	1.00 (0.91, 1.11)
No	1328/3910	34.0	1
Sewage Pond or Manure Lagoon Located near Home			
Yes	1134/3016	36.5	**1.22 (1.11, 1.35)**
No	1527/4777	32.0	1
Water Source			
Lake	4/15	26.7	0.94 (0.73, 1.21)
Dugout or reservoir	125/419	29.8	**0.78 (0.61, 0.98)**
Spring, river, or creak	117/306	38.2	1.11 (0.85, 1.46)
Shallow well water (less than 100ft)	507/1577	32.1	**0.86 (0.75, 0.99)**
Deep well water (more than 100ft)	654/1897	34.5	0.55 (0.84, 1.10)
Bottled water	872/2456	35.5	1
Another source	101/297	34.0	0.94 (0.73, 1.21)
Unknown	329/1006	32.7	0.89 (0.75, 1.04)

OR, odds ratio; CI, confidence interval. * Odds ratios that are significantly different from zero ($p < 0.05$) are shown in bold.

Table 3. Bivariable analysis of the association between individual factors and sinus problems.

	Sinus Problems		Unadjusted OR * (95% CI)
	Yes/Total	(%)	
Individual Factors			
Lifestyle Factors			
Smoking			
Current smoker	305/951	32.1	0.96 (0.82, 1.11)
Ex-smoker	1049/2868	36.6	**1.18 (1.07, 1.30)**
Never smoker	1394/4252	32.8	1
Alcohol Consumption			
More than 3 times a week	260/850	30.6	**0.83 (0.69, 0.99)**
1–3 times a week	637/1923	33.1	0.93 (0.80, 1.08)
Less than once a week	1355/3871	35.0	1.02 (0.89, 1.16)
Never	495/1435	34.5	1
Early Life Exposure			
Ever Lived on a Farm			
Yes	2245/6690	33.6	**0.88 (0.78, 1.00)**
No	508/1399	36.3	1
Lived on a Farm during First Year of Life			
Yes	1791/5452	32.9	**0.85 (0.77, 0.93)**
No	939/2574	36.5	1
Mother Smoking in Pregnancy			
Yes	472/1200	39.3	**1.31 (1.16, 1.50)**
No	1954/5972	32.7	1
Unknown	323/907	35.6	1.11 (0.96, 1.29)
Birth Weight			
<2500 g	197/433	45.5	**1.39 (1.13, 1.70)**
≥2500, <4000 g	1163/3113	37.4	1
≥4000 g	179/527	34.0	0.85 (0.70, 1.04)
Unknown	1150/3842	29.9	**0.70 (0.63, 0.78)**
Breastfed as a Child			
Yes	1257/3702	34.0	0.90 (0.80, 1.00)
No	804/2228	36.1	1
Unknown	648/2038	31.8	**0.80 (0.70, 0.91)**
Breastfed for 6 Months or Longer			
Yes	485/1440	33.7	0.88 (0.77, 1.01)
No	1101/3042	36.2	1
Unknown	1123/3486	32.2	**0.82 (0.74, 0.91)**
Occupational History			
Any Occupational History in Farm			
Yes	1113/3506	31.7	**0.81 (0.74, 0.89)**
No	1616/4498	35.9	1
Adult Farming Exposure Years			
0	1651/4506	35.8	1
>0, <30	444/1355	32.8	**0.86 (0.76, 0.98)**
≥30, <50	500/1534	32.6	**0.85 (0.75, 0.96)**
≥50	134/505	26.5	**0.63 (0.51, 0.77)**

Table 3. *Cont.*

	Sinus Problems		Unadjusted OR * (95% CI)
	Yes/Total	(%)	
Individual Factors			
Occupational Exposures			
Grain Dust			
Yes	1805/5431	33.2	**0.86 (0.78, 0.96)**
No	916/2535	36.1	1
Mine Dust			
Yes	151/438	34.5	0.98 (0.80, 1.20)
No	2570/7528	34.1	1
Asbestos Dust			
Yes	218/538	40.5	**1.29 (1.08, 1.54)**
No	2503/7428	33.7	1
Wood Dust			
Yes	1079/3073	35.1	1.04 (0.94, 1.14)
No	1642/4893	33.6	1
Livestock			
Yes	1393/4096	34.0	0.97 (0.88, 1.06)
No	1328/3870	34.3	1
Stubble Smoke			
Yes	1137/3204	35.5	1.09 (0.99, 1.20)
No	1584/4762	33.3	1
Diesel Fumes			
Yes	1598/4682	34.1	0.96 (0.87, 1.05)
No	1123/3284	34.2	1
Welding Fumes			
Yes	1048/3272	32.0	**0.82 (0.75, 0.90)**
No	1673/4694	35.6	1
Solvents			
Yes	1079/2828	38.2	**1.27 (1.15, 1.40)**
No	1642/5138	32.0	1
Oil or Gas Fumes			
Yes	636/1912	33.3	0.92 (0.83, 1.03)
No	2085/6054	34.4	1
Herbicides			
Yes	1408/4038	34.9	1.04 (0.95, 1.14)
No	1313/3928	33.4	1
Fungicides			
Yes	893/2615	34.1	0.97 (0.88, 1.07)
No	1828/5351	34.2	1
Insecticides			
Yes	1294/3593	36.0	**1.14 (1.04, 1.25)**
No	1427/4373	32.6	1
Mold			
Yes	1155/2761	41.8	**1.64 (1.49, 1.81)**
No	1566/5205	30.1	1
Radiation			
Yes	290/678	42.8	**1.48 (1.26, 1.74)**
No	2431/7288	33.4	1

Table 3. *Cont.*

	Sinus Problems		Unadjusted OR * (95% CI)
	Yes/Total	(%)	
Individual Factors			
Health Conditions			
House Dust Allergy			
Yes	645/1016	63.5	**4.09 (3.56, 4.69)**
No	2032/6848	29.7	1
Cat Allergy			
Yes	519/906	57.3	**2.99 (2.59, 3.45)**
No	2158/6958	31.0	1
Dog Allergy			
Yes	289/468	61.8	**3.39 (2.80, 4.12)**
No	2388/7396	32.3	1
Grass Allergy			
Yes	730/1243	58.7	**3.37 (2.97, 3.82)**
No	1947/6621	29.4	1
Pollen Allergy			
Yes	986/1663	59.3	**3.85 (3.43, 4.31)**
No	1691/6201	27.3	1
Mold Allergy			
Yes	856/1380	62.0	**4.16 (3.68, 4.69)**
No	1821/6484	28.1	1
Ear Infection in Past Year			
Yes	248/423	58.6	**2.85 (2.34, 3.46)**
No	2466/7520	32.8	1
Stomach Acidity or Reflux in Past Year			
Yes	566/1139	49.7	**2.08 (1.83, 2.36)**
No	2143/6788	31.6	1
Usual Cough			
Yes	540/1207	44.7	**1.66 (1.47, 1.88)**
No	2189/6822	32.1	1
Usual Phlegm			
Yes	529/1222	43.3	**1.55 (1.37, 1.75)**
No	2172/6721	32.3	1
Ever Wheeze			
Yes	1494/3304	45.2	**2.29 (2.08, 2.51)**
No	1261/4797	26.3	1
Ever Asthma			
Yes	459/787	58.3	**2.99 (2.57, 3.47)**
No	2296/7314	31.4	1
Ever Hay Fever			
Yes	659/967	68.1	**5.10 (4.39, 5.91)**
No	2095/7133	29.4	1
Number of Chronic Diseases			
0	1486/4575	32.5	1
1	806/2247	35.9	**1.15 (1.04, 1.28)**
≥2	463/1279	36.2	**1.17 (1.03, 1.33)**

Table 3. *Cont.*

	Sinus Problems		Unadjusted OR * (95% CI)
	Yes/Total	(%)	
Individual Factors			
Family History			
Father Lung Disease			
Yes	541/1236	43.8	**1.65 (1.46, 1.86)**
No	1884/5989	31.5	1
Unknown	328/870	37.7	**1.31 (1.13, 1.52)**
Mother Lung Disease			
Yes	404/872	46.3	**1.74 (1.51, 2.01)**
No	2145/6623	32.4	1
Unknown	206/605	34.0	1.07 (0.89, 1.27)
Brother/Sister Lung Disease			
Yes	411/858	47.9	**1.90 (1.65, 2.20)**
No	2057/6414	32.1	1
Unknown	286/825	34.7	1.10 (0.94, 1.28)

* Odds ratios that are significantly different from zero ($p < 0.05$) are shown in bold.

Table 4. Bivariable analysis of the association between individual factors and sinus problems.

	Sinus Problems		Unadjusted OR * (95% CI)
	Yes/Total	(%)	
Covariates			
Sex			
Male	1115/3984	28.0	1
Female	1640/4113	39.9	**1.69 (1.55, 1.85)**
Age (Years)			
18–45	665/1264	34.5	1
46–55	710/2025	35.1	1.03 (0.90, 1.17)
56–65	712/1915	37.2	1.11 (0.97, 1.27)
>65	668/2227	30.0	**0.80 (0.70, 0.92)**
Body Mass Index (kg/m^2)			
Normal (<25)	743/2301	32.3	1
Overweight ($\geq$25, <30)	1010/3143	32.1	0.98 (0.88, 1.10)
Obese ($\geq$30)	854/2258	37.8	**1.25 (1.11, 1.42)**
Education			
$\leq$Grade 12	1482/4825	30.7	**0.69 (0.63, 0.76)**
>Grade 12	1237/3186	38.8	1

* Odds ratios that are significantly different from zero ($p < 0.05$) are shown in bold.

The multivariable logistic regression analysis adjusted for covariates and households is presented in Table 5. The contextual factor farm location was significantly associated with decreased risk of sinus problems, while sewage pond located near home was associated with increased risk of sinus problems. Past smoker, low birth weight, occupational exposures to solvents or molds, some health conditions (house dust allergy, pollen allergy, mold allergy, ear infection in past year, stomach acidity or reflux in past year, ever wheeze, and ever hay fever), family histories (father lung disease, mother lung disease, brother/sister lung disease), female sex, and higher educational status were also identified as the significant determinants positively associated with sinus problems.

Table 5. Multivariable analysis of the dependency of sinus problems on contextual factors, individual factors, and covariates.

	Adjusted OR * (95% CI)
Contextual Factors	
Environmental	
Quadrant (Region)	
Southwest	1.10 (0.93, 1.31)
Southeast	0.96 (0.81, 1.14)
Northeast	0.95 (0.81, 1.11)
Northwest	1
Location of Home	
Farm	**0.83 (0.73, 0.94)**
Non-farm	1
Sewage Pond or Manure Lagoon Located near Home	
Yes	**1.19 (1.05, 1.34)**
No	1
Individual Factors	
Lifestyle Factors	
Smoking	
Current smoker	0.92 (0.76, 1.10)
Ex-smoker	**1.22 (1.08, 1.38)**
Never smoker	1
Early Life Exposure	
Birth Weight	
<2500 g	**1.66 (1.29, 2.13)**
≥2500, <4000 g	1
≥4000 g	1.08 (0.85, 1.38)
Unknown	0.90 (0.79, 1.03)
Occupational Exposures	
Solvents	
Yes	**1.35 (1.18, 1.53)**
No	1
Mold	
Yes	**1.32 (1.16, 1.50)**
No	1
Radiation	
Yes	0.95 (0.67, 1.35)
No	1
Health Conditions	
House Dust Allergy	
Yes	**1.98 (1.50, 2.61)**
No	1
Pollen Allergy	
Yes	**1.38 (1.16, 1.65)**
No	1
Mold Allergy	
Yes	**1.93 (1.55, 2.39)**
No	1

Table 5. *Cont.*

	Adjusted OR * (95% CI)
Individual Factors	
Ear Infection in Past Year	
Yes	**2.99 (2.28, 3.93)**
No	1
Stomach Acidity or Reflux in Past Year	
Yes	**2.37 (1.85, 3.02)**
No	1
Ever Wheeze	
Yes	**1.69 (1.51, 1.90)**
No	1
Ever Hay Fever	
Yes	**2.85 (2.36, 3.45)**
No	1
Family History	
Father Lung Disease	
Yes	**1.28 (1.10, 1.48)**
No	1
Unknown	**1.35 (1.09, 1.67)**
Mother Lung Disease	
Yes	**1.30 (1.10, 1.54)**
No	1
Unknown	0.99 (0.76, 1.29)
Brother/Sister Lung Disease	
Yes	**1.34 (1.12, 1.61)**
No	1
Unknown	1.08 (0.88, 1.32)
Covariates	
Sex	
Male	1
Female	**1.81 (1.61, 2.03)**
Age (Years)	
18–45	1
46–55	1.08 (0.92, 1.26)
56–65	**1.18 (1.00, 1.39)**
>65	0.99 (0.83, 1.17)
Education	
≤Grade 12	**0.76 (0.68, 0.86)**
>Grade 12	1
Significant Interactions (Please see Figure 1)	*p*-Value
Quadrant and Radiation	**0.010**
Birth Weight and Stomach Acidity or Reflux	**0.003**
House Dust Allergy and Mold Allergy	**0.003**
Stomach Acidity or Reflux and Ear Infection	**0.025**
Ever Hay Fever and Ear Infection	**0.041**

* Odds ratios that are significantly different from zero ($p < 0.05$) are shown in bold.

In this final model, five statistically significant interactions were observed (Table 5 and Figure 1). Radiation was a significant risk for sinus problems in all quadrant of Saskatchewan (Figure 1a). The association between birth weight and sinus problems completely differed depending on whether participants were with or without stomach acidity/reflux (Figure 1b). Among subjects without stomach acidity/reflux, lower birth weight indicated an increased risk compared with normal birth weight. In those with stomach acidity/reflux, however, lower birth weight was associated with decreased risk of sinus problems. Mold allergy was related to greater risk of sinus problems in subjects with and without house dust allergy (Figure 1c). Although the effect seemed to be blunted in the former, subjects who had both of these allergies were at a considerably higher risk. A similar tendency was observed in the interaction between stomach acidity/reflux and ear infection and in that between hay fever and ear infection as shown in Figure 1d,e, respectively.

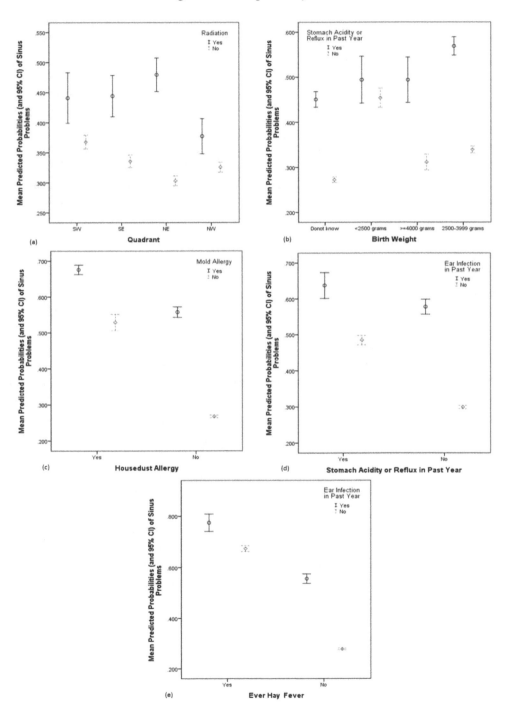

Figure 1. Mean predicted probabilities of sinus problems, illustrating the interactive associations among risk factors.

4. Discussion

In this large-scale cross-sectional study, we found living on a farm to be associated with a lower risk of sinus problems, whereas some other environmental and occupational exposures, health conditions such as allergy and stomach acidity/reflux, family history of lung disease, and female sex were associated with a higher risk of sinus problems. We also revealed some significant interactive effects between these factors on sinus problems, which have a reasonable physiological or pathological basis. We discuss below the factors associated with sinus problems systematically.

4.1. Environmental Factors

The present study indicated an inverse relationship between farm living and the prevalence of sinus problems. On the other hand, living near a sewage pond or manure lagoon was significantly associated with the prevalence of sinus problems even after multivariable adjustment. Dampness, indoor mold, any pets in home, and pesticides applied inside residence were not included in the multivariable model, whereas they were indicated to be risks of sinus problems in bivariable analyses.

Lower risk of allergic rhinitis in farm specific conditions has been reported by many previous studies [1,4,13,15]. It has been postulated that exposure to endotoxin might promote a skewing of the type I helper T cells (Th1)/type 2 helper T cells (Th2) balance toward non-allergic Th1 responses [1,4], thus protecting against allergies. The immune deviation into either Th1 or Th2 polarization is suggested to be established already at 5 years of age [4]. It is also well known that pregnancy and early life represent a biological window of opportunity for shaping subsequent immune reactivity [5,14]. The timing of exposure seems to be crucial and determines the exposure's beneficial or detrimental effects [5,7,10,12,14,16]. In the present study, farm residents were more likely to spend their first year of life on farm compared with non-farm residents. On the basis of this information, a high proportion of farm residents who had been exposed to farm specific conditions in their early life might experience the protective effect of living on a farm, via allergic sensitization and shaping subsequent immune responses.

Another possible explanation of the inverse association between living on a farm and sinus problems could relate to selective migration of less healthy residents from rural to urban areas. The subjects or their families may have stopped farming because of symptoms related to exposure. We could not rule out such a "healthy farmer effect" because of lack of information, although the proportion of the subjects who lived on a farm during their first year but not at the time of investigation were not different between subjects with and without sinus problems (47.6% vs. 50.0% in subjects who spent their early life on a farm, $p = 0.100$).

We could not find any previous studies showing the direct associations between sewage pond or manure lagoon located near home and the prevalence of sinus problems. In the present study, the subjects who lived near a sewage pond were more likely to report dampness (22.8% vs. 17.0%, $p < 0.001$) and/or indoor mildew odor (20.9% vs. 14.7%, $p < 0.001$), which both have been reported as risks of a variety of adverse respiratory health conditions including sinus problems [31,32]. Though these factors were not included in the multivariable model, there seems to be a need for more research to investigate whether or not these factors increase the risk of sinus problems.

4.2. Lifestyle

In the present study, compared to non-smokers, ex-smokers were significantly at a greater risk of sinus problems. Cigarette smoking can cause mucosal hyper-responsiveness, resulting in sinus symptoms and intensification of allergic reactions [2]. Adverse respiratory symptoms might make smokers quit smoking and contribute to the higher risk of ex-smokers.

4.3. Early Life Exposure

In a bivariable analysis, we observed that ever lived on a farm and lived on a farm during the first year of life were negatively associated with the prevalence of sinus problems, which supports the evidence of the hygiene hypothesis [4,10–12,15]. If the mother smoked during pregnancy, it was significantly associated with the increased risk of sinus problems, however, this variable was not significant at $p < 0.05$ in the multivariable analysis. In the final model, we found that low birth weight was associated with an increased risk of sinus problems, however, previous studies have reported conflicting results [33].

4.4. Occupational History and Exposures

A significant association was observed between occupational history related to farm work, adult farming exposure years, grain dust, asbestos dust, welding fumes, solvents, insecticides, mold or radiation, and sinus problems in bivariable analyses. Among them, solvents and mold were indicated to be risk factors by the multivariable analysis. Though there is limited information regarding the association between solvent and sinus problems, chemical exposures to paints, epoxies, and resins are known to produce nasal irritation [3]. Slager et al. reported that maintenance activities such as painting and repairing engines were significant predictors of rhinitis [3]. Mold is well known as one of the most common aeroallergens implicated in persistent allergic rhinitis [1,2], and this is consistent with the risk of mold allergy in this study. Although some previous studies reported that specific pesticides such as malathion and glyphosate might contribute to rhinitis in farmers [3,7], any variables regarding pesticides (i.e., insecticides, fungicides, and herbicides) were not retained in the final multivariable model in the current analysis. In the present study, an interactive effect was observed between radiation and quadrant on sinus problems, indicating that an occupational exposure associated with radiation was a significant risk for sinus problems in all quadrants. Some studies reported the post-radiotherapy rhinosinusitis in nasopharyngeal carcinoma patients [34], while there was no report showing the association between sinus problems and environmental or occupational exposure to radiation.

4.5. Health Conditions

House dust allergy, pollen allergy, mold allergy, ear infection, stomach acidity/reflux, wheeze, and hay fever were identified to be risk factors of sinus problems by multivariable analysis. Furthermore, some of these factors closely interacted with each other (i.e., house dust allergy and mold allergy, hay fever and ear infection, and stomach acidity/reflux and ear infection), with location of home (living on a farm and house dust allergy), and with birth weight (birth weight and stomach acidity/reflux).

The coexistence of gastro-esophageal reflux disease (GERD) and various respiratory disorders such as chronic rhinosinusitis or ear infection are reported by several past studies, although a causal link between them has so far not been sufficiently documented [35–38]. There are few studies showing the association between birth weight and stomach acidity/reflux. A national cohort study of more than 600,000 infants born in Sweden reported that preterm birth is associated with an increased risk of gastric acid-related disorders [39]. Another study using the same population suggested that preterm birth is also associated with a decreased risk of allergic rhinitis, in accordance with other previous studies [33]. However, the influence of stomach acidity/reflux was not considered in these previous studies, and there is no study in which the interactive effect between reflux and birth weight on sinus problems was investigated. In the present study, the association between birth weight and sinus problems completely differed depending on whether subjects were with or without stomach acidity/reflux; lower birth weight represented an increased risk in the subjects without reflux but a decreased risk in the subjects with reflux compared with normal birth weight. To our best knowledge, this is the first study reporting the interactive effect between birth weight and stomach acidity/reflux on the prevalence of sinus problems. Further studies are needed to confirm this finding.

4.6. Family History

In our study, there was no information on family history of sinus problems, however, the information on family history of lung disease (i.e., asthma, chronic bronchitis, and emphysema) was available. Hence, the association between family history of lung disease and sinus problems were investigated. Father, mother, and brother/sister lung disease were all significantly associated with the prevalence of sinus problems. Family history of asthma or allergic diseases have been reported to be a significant predictive factor of their children's status by many previous studies [1,4,5,10,11,18,40].

4.7. Other Risk Factors (Female Sex and Educational Status)

In the present study, female sex and higher educational status were significantly associated with an increased risk of sinus problems. Female sex has been indicated to be a risk factor of rhinitis, whereas the associations seemed to differ by atopic status and/or population age [4,5,18]. Matheson et al. showed that in subjects who were atopic in adult life, the incidence of rhinitis was higher in boys, but this higher incidence reversed in adult life when women had a higher risk than men; and in subjects without atopy in adult life, females had a consistently increased risk of rhinitis compared with males throughout life [5]. Hormonal factors are a possible explanation for these sex differences [5,41]. The higher risk of sinus problems in females in this study is consistent with the previous studies, because we investigated the incidence of every sinus problem in adult population.

On the other hand, the association between educational status and sinus problems is controversial. Tokunaga et al. reported that higher educational attainment indicated a higher risk of allergic rhinitis [42], whereas some studies have shown the inverse associations [3,40,43]. Educational status, however, seemed to reflect various other socioeconomic, environmental, and occupational factors, rather than to be an independent risk factor itself.

4.8. Limitation and Strengths of This Study

Our study had some limitations that are pertinent to all questionnaire-based cross-sectional studies. The questionnaire-derived information could result in recall bias, misclassification, and underestimation of the prevalence of sinus problems and its association with the factors. There was also the lack of data on the intensity and age of initial exposures to the factors as well as no objective measurements of allergy status such as skin prick positivity or serum Immunoglobulin E (IgE) levels. Therefore, it was not possible to distinguish between allergic and non-allergic sinus problems. The information was collected on sinus trouble but not separately as rhinitis, chronic rhinitis/sinusitis, nasal disorders, or sinus disorders.

The major strength of this study is the large sample size and extensive information which has been obtained on contextual and individual factors and important covariates via self-administered mail-out questionnaires. Because the population studied live in widespread locations in the four quadrants of the province, representing a wide range of geographical areas in Saskatchewan, a mail questionnaire survey seemed to be the best option. Other authors have discussed this issue and they have concluded that with the increasing cost of interviewing, a mail questionnaire surveys in widely spread geographical areas was the best [20,44].

5. Conclusions

In the present study, farm residents had a significantly lower risk of sinus problems than non-farm residents, likely due to exposure to farm specific environments in their early life. Some occupational exposures (solvents and mold) related to farm work, however, exactly associated with an increased risk of sinus problems. The timing and type of the farm exposures are likely responsible for determining the development of non-allergic sinus problems or protection against allergy. We also reported the interactive effect between birth weight and stomach acidity/reflux on the prevalence of sinus problems for the first time. Lower birth weight represented an increased risk in the subjects without reflux but a decreased risk in the subjects with reflux compared with normal birth weight. Further studies are needed to confirm this finding. Our findings provided further insights into the prevalence and determinants of sinus problems in the rural population.

Acknowledgments: This study was funded by a grant from the Canadian Institutes of Health Research "Saskatchewan Rural Health Study", Canadian Institutes of Health Research MOP-187209-POP-CCAA-11829, approved by the Biomedical Research Ethics Board (Bio# 09-56) of the University of Saskatchewan, Canada. The Saskatchewan Rural Health Study (SRHS) Team consists of: James Dosman (Designated Principal Investigator, University of Saskatchewan, Saskatoon, SK, Canada); Punam Pahwa (Co-principal Investigator, University of Saskatchewan, Saskatoon, SK, Canada); John Gordon (Co-principal Investigator, University of Saskatchewan, Saskatoon, SK, Canada); Yue Chen (University of Ottawa, Ottawa, ON, Canada); Roland Dyck (University of Saskatchewan, Saskatoon, SK, Canada); Louise Hagel (Project Manager, University of Saskatchewan, Saskatoon, SK, Canada); Bonnie Janzen (University of Saskatchewan, Saskatoon, SK, Canada); Chandima Karunanayake (University of Saskatchewan, Saskatoon, SK, Canada); Shelley Kirychuk (University of Saskatchewan, Saskatoon, SK, Canada); Niels Koehncke (University of Saskatchewan, Saskatoon, SK, Canada); Joshua Lawson (University of Saskatchewan, Saskatoon, SK, Canada); William Pickett (Queen's University, Kingston, ON, Canada); Roger Pitblado (Professor Emeritus, Laurentian University, Sudbury, ON, Canada); Donna Rennie (University of Saskatchewan, Saskatoon, SK, Canada); Ambikaipakan Senthilselvan, (University of Alberta, Edmonton, AB, Canada). We are grateful for the contributions of the rural municipality administrators and the community leaders of the towns included in the study who facilitated access to the study populations and to all of the participants who donated their time to complete and return the survey.

Author Contributions: A.K.-M. authored most of the paper, carried out the statistical analysis, reviewed the literature, reviewed the citations, and created the abstract and manuscript. J.A.D. and P.P. are the co-principal investigators of the SRHS. C.P.K., D.C.R., J.A.L., S.K., R.F.D., N.K., A.S., J.A.D., and P.P. contributed to grant writing, development of study design, questionnaire development, and study coordination. C.P.K., D.C.R., J.A.L., S.K., R.F.D., N.K., A.S., J.A.D., and P.P. provided input into the writing of the manuscript and edited the manuscript. C.P.K. managed the database. The Saskatchewan Rural Health Study Team members contributed during the grant writing and questionnaires development and with conducting the survey. All authors read and approved the final manuscript.

Conflicts of Interest: The authors declare no conflict of interest. The founding sponsors had no role in the design of the study; in the collection, analyses, or interpretation of data; in the writing of the manuscript, and in the decision to publish the results.

References

1. Wang, D.Y. Risk factors of allergic rhinitis: Genetic or environmental? *Ther. Clin. Risk Manag.* **2005**, *1*, 115–123. [CrossRef] [PubMed]

2. Dykewicz, M.S.; Hamilos, D.L. Rhinitis and sinusitis. *J. Allergy Clin. Immunol.* **2010**, *125*, S103–S115. [CrossRef] [PubMed]

3. Slager, R.E.; Simpson, S.L.; LeVan, T.D.; Poole, J.A.; Sandler, D.P.; Hoppin, J.A. Rhinitis associated with pesticide use among private pesticide applicators in the agricultural health study. *J. Toxicol. Environ. Health A* **2010**, *73*, 1382–1393. [CrossRef] [PubMed]

4. Eriksson, J.; Ekerljung, L.; Lötvall, J.; Pullerits, T.; Wennergren, G.; Rönmark, E.; Torén, K. Growing up on a farm leads to lifelong protection against allergic rhinitis. *Allergy* **2010**, *65*, 1397–1403. [CrossRef] [PubMed]

5. Matheson, M.C.; Dharmage, S.C.; Abramson, M.J.; Walters, E.H.; Sunyer, J.; de Marco, R.; Leynaert, B.; Heinrich, J.; Jarvis, D.; Norbäck, D.; et al. Early-life risk factors and incidence of rhinitis: Results from the European Community Respiratory Health Study—An international population-based cohort study. *J. Allergy Clin. Immunol.* **2011**, *128*, 816–823. [CrossRef] [PubMed]

6. Macdonald, K.I.; McNally, J.D.; Massoud, E. The health and resource utilization of Canadians with chronic rhinosinusitis. *Laryngoscope* **2009**, *119*, 184–189. [CrossRef] [PubMed]

7. Poole, J.A. Farming-associated environmental exposures and effect on atopic diseases. *Ann. Allergy Asthma Immunol.* **2012**, *109*, 93–98. [CrossRef] [PubMed]

8. Sundaresan, A.S.; Hirsch, A.G.; Storm, M.; Tan, B.K.; Kennedy, T.L.; Greene, J.S.; Kern, R.C.; Schwartz, B.S. Occupational and environmental risk factors for chronic rhinosinusitis: A systematic review. *Int. Forum Allergy Rhinol.* **2015**, *5*, 996–1003. [CrossRef] [PubMed]

9. Demos, K.; Sazakli, E.; Jelastopulu, E.; Charokopos, N.; Ellul, J.; Leotsinidis, M. Does farming have an effect on health status? A comparison study in West Greece. *Int. J. Environ. Res. Public Health* **2013**, *10*, 776–792. [CrossRef] [PubMed]

10. Riedler, J.; Braun-Fahrlander, C.; Eder, W.; Schreuer, M.; Waser, M.; Maisch, S.; Carr, D.; Schierl, R.; Nowak, D.; von Mutius, E.; et al. Exposure to farming in early life and development of asthma and allergy: A cross-sectional survey. *Lancet* **2001**, *358*, 1129–1133. [CrossRef]

11. Leynaert, B.; Neukirch, C.; Jarvis, D.; Chinn, S.; Burney, P.; Neukirch, F.; European Community Respiratory Health Survey. Does living on a farm during childhood protect against asthma, allergic rhinitis, and atopy in adulthood? *Am. J. Respir. Crit. Care Med.* **2001**, *164*, 1829–1834. [CrossRef] [PubMed]

12. Braun-Fahrlander, C.; Riedler, J.; Herz, U.; Eder, W.; Waser, M.; Grize, L.; Maisch, S.; Carr, D.; Gerlach, F.; Bufe, A.; et al. Environmental exposure to endotoxin and its relation to asthma in school-age children. *N. Engl. J. Med.* **2002**, *347*, 869–877. [CrossRef] [PubMed]

13. Waser, M.; Michels, K.B.; Bieli, C.; Flöistrup, H.; Pershagen, G.; von Mutius, E.; Ege, M.; Riedler, J.; Schram-Bijkerk, D.; Brunekreef, B.; et al. Inverse association of farm milk consumption with asthma and allergy in rural and suburban populations across Europe. *Clin. Exp. Allergy* **2007**, *37*, 661–670. [CrossRef] [PubMed]

14. Von Mutius, E.; Vercelli, D. Farm living: Effects on childhood asthma and allergy. *Nat. Rev. Immunol.* **2010**, *10*, 861–868. [CrossRef] [PubMed]

15. Smit, L.A.; Hooiveld, M.; van der Sman-de Beer, F.; Opstal-van Winden, A.W.; Beekhuizen, J.; Wouters, I.M.; Yzermans, C.J.; Heederik, D. Air pollution from livestock farms, and asthma, allergic rhinitis and COPD among neighbouring residents. *Occup. Environ. Med.* **2014**, *71*, 134–140. [CrossRef] [PubMed]

16. Brunekreef, B.; Von Mutius, E.; Wong, G.K.; Odhiambo, J.A.; Clayton, T.O.; ISAAC Phase Three Study Group. Early life exposure to farm animals and symptoms of asthma, rhinoconjunctivitis and eczema: An ISAAC Phase Three Study. *Int. J. Epidemiol.* **2012**, *41*, 753–761. [CrossRef] [PubMed]

17. Cooper, P.J.; Vaca, M.; Rodriguez, A.; Chico, M.E.; Santos, D.N.; Rodrigues, L.C.; Barreto, M.L. Hygiene, atopy and wheeze-eczema-rhinitis symptoms in schoolchildren from urban and rural Ecuador. *Thorax* **2014**, *69*, 232–239. [CrossRef] [PubMed]

18. Matheson, M.C.; Walters, E.H.; Simpson, J.A.; Wharton, C.L.; Ponsonby, A.L.; Johns, D.P.; Jenkins, M.A.; Giles, G.G.; Hopper, J.L.; Abramson, M.J.; et al. Relevance of the hygiene hypothesis to early vs. late onset allergic rhinitis. *Clin. Exp. Allergy* **2009**, *39*, 370–378. [CrossRef] [PubMed]

19. Pahwa, P.; Karunanayake, C.P.; Hagel, L.; Janzen, B.; Pickett, W.; Rennie, D.; Senthilselvan, A.; Lawson, J.; Kirychuk, S.; Dosman, J. The Saskatchewan rural health study: An application of a population health framework to understand respiratory health outcomes. *BMC Res. Notes* **2012**, *5*, 400. [CrossRef] [PubMed]

20. Dillman, D.A. *Mail and Internet Surveys: The Tailored Design Method*; John Wiley: Hoboken, NJ, USA, 2007.

21. Pickett, W.; Day, L.; Hagel, L.; Brison, R.J.; Marlenga, B.; Pahwa, P.; Koehncke, N.; Crowe, T.; Phyllis Snodgrass, P.; Dosman, J. The Saskatchewan Farm Injury Cohort: Rationale and methodology. *Public Health Rep.* **2008**, *123*, 567–575. [CrossRef] [PubMed]

22. Health Canada. *Strategies for Population Health: Investing in the Health of Canadians*; Health Canada: Ottawa, ON, Canada, 1994. Available online: http://publications.gc.ca/collections/Collection/H88-3-30-2001/pdfs/other/strat_e.pdf (accessed on 1 December 2017).

23. Statistics Canada. *Statistical Report on the Health of Canadians*; Statistics Canada: Ottawa, ON, Canada, 1999. Available online: http://www.statcan.gc.ca/pub/82-570-x/4227734-eng.pdf (accessed on 1 December 2017).

24. Health Canada. *Toward a Healthy Future: Second Report on the Health of Canadians*; Health Canada: Ottawa, ON, Canada, 1999. Available online: http://publications.gc.ca/collections/Collection/H39-468-1999E.pdf (accessed on 1 December 2017).

25. Desrosiers, M.; Evans, G.A.; Keith, P.K.; Wright, E.D.; Kaplan, A.; Bouchard, J.; Ciavarella, A.; Doyle, P.W.; Javer, A.R.; Leith, E.S.; et al. Canadian clinical practice guidelines for acute and chronic rhinosinusitis. *Allergy Asthma Clin. Immunol.* **2011**, *7*, 2. [CrossRef] [PubMed]

26. Statistics Canada. *National Population Health Survey Household Component: Documentation for the Derived Variables and the Constant Longitudinal Variables*; Statistics Canada: Ottawa, ON, Canada. Available online: http://www23.statcan.gc.ca/imdb-bmdi/pub/document/3225_D10_T9_V3-eng.pdf (accessed on 1 December 2017).

27. Human Resources and Skills Development Canada, the Public Health Agency of Canada and Indian and Northern Affairs Canada. *The Well-Being of Canada's Young Children: Government of Canada Report*; Government of Canada: Ottawa, ON, Canada, 2011. Available online: http://www.dpe-agje-ecd-elcc.ca/eng/ecd/well-being/sp_1027_04_12_eng.pdf (accessed on 1 December 2017).

28. Martin, J.A.; Hamilton, B.E.; Osterman, M.J.; Curtin, S.C.; Mathews, T.J. *Births: Final Data for 2012*; National Vital Statistics Reports; National Center for Health Statistics: Hyattsville, MD, USA, 2013; Volume 62. Available online: https://www.cdc.gov/nchs/data/nvsr/nvsr62/nvsr62_09.pdf (accessed on 1 December 2017).

29. Pan, W. Akaike's information criterion in generalized estimating equations. *Biometrics* **2001**, *57*, 120–125. [CrossRef] [PubMed]

30. Hardin, J.W.; Hilbe, J.M. *Generalized Estimating Equations*; Chapman & Hall/CRC: Boca Raton, FL, USA, 2003.

31. Fisk, W.J.; Eliseeva, E.A.; Mendell, M.J. Association of residential dampness and mold with respiratory tract infections and bronchitis: A meta-analysis. *Environ. Health* **2010**, *9*, 72. [CrossRef] [PubMed]

32. Thrasher, J.D.; Gray, M.R.; Kilburn, K.H.; Dennis, D.P.; Yu, A. A water-damaged home and health of occupants: A case study. *J. Environ. Public Health* **2012**, *2012*, 312836. [CrossRef] [PubMed]

33. Crump, C.; Sundquist, K.; Sundquist, J.; Winkleby, M.A. Gestational age at birth and risk of allergic rhinitis in young adulthood. *J. Allergy Clin. Immunol.* **2011**, *127*, 1173–1179. [CrossRef] [PubMed]

34. Deng, Z.Y.; Tang, A.Z. Bacteriology of postradiotherapy chronic rhinosinusitis in nasopharyngeal carcinoma patients and chronic rhinosinusitis. *Eur. Arch. Otorhinolaryngol.* **2009**, *266*, 1403–1407. [CrossRef] [PubMed]

35. Miura, M.S.; Mascaro, M.; Rosenfeld, R.M. Association between otitis media and gastroesophageal reflux: A systematic review. *Otolaryngol. Head Neck Surg.* **2012**, *146*, 345–352. [CrossRef] [PubMed]

36. Sone, M.; Kato, T.; Nakashima, T. Current concepts of otitis media in adults as a reflux-related disease. *Otol. Neurotol.* **2013**, *34*, 1013–1017. [CrossRef] [PubMed]

37. Katle, E.J.; Hatlebakk, J.G.; Steinsvag, S. Gastroesophageal reflux and rhinosinusitis. *Curr. Allergy Asthma Rep.* **2013**, *13*, 218–223. [CrossRef] [PubMed]

38. Bohnhorst, I.; Jawad, S.; Lange, B.; Kjeldsen, J.; Hansen, J.M.; Kjeldsen, A.D. Prevalence of chronic rhinosinusitis in a population of patients with gastroesophageal reflux disease. *Am. J. Rhinol. Allergy* **2015**, *29*, e70–e74. [CrossRef] [PubMed]

39. Crump, C.; Winkleby, M.A.; Sundquist, J.; Sundquist, K. Gestational age at birth and risk of gastric acid-related disorders in young adulthood. *Ann. Epidemiol.* **2012**, *22*, 233–238. [CrossRef] [PubMed]

40. Shpakou, A.; Brozek, G.; Stryzhak, A.; Neviartovich, T.; Zejda, J. Allergic diseases and respiratory symptoms in urban and rural children in Grodno Region (Belarus). *Pediatr. Allergy Immunol.* **2012**, *23*, 339–346. [CrossRef] [PubMed]

41. Govaere, E.; Van Gysel, D.; Massa, G.; Verhamme, K.M.; Doli, E.; De Baets, F. The influence of age and gender on sensitization to aero-allergens. *Pediatr. Allergy Immunol.* **2007**, *18*, 671–678. [CrossRef] [PubMed]

42. Tokunaga, T.; Ninomiya, T.; Osawa, Y.; Imoto, Y.; Ito, Y.; Takabayashi, T.; Narita, N.; Kijima, A.; Murota, H.; Katayama, I.; et al. Factors associated with the development and remission of allergic diseases in an epidemiological survey of high school students in Japan. *Am. J. Rhinol. Allergy* **2015**, *29*, 94–99. [CrossRef] [PubMed]

43. Kilty, S.J.; McDonald, J.T.; Johnson, S.; Al-Mutairi, D. Socioeconomic status: A disease modifier of chronic rhinosinusitis? *Rhinology* **2011**, *49*, 533–537. [CrossRef] [PubMed]

44. Hox, J.J.; De Leeuw, E.D. A comparison of nonresponse in mail, telephone, and face-to-face surveys. *Qual. Quant.* **1994**, *28*, 329–344. Available online: https://link.springer.com/article/10.1007/BF01097014 (accessed on 3 December 2017). [CrossRef]

14

Rhinosinutis and Asthma in Children

Amelia Licari [iD], **Ilaria Brambilla, Riccardo Castagnoli, Alessia Marseglia, Valeria Paganelli** [iD], **Thomas Foiadelli** [iD] **and Gian Luigi Marseglia** * [iD]

Pediatric Clinic, University of Pavia, Fondazione IRCCS Policlinico San Matteo, 27100 Pavia, Italy; a.licari@smatteo.pv.it (A.L.); i.brambilla@smatteo.pv.it (I.B.); riccardo.castagnoli@yahoo.it (R.C.); alessiamarseglia@gmail.com (A.M.); vale.paganelli@gmail.com (V.P.); thomas.foiadelli@gmail.com (T.F.)
* Correspondence: gl.marseglia@smatteo.pv.it

Abstract: Rhinosinusitis and asthma are two comorbid conditions that lead to pathological and clinical diseases affecting the respiratory tract. They are connected by significant anatomical, epidemiological, pathophysiological, and clinical evidence, and also share therapeutic principles. The aim of this review is to provide an updated overview of the existing link between rhinosinusitis and asthma focusing on the pediatric age.

Keywords: rhinosinusitis; asthma; children

1. Introduction

Rhinosinusitis and asthma represent a major public health problem, because of their frequency and their impact on quality of life, school performance and economic burden [1]. According to the latest European Position Paper on Rhinosinusitis and Nasal Polyps, pediatric rhinosinusitis is defined as an inflammation of the nose and the paranasal sinuses characterized by two or more symptoms. These symptoms include nasal blockage, nasal obstruction, nasal congestion, or nasal discharge (anterior or posterior nasal drip), in combination or not with facial pain, facial pressure and coughing; these can be accompanied by either endoscopic signs of nasal polyps (with mucopurulent discharge primarily from the middle meatus and edema), mucosal obstruction primarily in the middle meatus, or computed tomography (CT) changes (as mucosal changes within the ostiomeatal complex or sinuses) [2].

Acute rhinosinusitis (ARS) in children is defined as a sinonasal inflammation lasting <12 weeks and is associated with the sudden onset of symptoms [2]. The vast majority of ARS is due to acute upper airway infections (viruses accounting for up to 90% of the causative agents) and might be aggravated by underlying allergic conditions (i.e., allergic rhinitis) [2].

We usually refer to chronic rhinosinusitis (CRS) when the disease lasts $\geq$12 weeks without the complete resolution of symptoms [2]. Compared with adults, coughing is a much more significant symptom in children with CRS than a decreased sense of smell. CRS in children may also coexist or be exacerbated by other widespread conditions such as allergic rhinitis, adenoid disease, and gastroesophageal reflux [2]. CRS is often characterized by periods of remission and exacerbation, with a significant impact on patient quality of life (QoL) [3]. CRS is broadly classified into two major phenotypes, based on nasal endoscopic and CT findings: CRS with nasal polyposis (CRSwNP) and CRS *sine* nasal polyposis (CRSsNP) [2].

Recent data have demonstrated that CRS affects approximately 5–15% of the general population in both Europe and the United States [4]. Nasal polyposis (NP) is more frequently seen in men than in women [5], and in adolescents or elderly and asthmatic subjects [6]; it is less common in childhood [7,8]. NP may be either isolated or associated with other medical conditions. Isolated NP in children is a rare condition, representing an alert sign for other underlying systemic diseases (including cystic fibrosis, immunodeficiencies, and primary ciliary dyskinesia) [9].

Pediatric severe chronic upper airway disease (P-SCUAD) is a novel term introduced to define difficult-to-treat cases, characterized by the persistence of upper airway inflammation and symptoms despite correct diagnosis and management [10]. These cases often show a negative impact on quality of life, social functioning, and school or work performance [11]. Although the definition and the pathogenesis of SCUAD in the pediatric population still need to be better clarified, it seems that the presence of important comorbidities, such as adenoid hypertrophy, allergic rhinitis (AR), and asthma, may have an impact on clinical outcomes and contribute to the lack of disease control in CRS patients [10,11]. Adenoids may act as a bacterial reservoir, as well as an active immunological organ in the context of CRS in children [12]. Moreover, emerging evidence has shown that adenoidectomy is effective in controlling symptoms in a proportion of children with CRS [13]. The evidence of an increased incidence of atopic predisposition in pediatric patients with rhinosinusitis, as well as the correlation between allergies and the severity of a sinus disease, have long been supported as a possible causal relationship between CRS and AR [14]. However, few data are available to prove a clear and definitive relationship, especially in children, and it seems that AR is not a trigger for CRS, but rather a comorbidity [14].

Asthma is defined as a heterogeneous condition, with the specific hallmark of chronic airway inflammation. It commonly manifests with symptoms such as coughing, wheezing, shortness of breath and chest tightness, which may change over time and in intensity due to airflow limitation in respiratory airways [15]. Patients can experience episodic flare-ups (exacerbations) that may be life-threatening, usually triggered by factors such as exercise, allergen exposure, weather, or viral infections, and represent a major health problem to patients [15].

The aim of this review is to provide an updated overview on the existing link between rhinosinusitis and asthma focusing on pediatric age.

2. Rhinosinusitis and Asthma in Children

Strong anatomical, epidemiological, pathophysiological, clinical, and therapeutic evidence has recently been revealed regarding the link between upper and lower airways, changing the global pathogenic view of respiratory diseases. The term "united airway disease (UAD)" is used to define this complex interplay [16,17].

2.1. Anatomical Evidence

The respiratory apparatus is anatomically divided into the upper and lower respiratory tracts and has the function of air conduction and gas exchange [6]. Although considered as different entities, the nose and the lung share several microscopic and macroscopic similarities [6]. Histologically, both nose and bronchi are composed of pseudostratified respiratory epithelium with columnar ciliated cells. The basement membrane and ciliary epithelium with glands and goblet cells are present through the whole respiratory tree, all the way to the passage in the respiratory bronchioles with the air cells [16]. This complex anatomical structure makes it necessary to humidify, temper, filter, and supply the air with nitric oxide before entering the gas-exchange region of the lung, protecting the lower respiratory tract from potentially harmful external agents. Rhinosinusitis causes the loss of nasal breathing, a potential trigger for bronchial disorders due to the inhalation of cold and dry air [18]. In addition, the air conduction system plays a central role in protecting the lower tract from inhaled foreign substances, by avoiding the passage of particles of 5–10 μm in diameter [18]. In contrast, mouth breathing leads to increased concentrations of inhaled aeroallergens that may reach the lower respiratory tract, potentially inducing a bronchoconstriction in asthmatic subjects. The communication between the nose and bronchi also seems to be implemented via mechanisms such as neural reflexes and systemic pathways [18].

2.2. Epidemiogical Evidence

There is increasing epidemiological evidence linking asthma to CRS in adults, especially eosinophilic asthma phenotypes and CRSwNP. Adult asthmatic patients, especially those with severe asthma, often have CRSwNP [19]. The presence of NP is associated with the severity of asthma, ranging from 10–30% in mild asthma to 70–90% in severe asthma and regardless of smoking status [20,21]. In the European Unbiased Biomarkers for the Prediction of Respiratory Disease Outcomes (UBIOPRED) cohort of severe asthma, a high incidence of upper airway symptoms was observed, with the presence of NP in 25% of adult subjects [21]. The impact of upper airway comorbidities on asthma severity and control was also reported in the US Severe Asthma Research Program (SARP) study and in the UK Difficult Asthma National Registry [22]. Epidemiological examinations and evidence-based studies are often lacking in the pediatric population. It was reported that 27% of a series of pediatric patients admitted with status asthmaticus had radiological evidence of rhinosinusitis [23], while in another study, 44% of 128 asthmatic children had evidence of rhinosinusitis upon endoscopic examination [24]. Furthermore, an asymptomatic "occult" sinusal involvement, diagnosed with nasal endoscopy, was demonstrated in 7.5% of an uncontrolled asthmatic children population [25]. Fewer studies have investigated whether asthma affects the upper airways. Dejima et al. showed that children with asthma have worse surgical outcomes after sinus surgery and/or adenoidectomy compared with non-asthmatic children [26]. The impact of upper airway pathology on asthma severity and control was demonstrated in the setting of pediatric non-severe asthma: in pre-school children, untreated or undiagnosed upper airways obstruction, often due to rhinosinusitis and concomitant adenoid hypertrophy, may worsen the obstructive pathology of the lower airways [27]. This data has not yet been confirmed for pediatric studies on severe asthma; the cluster analysis of pediatric SARP reported a higher incidence of comorbidities in cluster 3: the main comorbidities found increased bronchial hyperresponsiveness and lower lung function [28]. This may suggest that phenotypes in children differ from those in adults; they are also known to rapidly change over time.

2.3. Pathophysiological Mechanisms

Asthma and CRS are both heterogeneous disorders with a complex pathophysiology, sharing the common type 2 inflammatory pattern, including Th2 cell induction, interleukin (IL)-5 and IL-13 production, and eosinophilic infiltration [18,29]. A direct relationship between upper (nasal) and lower inflammation was observed in an adult population [30].

Few studies directly investigated concomitant upper and lower inflammation in children. Riccio et al. showed the presence of a typical Th2 cytokine response (increased IL-4 and tumor necrosis factor-α (TNF-α)) in the rhinosinusal lavage in allergic asthmatic children with rhinosinusitis [31]. On the other hand, a reversal of the cytokine pattern from a Th2 to a Th1 profile in both allergic and non-allergic children has been observed after medical treatment of CRS: Tosca et al. looked at the change in levels of IL-4 and interferon-γ (IFN-γ) in rhinosinusal lavage fluid in children with asthma and CRS after a 14-day treatment of oral antibiotics and intranasal steroids and a 10-day treatment of oral steroids. They demonstrated a significant decrease in IL-4 and a significant increase in IFN-γ in allergic study participants, and a significant decrease in IL-4 and a non-significant increase in IFN-γ in non-allergic study participants after the treatment [32]. The inflammatory response in the sinus and adenoid tissues of children with CRS and asthma has been observed as quantitatively amplified by Anfuso et al.: children with CRS and asthma had significantly higher sinus levels of TNF-α as well as adenoid levels of epidermal growth factor, eotaxin, fibroblast growth factor-2, growth-related oncogene, and platelet-derived growth factor-AA compared with children with CRS and without asthma [33].

According to the concept of "united airways disease", airway inflammation may start at one site and extend to other sections eventually, and vice versa. Besides the extension by contiguity, airway inflammation is sustained by a complex interplay among several immunological mechanisms that take place both inside and outside the respiratory system, even involving the bone marrow [34]. In an experimental murine model of eosinophilic asthma triggered by *Aspergillus fumigatus* sensitization, it was demonstrated that, after intranasal allergen exposure, basophils and Th2 lymphocytes circulate and migrate significantly to several sites, including the bronchial airways, after being released from the storage pools in the bone marrow [35,36]. Thus, triggering inflammation in the airways may stimulate the bone marrow to produce inflammatory cells and mediators that have an effect on respiratory sites other than those affected initially.

Finally, altered breathing patterns, nasal, pharyngeal, and bronchial reflexes, post-nasal drip, and inhalation of polluted or cold air represent other mechanisms that may further exacerbate the inflammatory disease from upper to lower airways, although they did not end up being the main determinant of comorbidity between CRS and asthma [37].

A better definition of inflammatory pathways of both childhood CRS and asthma is needed in order to recognize the linked pathophysiologic mechanisms of both diseases.

2.4. Clinical and Therapeutic Management

The impact of the presence and severity of upper airway pathology on both asthma severity and control has been demonstrated in several studies [38,39]. In particular, reduced asthma control increased airway obstruction and impaired QoL are the main items in asthmatic patients with CRS [3,38–40]. On the other hand, previous pediatric studies focused on asthma outcomes when rhinosinusitis is treated pharmacologically [41]. An improvement of asthmatic symptoms, lung function and airway hyperresponsiveness has been more recently confirmed after rhinosinusitis therapy in children with both diseases [31,42]; in particular, an improvement in both asthma QoL and control has been experienced in patients presenting with CRS refractory to medical therapy and coexistent asthma after endoscopic sinus surgery (ESS) procedures [43].

CRS and NP have also been both identified as independent risk factors for frequent asthma exacerbations in adults [44,45]. In the large SARP cohort study, CRSwNP were significantly associated with exacerbation frequency [46]. Subsequently, CRS symptom severity has been associated with asthma-related oral corticosteroid use [47].

Early identification of an upper airway disease is crucial for asthmatic patients at risk of more severe disease. Thus, an ear, nose, and throat (ENT) specialist evaluation with a nasal endoscopy and imaging is mandatory to confirm or rule out the clinical suspicion of sino-nasal involvement. As in adults, untreated sinus disease may also contribute to unstable asthma control in childhood. Thus, children with difficult-to-treat or severe asthma should be actively screened for comorbid disorders, in particular those involving the upper airways. Finally, all patients with uncontrolled asthma should be assessed for the possibility of upper airway disease, even in the case of minimal or absent symptoms [48].

Diagnostic biomarkers have been proposed as indicators of type 2 inflammation, such as serum total immunoglobulin E (IgE), eosinophilic cationic protein (ECP), eosinophils, and cytokines IL-4, IL-5 and IL-13, all detectable in blood and from now on in nasal secretions [34]. Higher levels of mucosal and blood eosinophils (together with comorbid asthma), IgE, ECP, and IL-5 have been correlated with the recurrence of the nasal disease, acting as prognostic biomarkers in CRSwNP [49,50]. Furthermore, the presence of *Staphylococcus aureus* and its enterotoxin-specific IgE has also been proposed as a risk factor for co-morbid asthma and for recurrence of NP after surgery [51].

As for asthma, achieving and maintaining the clinical control of the disease is the primary goal of a CRS treatment. Control is defined as a disease state in which patients exhibit negligible symptoms with the minimal effective local therapy, in the presence of a healthy or almost healthy nasal mucosa, as stated in the latest European Guidelines on Sinusitis and Nasal Polyposis (EPOS) [2]. Corticosteroids, and especially topical corticosteroids, in conjunction with nasal saline irrigation represent the mainstay of treatment for patients with CRSwNP or CRSsNP, even at the pediatric age, while the use of systemic corticosteroid therapy is burdened by a significant risk of side effects, such as insomnia, weight gain, gastrointestinal symptoms, adrenal suppression, osteoporosis, steroid-induced diabetes mellitus, and growth retardation in children, especially for prolonged therapy [2]. Other therapies, such as antibiotics, antihistamines, and leukotriene receptor antagonists, have not yet proven to be effective in reducing signs and symptoms of CRSwNP [2]. In case of failure of medical therapy, functional ESS might be indicated with satisfactory but temporary results [2]. Recurrence of disease after surgery has been reported to be as high as 80%, in particular in patients with CRSwNP and increased eosinophil counts, IL-5 and IgE in nasal tissue [52]. Therefore, surgery must always be accompanied by medical therapy, since topical corticosteroids may slow down the recurrence of mucosal inflammation.

Despite all possible therapeutic measures, a subgroup of patients, characterized by severe and recurrent CRSwNP and comorbid asthma and identified by a type 2 immune response (IgE, eosinophils, IL-5 and IL-4/IL-13), may remain uncontrolled and require further innovative therapy. For those patients, biological agents may represent a future valuable alternative, as they can simultaneously control symptoms of both upper and lower airways [53]. While anti-IgE and anti-IL-5 monoclonal antibodies now have an established position in the therapeutic management of severe asthma, an indication for biologics in chronic uncontrolled upper airway diseases has not yet been provided. However, monoclonal antibodies against IgE, IL-5, and IL-4 or IL-13 pathways (omalizumab, mepolizumab, and dupilumab) have been tested with promising results in recent proof-of-concept studies performed in adult patients with CRSwNP with or without asthma; the first adult studies on phase III of these biotherapeutics are still running and may disclose new and significant treatment options to target both upper and lower airway disease [43].

As for precision medicine in asthma, a step forward towards the tailored management and therapy of patients with chronic upper airway inflammation has been recently proposed, with the aim of improving care and preventing asthma [54]; a dedicated approach to the pediatric age is still lacking and may represent a future area of research.

3. Conclusions

Rhinosinusitis and asthma are closely related to each other in many aspects, sharing not only common pathophysiological mechanisms but also therapeutic principles. As in adults, a cluster of chronic upper airway comorbidities is also recognized in childhood asthma, including chronic rhinosinusitis. Undiagnosed and untreated chronic rhinosinusitis may contribute to worsen asthma control and complicate diagnostic and therapeutic management of asthmatic patients. Early recognition of upper airway disease in asthmatic patients is also crucial to identify patients at risk of more severe disease. The possibility of upper airway disease should be ruled out in all patients with uncontrolled or troublesome asthma, even in the case of minimal or absent symptoms.

Acknowledgments: This manuscript has not received funding. The authors have no relevant affiliations or financial involvement with any organization or entity with a financial interest in or financial conflict with the subject matter or materials discussed in the manuscript. This includes employment, consultancies, honoraria, stock ownership or options, expert testimony, grants or patents received or pending, or royalties.

Author Contributions: I.B., A.M., V.P. and T.F. reviewed the literature, A.L. and R.C. drafted the first version of the manuscript; A.L. and G.L.M. critically revised the final version of the manuscript. All of authors read and approved the final manuscript.

Conflicts of Interest: The authors declare no conflict of interest.

References

1. Giavina-Bianchi, P.; Aun, M.V.; Takejima, P.; Kalil, J.; Agondi, R.C. United airway disease: Current perspectives. *J. Asthma Allergy* **2016**, *9*, 93–100. [CrossRef] [PubMed]
2. Fokkens, W.J.; Lund, V.J.; Mullol, J.; Bachert, C.; Alobid, I.; Baroody, F.; Cohen, N.; Cervin, A.; Douglas, R.; Gevaert, P.; et al. European Position Paper on Rhinosinusitis and Nasal Polyps 2012. *Rhinol. Suppl.* **2012**, *23*, 1–299.
3. Huang, C.C.; Chang, P.H.; Wu, P.W.; Wang, C.H.; Fu, C.H.; Huang, C.C.; Tseng, H.J.; Lee, T.J. Impact of nasal symptoms on the evaluation of asthma control. *Medicine* **2017**, *96*, e6147. [CrossRef] [PubMed]
4. Johansson, L.; Akerlund, A.; Holmberg, K.; Melén, I.; Bende, M. Prevalence of nasal polyps in adults: The Skövde population-based study. *Ann. Otol. Rhinol. Laryngol.* **2003**, *112*, 625–629. [CrossRef] [PubMed]

5. Chaaban, M.R.; Walsh, E.M.; Woodworth, B.A. Epidemiology and differential diagnosis of nasal polyps. *Am. J. Rhinol. Allergy* **2013**, *27*, 473–478. [CrossRef] [PubMed]

6. Marseglia, G.L.; Merli, P.; Caimmi, D.; Licari, A.; Labó, E.; Marseglia, A.; Ciprandi, G.; La Rosa, M. Nasal disease and asthma. *Int. J. Immunopathol. Pharmacol.* **2011**, *24*, 7–12. [CrossRef] [PubMed]

7. Marseglia, G.L.; Caimmi, S.; Marseglia, A.; Poddighe, D.; Leone, M.; Caimmi, D.; Ciprandi, G.; Castellazzi, A.M. Rhinosinusitis and asthma. *Int. J. Immunopathol. Pharmacol.* **2010**, *23*, 29–31. [PubMed]

8. Caimmi, D.; Matti, E.; Pelizzo, G.; Marseglia, A.; Caimmi, S.; Labò, E.; Licari, A.; Pagella, F.; Castellazzi, A.M.; Pusateri, A.; et al. Nasal polyposis in children. *J. Biol. Regul. Homeost. Agents* **2012**, *26*, S77–S83. [PubMed]

9. Licari, A.; Caimmi, S.; Bosa, L.; Marseglia, A.; Marseglia, G.L.; Caimmi, D. Rhinosinusitis and asthma: A very long engagement. *Int. J. Immunopathol. Pharmacol.* **2014**, *27*, 499–508. [CrossRef] [PubMed]

10. Prokopakis, E.P.; Kalogjera, L.; Karatzanis, A.D. Pediatric Severe Chronic Upper Airway Disease (P-SCUAD). *Curr. Allergy Asthma Rep.* **2015**, *15*, 68. [CrossRef] [PubMed]

11. Karatzanis, A.; Kalogjera, L.; Scadding, G.; Velegrakis, S.; Kawauchi, H.; Cingi, C.; Prokopakis, E. Severe Chronic Upper Airway Disease (SCUAD) in children. Definition issues and requirements. *Int. J. Pediatr. Otorhinolaryngol.* **2015**, *79*, 965–968. [CrossRef] [PubMed]

12. Brambilla, I.; Pusateri, A.; Pagella, F.; Caimmi, D.; Caimmi, S.; Licari, A.; Barberi, S.; Castellazzi, A.M.; Marseglia, G.L. Adenoids in children: Advances in immunology, diagnosis, and surgery. *Clin. Anat.* **2014**, *27*, 346–352. [CrossRef] [PubMed]

13. Shin, K.S.; Cho, S.H.; Kim, K.R.; Tae, K.; Lee, S.H.; Park, C.W.; Jeong, J.H. The role of adenoids in pediatric rhinosinusitis. *Int. J. Pediatr. Otorhinolaryngol.* **2008**, *72*, 1643–1650. [CrossRef] [PubMed]

14. Georgalas, C.; Vlastos, I.; Picavet, V.; van Drunen, C.; Garas, G.; Prokopakis, E. Is chronic rhinosinusitis related to allergic rhinitis in adults and children? Applying epidemiological guidelines for causation. *Allergy* **2014**, *69*, 828–833. [CrossRef] [PubMed]

15. Global Initiative for Asthma. Global Strategy for Asthma Management and Prevention. 2017. Available online: www.ginasthma.org (accessed on 3 December 2017).

16. Licari, A.; Castagnoli, R.; Denicolò, C.F.; Rossini, L.; Marseglia, A.; Marseglia, G.L. The Nose and the Lung: United Airway Disease? *Front. Pediatr.* **2017**, *5*, 44. [CrossRef] [PubMed]

17. Hellings, P.W.; Prokopakis, E.P. Global airway disease beyond allergy. *Curr. Allergy Asthma Rep.* **2010**, *10*, 143–149. [CrossRef] [PubMed]

18. Ciprandi, G.; Caimmi, D.; Miraglia Del Giudice, M.; La Rosa, M.; Salpietro, C.; Marseglia, G.L. Recent developments in united airways disease. *Allergy Asthma Immunol. Res.* **2012**, *4*, 171–177. [CrossRef] [PubMed]

19. Jarvis, D.; Newson, R.; Lotvall, J.; Hastan, D.; Tomassen, P.; Keil, T.; Gjomarkaj, M.; Forsberg, B.; Gunnbjornsdottir, M.; Minov, J.; et al. Asthma in adults and its association with chronic rhinosinusitis: The GA2LEN survey in Europe. *Allergy* **2012**, *67*, 91–98. [CrossRef] [PubMed]

20. Shaw, D.E.; Sousa, A.R.; Fowler, S.J.; Fleming, L.J.; Roberts, G.; Corfield, J.; Pandis, I.; Bansal, A.T.; Bel, E.H.; Auffray, C.; et al. Clinical and inflammatory characteristics of the European U-BIOPRED adult severe asthma cohort. *Eur. Respir. J.* **2015**, *46*, 1308–1321. [CrossRef] [PubMed]

21. Lin, D.C.; Chandra, R.K.; Tan, B.K.; Zirkle, W.; Conley, D.B.; Grammer, L.C.; Kern, R.C.; Schleimer, R.P.; Peters, A.T. Association between severity of asthma and degree of chronic rhinosinusitis. *Am. J. Rhinol. Allergy* **2011**, *25*, 205–208. [CrossRef] [PubMed]

22. Sweeney, J.; Patterson, C.C.; Menzies-Gow, A.; Niven, R.M.; Mansur, A.H.; Bucknall, C.; Chaudhuri, R.; Price, D.; Brightling, C.E.; Heaney, L.G.; et al. Comorbidity in severe asthma requiring systemic corticosteroid therapy: Cross-sectional data from the Optimum Patient Care Research Database and the British Thoracic Difficult Asthma Registry. *Thorax* **2016**, *71*, 339–346. [CrossRef] [PubMed]

23. Smart, B.A.; Slavin, R.G. Rhinitis and pediatric asthma. *Immunol. Allergy Clin. N. Am.* **2005**, *25*, 67–82. [CrossRef] [PubMed]

24. Tosca, M.A.; Riccio, A.M.; Marseglia, G.L.; Caligo, G.; Pallestrini, E.; Ameli, F.; Mira, E.; Castelnuovo, P.; Pagella, F.; Ricci, A.; et al. Nasal endoscopy in asthmatic children: Assessment of rhinosinusitis and adenoiditis incidence, correlations with cytology and microbiology. *Clin. Exp. Allergy* **2001**, *31*, 609–615. [CrossRef] [PubMed]

25. Marseglia, G.L.; Caimmi, S.; Marseglia, A.; Pagella, F.; Ciprandi, G.; La Rosa, M.; Leonardi, S.; Miraglia Del Giudice, M.; Caimmi, D. Occult sinusitis may be a key feature for non-controlled asthma in children. *J. Biol. Regul. Homeost. Agents* **2012**, *26*, S125–S131. [PubMed]

26. Dejima, K.; Hama, T.; Miyazaki, M.; Yasuda, S.; Fukushima, K.; Oshima, A.; Yasuda, M.; Hisa, Y. A clinical study of endoscopic sinus surgery for sinusitis in patients with bronchial asthma. *Int. Arch. Allergy Immunol.* **2005**, *138*, 97–104. [CrossRef] [PubMed]

27. Marseglia, G.L.; Caimmi, D.; Pagella, F.; Matti, E.; Labó, E.; Licari, A.; Salpietro, A.; Pelizzo, G.; Castellazzi, A.M. Adenoids during childhood: The facts. *Int. J. Immunopathol. Pharmacol.* **2011**, *24*, 1–5. [CrossRef] [PubMed]

28. Fleming, L.; Murray, C.; Bansal, A.T.; Hashimoto, S.; Bisgaard, H.; Bush, A.; Frey, U.; Hedlin, G.; Singer, F.; van Aalderen, W.M.; et al. The burden of severe asthma in childhood and adolescence: Results from the paediatric U-BIOPRED cohorts. *Eur. Respir. J.* **2015**, *46*, 1322–1333. [CrossRef] [PubMed]

29. Håkansson, K.; Bachert, C.; Konge, L.; Thomsen, S.F.; Pedersen, A.E.; Poulsen, S.S.; Martin-Bertelsen, T.; Winther, O.; Backer, V.; von Buchwald, C. Airway Inflammation in Chronic Rhinosinusitis with Nasal Polyps and Asthma: The United Airways Concept Further Supported. *PLoS ONE* **2015**, *10*, e0127228. [CrossRef] [PubMed]

30. ten Brinke, A.; Grootendorst, D.C.; Schmidt, J.T.; De Bruïne, F.T.; van Buchem, M.A.; Sterk, P.J.; Rabe, K.F.; Bel, E.H. Chronic sinusitis in severe asthma is related to sputum eosinophilia. *J. Allergy Clin. Immunol.* **2002**, *109*, 621–626. [CrossRef] [PubMed]

31. Riccio, A.M.; Tosca, M.A.; Cosentino, C.; Pallestrini, E.; Ameli, F.; Canonica, G.W.; Ciprandi, G. Cytokine pattern in allergic and non-allergic chronic rhinosinusitis in asthmatic children. *Clin. Exp. Allergy* **2002**, *32*, 422–426. [CrossRef] [PubMed]

32. Tosca, M.A.; Cosentino, C.; Pallestrini, E.; Riccio, A.M.; Milanese, M.; Canonica, G.W.; Ciprandi, G. Medical treatment reverses cytokine pattern in allergic and nonallergic chronic rhinosinusitis in asthmatic children. *Pediatr. Allergy Immunol.* **2003**, *14*, 238–241. [CrossRef] [PubMed]

33. Anfuso, A.; Ramadan, H.; Terrell, A.; Demirdag, Y.; Walton, C.; Skoner, D.P.; Piedimonte, G. Sinus and adenoid inflammation in children with chronic rhinosinusitis and asthma. *Ann. Allergy Asthma Immunol.* **2015**, *114*, 103–110. [CrossRef] [PubMed]

34. Licari, A.; Brambilla, I.; De Filippo, M.; Poddighe, D.; Castagnoli, R.; Marseglia, G.L. The role of upper airway pathology as a co-morbidity in severe asthma. *Expert Rev. Respir. Med.* **2017**, *11*, 855–865. [CrossRef] [PubMed]

35. Mathias, C.B.; Freyschmidt, E.J.; Caplan, B.; Jones, T.; Poddighe, D.; Xing, W.; Harrison, K.L.; Gurish, M.F.; Oettgen, H.C. IgE influences the number and function of mature mast cells, but not progenitor recruitment in allergic pulmonary inflammation. *J. Immunol.* **2009**, *182*, 2416–2424. [CrossRef] [PubMed]

36. Poddighe, D.; Mathias, C.B.; Freyschmidt, E.J.; Kombe, D.; Caplan, B.; Marseglia, G.L.; Oettgen, H.C. Basophils are rapidly mobilized following initial aeroallergen encounter in naïve mice and provide a priming source of IL-4 in adaptive immune responses. *J. Biol. Regul. Homeost. Agents* **2014**, *28*, 91–103. [PubMed]

37. Braunstahl, G.J.; Fokkens, W. Nasal involvement in allergic asthma. *Allergy* **2003**, *58*, 1235–1243. [CrossRef] [PubMed]

38. Amelink, M.; de Groot, J.C.; de Nijs, S.B.; Lutter, R.; Zwinderman, A.H.; Sterk, P.J.; ten Brinke, A.; Bel, E.H. Severe adult-onset asthma: A distinct phenotype. *J. Allergy Clin. Immunol.* **2013**, *132*, 336–341. [CrossRef] [PubMed]

39. Phillips, K.M.; Hoehle, L.P.; Bergmark, R.W.; Campbell, A.P.; Caradonna, D.S.; Gray, S.T.; Sedaghat, A.R. Chronic rhinosinusitis severity is associated with need for asthma-related systemic corticosteroids. *Rhinology* **2017**, *55*, 211–217. [CrossRef] [PubMed]

40. Ek, A.; Middelveld, R.J.; Bertilsson, H.; Bjerg, A.; Ekerljung, L.; Malinovschi, A.; Stjärne, P.; Larsson, K.; Dahlén, S.E.; Janson, C. Chronic rhinosinusitis in asthma is a negative predictor of quality of life: Results from the Swedish GA(2)LEN survey. *Allergy* **2013**, *68*, 1314–1321. [CrossRef] [PubMed]

41. Lai, L.; Hopp, R.J.; Lusk, R.P. Pediatric chronic sinusitis and asthma: A review. *J. Asthma* **2006**, *43*, 719–725. [CrossRef] [PubMed]

42. Tosca, M.A.; Cosentino, C.; Pallestrini, E.; Caligo, G.; Milanese, M.; Ciprandi, G. Improvement of clinical and immunopathologic parameters in asthmatic children treated for concomitant chronic rhinosinusitis. *Ann. Allergy Asthma Immunol.* **2003**, *91*, 71–78. [CrossRef]

43. Schlosser, R.J.; Smith, T.L.; Mace, J.; Soler, Z.M. Asthma quality of life and control after sinus surgery in patients with chronic rhinosinusitis. *Allergy* **2017**, *72*, 483–491. [CrossRef] [PubMed]

44. Ten Brinke, A.; Sterk, P.J.; Masclee, A.A.; Spinhoven, P.; Schmidt, J.T.; Zwinderman, A.H.; Rabe, K.F.; Bel, E.H. Risk factors of frequent exacerbations in difficult-to-treat asthma. *Eur. Respir. J.* **2005**, *26*, 812–818. [CrossRef] [PubMed]

45. Loymans, R.J.; Honkoop, P.J.; Termeer, E.H.; Snoeck-Stroband, J.B.; Assendelft, W.J.; Schermer, T.R.; Chung, K.F.; Sousa, A.R.; Sterk, P.J.; Reddel, H.K.; et al. Identifying patients at risk for severe exacerbations of asthma: Development and external validation of a multivariable prediction model. *Thorax* **2016**, *71*, 838–846. [CrossRef] [PubMed]

46. Teague, W.G.; Phillips, B.R.; Fahy, J.V.; Wenzel, S.E.; Fitzpatrick, A.M.; Moore, W.C.; Hastie, A.T.; Bleecker, E.R.; Meyers, D.A.; Peters, S.P.; et al. Baseline Features of the Severe Asthma Research Program (SARP III) Cohort: Differences with Age. *J. Allergy Clin. Immunol. Pract.* **2018**, *6*, 545.e4–554.e4. [CrossRef] [PubMed]

47. Phillips, K.M.; Hoehle, L.P.; Caradonna, D.S.; Gray, S.T.; Sedaghat, A.R. Association of severity of chronic rhinosinusitis with degree of comorbid asthma control. *Ann. Allergy Asthma Immunol.* **2016**, *117*, 651–654. [CrossRef] [PubMed]

48. Chung, K.F.; Wenzel, S.E.; Brozek, J.L.; Bush, A.; Castro, M.; Sterk, P.J.; Adcock, I.M.; Bateman, E.D.; Bel, E.H.; Bleecker, E.R.; et al. International ERS/ATS guidelines on definition, evaluation and treatment of severe asthma. *Eur. Respir. J.* **2014**, *43*, 343–373. [CrossRef] [PubMed]

49. Jonstam, K.; Westman, M.; Holtappels, G.; Holweg, C.T.J.; Bachert, C. Serum periostin, IgE, and SE-IgE can be used as biomarkers to identify moderate to severe chronic rhinosinusitis with nasal polyps. *J. Allergy Clin. Immunol.* **2017**, *140*, 1705.e3–1708.e3. [CrossRef] [PubMed]

50. Chen, F.; Hong, H.; Sun, Y.; Hu, X.; Zhang, J.; Xu, G.; Zhao, W.; Li, H.; Shi, J. Nasal interleukin 25 as a novel biomarker for patients with chronic rhinosinusitis with nasal polyps and airway hypersensitiveness: A pilot study. *Ann. Allergy Asthma Immunol.* **2017**, *119*, 310.e2–316.e2. [CrossRef] [PubMed]

51. Bachert, C.; Zhang, N.; Krysko, O.; van Crombruggen, K.; Gevaert, E. Nasal polyposis and asthma: A mechanistic paradigm focusing on *Staphylococcus aureus*. In *The Nose and Sinuses in Respiratory Disorders (ERS Monograph)*; Bachert, C., Bourdin, A., Chanez, P., Eds.; European Respiratory Society: Sheffield, UK, 2017; pp. 122–137.

52. Van Zele, T.; Holtappels, G.; Gevaert, P.; Bachert, C. Differences in initial immunoprofiles between recurrent and nonrecurrent chronic rhinosinusitis with nasal polyps. *Am. J. Rhinol. Allergy* **2014**, *28*, 192–198. [CrossRef] [PubMed]

53. Bachert, C.; Gevaert, P.; Hellings, P. Biotherapeutics in Chronic Rhinosinusitis with and without Nasal Polyps. *J. Allergy Clin. Immunol. Pract.* **2017**, *5*, 1512–1516. [CrossRef] [PubMed]

54. Hellings, P.W.; Akdis, C.A.; Bachert, C.; Bousquet, J.; Pugin, B.; Adriaensen, G.; Advani, R.; Agache, I.; Anjo, C.; Anmolsingh, R.; et al. EUFOREA Rhinology Research Forum 2016: Report of the brainstorming sessions on needs and priorities in rhinitis and rhinosinusitis. *Rhinology* **2017**, *55*, 202–210. [CrossRef] [PubMed]

15

An Overview of Surgical Approaches to Pediatric Chronic Sinusitis for Primary Care Providers

Ryan K. Sewell

Department of Otolaryngology-Head and Neck Surgery, University of Nebraska Medical Center, 981225 UNMC, Omaha, NE 68198-1225, USA; ryan.sewell@unmc.edu

Abstract: Pediatric chronic rhinosinusitis is a common condition amongst pediatric patients. Despite its prevalence, debate continues regarding the best treatment strategies. The current paper examines the literature as it pertains to the surgical management of pediatric chronic rhinosinusitis. Adenoidectomy remains the mainstay in the initial surgical management. Both maxillary sinus irrigation and balloon dilation of the sinuses have been studied with disagreement as to the timing and patient selection for those procedures. Functional endoscopic sinus surgery is an accepted treatment modality, especially in initial surgical failures. Further studies will be needed to better delineate patient selection and timing of specific surgical techniques.

Keywords: pediatric chronic rhinosinusitis; adenoidectomy; maxillary sinus irrigation; balloon catheter sinuplasty; functional endoscopic sinus surgery

1. Introduction

Pediatric chronic rhinosinusitis (PCRS) is a common condition encountered in clinical practice. A recent study by Gilani and Shin found 2.1% of ambulatory health care visits involving patients younger than 20 years of age included a diagnosis for PCRS [1]. Despite its prevalence, appropriate treatment remains elusive. Multiple consensus statements are present in the literature, each providing a somewhat different recommendation on the best practices as it pertains to the treatment of PCRS [2–4].

Adding to the uncertainty regarding the treatment is the definition. While specifics may vary, definitions often include 90 days of continuous symptoms (purulent rhinorrhea, nasal obstruction, facial pain/pressure, cough) and endoscopic findings of edema, purulent rhinorrhea, or polyps and/or CT findings of mucosal changes in the sinuses or ostiomeatal complex [2,3]. Pediatric patients present unique challenges when making a diagnosis based on the above criteria. The ability of a child to cooperate with nasal endoscopy or CT can be beyond their developmental capabilities. In addition, his or her ability to identify pain/pressure or nasal obstruction can also be difficult.

After making the diagnosis of PCRS, treatment recommendations can vary based on the source utilized. It is accepted that surgical approaches are indicated after failure of maximal medical therapy. What constitutes maximal medical therapy, however, differs in the literature. It is beyond the scope of the current paper to further define maximal medical therapy. It is also beyond the scope of this paper to examine the treatment of pediatric patients with certain conditions, such as cystic fibrosis or ciliary dyskinesia, which will predispose them to PCRS. The current paper seeks to examine the current literature as it pertains to the surgical management of PCRS.

2. Adenoidectomy

The adenoids are felt to be a bacterial reservoir in PCRS [4]. Adenoidectomy is therefore a commonly performed procedure in the treatment of PCRS. A pediatric clinical consensus statement provided strong support for the use of adenoidectomy in patients under 6 years of age with less consensus for patients aged 6–12 years of age [2]. Agreement was reached that it can be effective even when done as a standalone procedure [2].

It is also a largely successful operation for PCRS. When adenoidectomy is examined alone in the treatment of PCRS, a meta-analysis showed 69.3% of patients showed an improvement in symptoms [5]. The relatively high success rate and routine nature of the surgery make it a mainstay in the treatment of medically refractory PCRS. A recent survey of both American Society of Pediatric Otolaryngology (ASPO) and American Rhinologic Society (ARS) members reveals it is indeed a commonly employed tool. A total of 94% of respondents include adenoidectomy in the initial surgical management of PCRS [6]. Any surgical management of PCRS, especially in children under age six, should include consideration of adenoidectomy.

Adenoidectomy is a relatively simple operation with minimal morbidity. Multiple techniques exist for adenoidectomy, including curette, electrocautery, microdebrider, and coblator. A recent study compared electrocautery, microdebrider, and coblator [7]. It found electrocautery to be associated with a lower cost and comparable complication rate to the other techniques. A previous meta-analysis compared electrocautery to curettage [8]. It found electrocautery to be associated with decreased intraoperative hemorrhage and time. These studies indicate that suction electrocautery remains the most cost-effective option with comparable to decreased risk profiles when compared to other techniques.

3. Maxillary Sinus Irrigation

An adjunct procedure to adenoidectomy is maxillary sinus puncture and irrigation. A recent study showed it is used in 18% of cases as an addition to adenoidectomy in the initial treatment of PCRS [6]. The goal of this procedure is twofold. One, it is meant to obtain cultures to help direct antibiotic therapy. When compared to endoscopically guided middle meatal cultures with antral biopsy, both were equally effective in obtaining cultures [9]. The second goal of the procedure is therapeutic as it also allows for the irrigation of the trapped mucous within the sinus [9].

Various techniques for this procedure have been described. An inferior meatal puncture can be done by creating a new opening into the maxillary sinus through the inferior meatus. This does not involve the access of any anatomic openings but rather creates a new one. It can also be done using endoscopic guidance using a 45 degree needle through the middle meatus [10]. A more recent procedure involves the use a sinus balloon catheter [11]. This technique involves accessing the maxillary sinus via the middle meatus using endoscopic guidance. Entry into the maxillary sinus is confirmed via transillumination. The authors propose several advantages of the catheter, including no alteration of the normal anatomy and confirmation of entry into the maxillary sinus [11].

A study by Ramadan and Cost showed adding maxillary sinus puncture and irrigation with adenoidectomy improved outcomes when compared to adenoidectomy alone [10]. The authors in this paper utilized a needle to access the maxillary sinus via the middle meatus. At one year, 60.7% of the adenoidectomy alone group showed improvement compared to 87.5% of the adenoidectomy and irrigation group [10].

Maxillary sinus irrigation does carry increased surgical risk, however, when compared to adenoidectomy alone. All techniques carry some risk of epistaxis, pseudoproptosis, and orbital hemorrhage. These complication risks, and the desire to be less aggressive in the surgical management of PCRS, may explain why this is not commonly employed in the initial surgical management of PCRS.

4. Balloon Catheter Sinuplasty

Balloon catheters are a relatively new addition to the treatment armamentarium for PCRS. It involves a similar procedure described above to irrigate the sinus via placement of a catheter through the natural ostium into the sinus. While in its infancy the guidewire position was confirmed radiographically, this is generally no longer required with the addition of the lighted guidewires (transillumination). Dilation is added via a balloon (diameter can vary) to widen a sinus ostium.

The goals of balloon catheter sinuplasty (BCS) are to restore sinus ventilation and drainage pathways while preserving mucosa. It is performed as an adjunct to adenoidectomy in approximately 10% of surgeries for the initial management of PCRS [6].

The procedure is considered minimally invasive as it does not require the removal of any tissue from the patient. The minimally invasive nature of the procedure makes it attractive for PCRS. It does have some limitations. It is typically performed with endoscopic guidance, but placement of the guidewire lateral to the uncinate is done blindly. If accessory ostia are present, these can be inadvertently dilated. The relatively small size of the middle meatus in children can also predispose them to synechia formation.

Studies have shown it to be an effective tool in both the initial treatment of PCRS as well as in patients who have failed adenoidectomy [12,13]. In the initial management of PCRS, BCS, and adenoidectomy was noted to improve symptoms in 80% of patients [12]. It was technically feasible with over 90% of sinuses successfully cannulated. The success rate remained around 80% when revision cases were examined [13]. No complications were noted in either study.

The ultimate efficacy of BCS remains debated [14]. No clinical consensus could be reached regarding its effectiveness [2]. A recent American Academy of Otolaryngology Head and Neck Surgery clinical consensus statement regarding balloon dilation excluded recommendations related to patients under 18 [15]. Thottam et al. compared traditional sinus surgery to BCS with traditional ethmoidectomy [16]. They found similar success rates between the two procedures. The addition of the traditional ethmoidectomy in this study lessens the minimally invasive advantages of BCS and illustrates the limitation BCS offers to address ethmoid disease. Future studies will be needed to better define what role BCS should occupy in the treatment of PCRS.

5. Endoscpic Sinus Surgery

Endoscopic sinus surgery (ESS) is an important tool in the treatment of PCRS. The goals of endoscopic sinus surgery (for all patients) are twofold: open natural sinus pathways and preserve mucosa [3]. While it is utilized in the initial management of PCRS (8%), it is performed nearly 90% of the time when operating after initial surgical management (e.g., adenoidectomy) fails [6].

ESS, when used in appropriate patients, is an effective treatment [2]. A PubMed review of 11 articles regarding ESS outcomes showed a success rate of 82–100% [17]. A second meta-analysis examining the impact ESS has on quality of life measures for pediatric patients with PCRS showed a benefit [17]. The meta-analysis included 15 studies involving 1301 treated patients. They found reported ESS improves the quality of life in 71–100% of operated children [18].

The risks of ESS, however, can be serious. The risks of major complications are low but carry significant morbidity. The PubMed review found a complication rate of 1.4% (6/440). The complications included two orbital entries, two periorbital ecchymosis, one severe bleeding, and one orbital fat extrusion [17]. A second study found the risk of major complications (bleeding, cerebral spinal fluid leak, and meningitis) was 0.6% [18].

Concerns initially existed regarding the potential effects on facial growth. Bothwell et al. compared 67 children, 46 who had undergone ESS and 21 who had not had any surgery. No significant difference was noted in facial growth was seen between the two groups [19]. In sum, concerns regarding facial growth have been "unsubstantiated" [14].

Pediatric patients also present a unique dilemma regarding the appropriate post op management. In adult patients, the surgical area is typically endoscopically debrided under local anesthesia. In older children, debridement can be performed awake. In younger children, however, this is generally not possible. Several studies have looked at the utility of a 'second look' procedure in children. Walner et al. did not find an increased risk of a revision ESS in patients who did not have a debridement when compared to those who did [20]. It is not felt debridement is routinely necessary for pediatric ESS patients [2].

The high success rate but risk of serious complications (albeit rare) in ESS creates a clinical dilemma. Agreement exists that ESS is the treatment of choice if initial surgical management fails [6]. The relatively high success rates of adenoidectomy alone make any decision to include ESS in the initial surgical management a difficult one. The clinical consensus statement agrees, concluding that while ESS is effective it should be reserved until after adenoidectomy [2].

6. Conclusions

PCRS presents multiple diagnostic and clinical challenges. Despite the prevalence of PCRS, the optimal management protocol, both medical and surgical, remains elusive. Agreement exists that surgery should be reserved for patients who fail medical management. Agreement also exists that for children under age 6 the initial surgical management should include adenoidectomy. ESS is an effective surgical option and is the treatment of choice for surgical failures. The use of other procedures (e.g., maxillary irrigation, balloon sinuplasty) in the initial management of PCRS is currently debated in the literature. Further studies are needed to determine the timing and patient selection for specific surgical techniques.

Conflicts of Interest: The author declares no conflict of interest.

References

1. Gilani, S.; Shin, J. The Burden and Visit Prevalence of Pediatric Chronic Rhinosinusitis. *Otolaryngol. Head Neck Surg.* **2017**, *157*, 1048–1052. [CrossRef] [PubMed]
2. Brietzke, S.E.; Shin, J.J.; Choi, S.; Lee, J.T.; Parikh, S.R.; Pena, M.; Prager, J.D.; Ramadan, H.; Veling, M.; Corrigan, M.; et al. Clinical consensus statement: Pediatric chronic rhinosinusitis. *Otolaryngol. Head Neck Surg.* **2014**, *151*, 542–553. [CrossRef] [PubMed]
3. Fokkens, W.J.; Lund, V.J.; Mullol, J.; Bachert, C.; Alobid, I.; Baroody, F.; Cohen, N.; Cervin, A.; Douglas, R.; Gevaert, P.; et al. EPOS 2012: European position paper on rhinosinusitis and nasal polyps 2012. *Rhinology* **2012**, *50*, 1–12. [PubMed]
4. Orlandi, R.R.; Kingdom, T.T.; Hwang, P.H.; Smith, T.L.; Alt, J.A.; Baroody, F.M.; Batra, P.S.; Bernal-Sprekelsen, M.; Bhattacharyya, N.; Chandra, R.K.; et al. International consensus statement on allergy and rhinology: Rhinosinusitis. *Int. Forum Allergy Rhinol.* **2016**, *6*, S22–S209. [CrossRef] [PubMed]
5. Brietzke, S.E.; Brigger, M.T. Adenoidectomy outcomes in pediatric rhinosinusitis: A meta-analysis. *Int. J. Ped. Otorhinolaryngol.* **2008**, *72*, 1541–1545. [CrossRef] [PubMed]
6. Beswick, D.M.; Messner, A.H.; Hwang, P.H. Pediatric chronic rhinosinusitis management in rhinologists and pediatric otolaryngologists. *Ann. Otol. Rhinol. Laryngol.* **2017**, *126*, 634–639. [CrossRef] [PubMed]
7. Sjogren, P.P.; Thomas, A.J.; Hunter, B.N.; Butterfield, J.; Gale, C.; Meier, J.D. Comparison of Pediatric Adenoidectomy Techniques. *Laryngoscope* **2018**, *128*, 745–749. [CrossRef] [PubMed]
8. Reed, J.; Sridhara, S.; Breitzke, S.E. Electrocautery adenoidectomy outcomes: A meta-analysis. *Otolaryngol. Head Neck Surg.* **2009**, *140*, 148–153. [CrossRef] [PubMed]
9. Deckard, N.A.; Kruper, G.J.; Bui, T.; Coticchia, J. Comparison of two minimally invasive techniques for treating chronic rhinosinusitis in the pediatric population. *Int. J. Pediatr. Otorhinolaryngol.* **2011**, *75*, 1296–1300. [CrossRef] [PubMed]
10. Ramadan, H.H.; Cost, J.L. Outcome of Adenoidectomy with Maxillary Sinus Wash for Chronic Rhinosinusitis in Children. *Laryngoscope* **2008**, *118*, 871–873. [CrossRef] [PubMed]
11. Zeiders, J.W.; Dahya, Z.J. Antral lavage using the Luma transillumination wire and vortex irrigator—A safe and effective advance in treating pediatric sinusitis. *Int. J. Pediatr. Otorhinolaryngol.* **2011**, *75*, 461–463. [CrossRef] [PubMed]
12. Ramadan, H.H.; Terrell, A.M. Balloon Catheter Sinuplasty and Adenoidectomy in Children with Chronic Rhinosinusitis. *Ann. Otol. Rhinol. Laryngol.* **2010**, *119*, 578–582. [CrossRef] [PubMed]
13. Ramadan, H.H.; Bueller, H.; Hster, S.T.; Terrell, A.M. Sinus Balloon Catheter Dilation after Adenoidectomy Failure for Children with Chronic Rhinosinusitis. *Arch. Otolaryngol. Head Neck Surg.* **2012**, *138*, 635–638. [CrossRef] [PubMed]

14. Sedaghat, A.R.; Cunningham, M.J. Does Balloon Catheter Sinuplasty Have a Role in Surgical Management of Pediatric Sinus Disease. *Laryngoscope* **2011**, *121*, 2053–2054. [CrossRef] [PubMed]

15. Piccirillo, J.F.; Payne, S.C.; Rosenfeld, R.M.; Baroody, F.M.; Batra, P.S.; DelGaudio, J.M.; Edelstein, D.R.; Lane, A.P.; Luong, A.U.; Manes, R.P.; et al. Clinical Consensus Statement: Balloon Dilation of the Sinuses. *Otolaryngol. Head Neck Surg.* **2018**, *158*, 203–214. [CrossRef] [PubMed]

16. Thottam, P.S.; Metz, C.M.; Kieu, M.C.; Dworkin, J.; Jagini, J.; Bangiyev, J.N.; Mehta, D. Functional Endoscopic Sinus Surgery Versus Balloon Sinuplasty with Ethmoidectomy: A 2-year Analysis in Pediatric Chronic Rhinosinusitis. *Indian J. Otolaryngol. Head Neck Surg.* **2016**, *68*, 300–306. [CrossRef] [PubMed]

17. Markary, C.A.; Ramadan, H.H. The Role of Sinus Surgery in Children. *Laryngoscope* **2013**, *123*, 1348–1352. [CrossRef] [PubMed]

18. Vlastarakos, P.V.; Fetta, M.; Segas, J.V.; Maragoudakis, P.; Nikolopoulos, T.P. Functional Endoscopic Sinus Surgery Improves Sinus-Related Symptoms and Quality of Life in Children with Chronic Rhinosinusitis: A Systematic Analysis and Meta-Analysis of Published Interventional Studies. *Clin. Pediatr.* **2013**, *52*, 1091–1097. [CrossRef] [PubMed]

19. Bothwell, M.R.; Piccirillo, J.F.; Lusk, R.P.; Ridenour, B.D. Long-term outcome of facial growth after functional endoscopic sinus surgery. *Otolaryngol. Head Neck Surg.* **2002**, *126*, 628–634. [CrossRef] [PubMed]

20. Walner, D.L.; Falciglia, M.; Willging, J.P.; Myer, C.M., 3rd. The role of second-look nasal endoscopy after pediatric functional endoscopic sinus surgery. *Arch. Otolaryngol. Head Neck Surg.* **1998**, *124*, 425–428. [CrossRef] [PubMed]

16

Complications of Short-Course Oral Corticosteroids for Eosinophilic Chronic Rhinosinusitis during Long-Term Follow-Up

Remi Motegi, Shin Ito, Hirotomo Homma, Noritsugu Ono, Hiroko Okada, Yoshinobu Kidokoro, Akihito Shiozawa and Katsuhisa Ikeda *

Department of Otorhinolaryngology, Juntendo University Faculty of Medicine, 2-1-1 Hongo, Bunkyo-ku, Tokyo 113-8421, Japan; rhibiya@juntendo.ac.jp (R.M.); shin709@juntendo.ac.jp (S.I.); h-honma@juntendo.ac.jp (H.H.); nori-o@juntendo.ac.jp (N.O.); hiokada@juntendo.ac.jp (H.O.); ykidoko@juntendo.ac.jp (Y.K.); ashioza@juntendo.ac.jp (A.S.)
* Correspondence: ike@juntendo.ac.jp

Abstract: The literature strongly recommends the use of oral corticosteroids in the management of patients with eosinophilic chronic rhinosinusitis (CRS) with nasal polyps. Although potential complications associated with the long-term use of oral corticosteroids for the treatment of CRS have been suggested, no studies have described these effects in detail. Forty-three patients with a mean age of 51 years with eosinophilic CRS were retrospectively evaluated after surgery. Short-course oral prednisolone (PSL, 0.5 mg/kg of body weight) was provided for one week when anosmia and eosinophilic mucin and/or nasal polyps were present. The postoperative follow-up period ranged from 12 to 108 months (average: 62 months). HbA1C showed normal ranges in all except one patient, who had a diabetic pattern of HbA1C of 6.5%. Five patients had serum cortisol levels below the cutoff value. However, re-examination of the serum cortisol and adrenocorticotropic hormone stimulation test showed normal ranges in all five patients who had initially shown abnormal values of serum cortisol. Thus, adrenal insufficiency in all the patients was negligible. Five (3 women and 2 men) out of the 15 patients (6 women and 9 men) who participated in bone mineral density measurement showed significant reductions, suggesting the presence of osteoporosis. Patients taking long-term and repeated short-course use of oral corticosteroids for refractory nasal polyps of eosinophilic CRS are likely to have a potentially increased risk for osteoporosis.

Keywords: eosinophilic chronic rhinosinusitis; nasal polyps; oral corticosteroid; osteoporosis; bone mineral density; cortisol; postoperative follow-up

1. Introduction

Chronic rhinosinusitis (CRS) is defined as persistent inflammation of the nasal and paranasal cavity mucosa lasting three or more months [1]. Based on an epidemiological study in the United States, about 29.2 million adults (prevalence: 14.2%) have CRS. The prevalence and medical costs of CRS are increasing and have become an important social issue [2]. The histomorphological patterns of chronic rhinosinusitis with nasal polyps are characterized by the predominance of eosinophils and mixed mononuclear cells but a relative paucity of neutrophils [3], and therefore can be designated as eosinophilic CRS. Mucosal infiltration with eosinophils in CRS with nasal polyps may have a poorer surgical outcome and is frequently associated with bronchial asthma [4].

Eosinophilic CRS is characterized by eosinophilic inflammation driven by Th2 cytokines [5]. Since glucocorticosteroids have potent anti-inflammatory effects, including decreasing inflammation mediated by eosinophils [6,7], they are the most common first-line treatment for CRS with nasal polyps [8]. Placebo-controlled studies showed that topical corticosteroid therapy reduced the recurrence of polyps after surgery [9,10]. However, since topical corticosteroid therapy is not effective in all patients, systemic glucocorticosteroids are sometimes used. A randomized, controlled, double-blind study demonstrated improved nasal symptom scores when compared to the placebo with a 14-day treatment with 50 mg prednisolone (PSL) [11]. Although short courses of 5–14 days of oral corticosteroids are recommended for safe use in CRS with nasal polyps [8], repeated or prolonged use of oral steroids may be associated with an increased risk of systemic side effects [12]. Other studies with level-2 evidence showed positive changes in the majority of the parameters evaluated [11,13,14]. Thus, analysis of the data supports the use of oral steroids in patients with CRS and with nasal polyps for immediate and short-term periods.

The anti-inflammatory effects of oral steroids cannot be separated from their metabolic effects. Repeated or prolonged use of oral steroids may be associated with an enhanced risk of systemic side effects. At three to six months after the end of the oral steroid treatment period for CRS, increases in insomnia and gastrointestinal disturbance have been suggested as adverse effects [11,13,15]. Potential complications associated with the long-term use of oral corticosteroids for the treatment of CRS have been suggested [16]. The prevalence of adrenal insufficiency and low bone mass were recognized in patients with CRS with nasal polyps taking oral steroids [17,18]. Conversely, no systemic or local side effects of steroid treatment were seen in any patients [14,19]. Thus, whether the long-term use of oral corticosteroid for the treatment of eosinophilic CRS causes adverse effects is still controversial. In general, the main adverse effects of corticosteroid oral treatment include disturbance in glucose metabolism, suppression of the hypothalamic pituitary adrenal axis, osteoporosis or changes in bone mineral density (BMD), growth retardation in children, and cataracts and glaucoma [12,20,21].

In the present study, we evaluated the systemic adverse effects during long-term follow-up with intermittent and repeated short-course use of oral corticosteroids in refractory nasal polyps of eosinophilic CRS. Moreover, to evaluate the prevalence of adverse systemic effects during long-term follow-up, we calculated the relationship between the cumulative doses of PSL and the presence of osteoporosis in addition to the risk factors for osteoporosis.

2. Materials and Method

2.1. Patients

This study of a series of cases was approved by the ethics committee of the Juntendo University Faculty of Medicine. The study was conducted in accordance with the Declaration of Helsinki, and the protocol was approved by the Ethics Committee of 17-180 (Project identification code). All subjects entered the study after providing informed consent.

Eosinophilic CRS was diagnosed based on the criteria of the Japanese Epidemiological survey of Refractory Eosinophilic Chronic Rhinosinusitis Study (JESREC) study [22]. Patients with specific types of CRS with nasal polyps, including aspirin sensitivity and cystic fibrosis, were excluded. Patients with eosinophilic CRS requiring oral corticosteroids postoperatively were recruited from the Department of Otorhinolaryngology of the Juntendo University Faculty of Medicine and the study was conducted between January 2007 and October 2016.

2.2. Study Protocol

Endoscopic sinus surgery was performed under general anesthesia according to our previous paper [23]. We used standard postoperative management as follows. All patients received an intranasal corticosteroid preparation of two puffs of fluticasone (100 μg) daily in each nostril as well as a saline nasal douche after surgery. A short-course of oral PSL (0.5 mg/kg of body weight) was prescribed for 5–10 days when anosmia and eosinophilic mucin and/or nasal polyps were present. Furthermore, levofloxacin (200 mg) was orally administered twice per day when massive, purulent nasal discharge occurred.

2.3. Outcome Measures

Details of the dose and duration of oral corticosteroid therapy were obtained for each patient from their clinical records. Lifetime cumulative doses of PSL were calculated, plus duration of therapy as the total period that continuous or intermittent corticosteroids had been taken. The criteria for diagnosing glucocorticoid-induced diabetes mellitus was defined as a fasting blood glucose level of ≥ 6.9 mmol/mol and HbA1c ≥ 65 mmol/mol [24]. The cutoff value for serum cortisol in the morning, used to define adrenal insufficiency, was 4.5 µg/dL. A rapid adrenocorticotropic hormone (ACTH test) was performed by measuring the serum cortisol concentrations immediately before and 30 and/or 60 min after the intravenous injection of cosyntropin (Cortrosyn; 0.25 mg). A normal response to the rapid ACTH test was defined as an increase in the serum cortisol concentration of at least 550 nmol/L (20 µg/dL). Bone mineral density (BMD) was measured at the anterior-posterior lumbar spine (L2–L4) by dual energy X-ray absorptiometry (Hologic Discovery A QDR, Hologic, Inc., Marlborough, MA, USA) using the same scanner for all patients. Lumbar spine BMD was computed from vertebrae that were unaffected by bone fracture or osteoarthritis using regression analysis [25]. BMD was expressed in absolute values as a T score and Z score matched for race and sex from peak bone mass (T score) or matched for age (Z score). Osteoporosis was defined as a T score of less than −2.5.

2.4. Statistical Analysis

The data were expressed as the mean $\pm$ S.D. Statistical analyses were evaluated using StatMate IV for Windows. One-way analysis of variance (ANOVA) followed by Fisher's exact test were used for 2-group comparison of age, body mass index, peripheral blood eosinophil, cumulative PSL dose, or duration of an oral corticosteroid. Pearson's chi-square test was used for 2-group comparison of gender. Pearson's correlation coefficient was used to examine the relationship between cumulative PSL and BMD. Differences were considered to be significant if $p < 0.05$.

3. Results

Forty-three patients with eosinophilic CRS requiring oral corticosteroids postoperatively (26 males and 17 females, ranging from 22 to 73 years, mean age of 51 years) were enrolled between January 2007 and October 2016. All 43 patients with eosinophilic CRS were taking frequent intermittent courses of an oral corticosteroid. The cumulative PSL dose ranged from 2.5 g to 22.7 g (mean: 12.8 g), with a duration of administration of 12 to 108 months (mean: 62 months), and daily dose of 5 to 30 mg.

The demographic and baseline clinical profiles are shown in Table 1. The proportion of male patients was 60%. Blood examination was performed before the administration of oral corticosteroids and demonstrated a mean total Immunoglobulin E of 387 IU/mL and a mean eosinophil of 8.7%. The comorbidity of allergic rhinitis and bronchial asthma was found to be 23 and 58%, respectively.

Table 1. Baseline demographics and clinical information (n = 43 patients).

Baseline Demographics and Clinical Information	
Male, no. (%)	26 (60)
Age, mean (min., max.)	51 (22, 73)
Serum eosinophil (%), mean (min., max.)	8.7 (0.3, 19.1)
Total IgE (IU/ml), mean (min., max.)	387 (18, 2288)
History of bronchial asthma, no. (%)	18 (42)
History of allergic rhinitis, no. (%)	10 (23)
History of eosinophilic otitis media, no. (%)	3 (0.7)

The distributions of HbA1c, serum cortisol level, and BMD are shown in Figure 1. HbA1c showed normal ranges in all except one patient. The patient revealed glucocorticoid-induced diabetes mellitus based on a fasting blood glucose of 126 mg/dL and a HbA1C of 6.5 mmol/mol. Five of the 19 patients had serum cortisol levels below the cutoff value. However, re-examination of the serum cortisol and

ACTH stimulation test showed normal ranges for all five patients initially showing abnormal values of serum cortisol. Thus, the adrenal insufficiency in all patients was negligible.

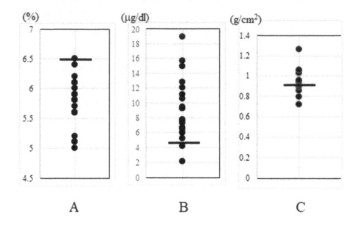

Figure 1. Scatterplots of (**A**) HgA1c, (**B**) serum cortisol, and (**C**) bone mineral density. Horizontal bars denote the normal limit.

Five (3 women and 2 men) of the 15 patients (6 women and 9 men) who participated in BMD measurement showed a significant reduction (33.3%) in bone density, suggesting the presence of osteoporosis. No vertebral fracture was observed in the present study. There were no significant differences in age, sex, peripheral blood eosinophil, cumulative PSL dose, or duration of oral corticosteroid between the groups with or without the presence of osteoporosis (Table 2). However, a significant increase in body mass index was observed in the group with the presence of osteoporosis but not in those without osteoporosis ($p < 0.01$). The cumulative PSL dose tended to be related to the reduction in BMD, but not significantly (Figure 2, $r = -0.28$, $p = 0.434$).

Table 2. Risk factors of osteoporosis.

	n	Osteoroporosis(+)	Osteoroporosis(−)
Age, mean (SD)	15	53.0 (11.5)	50.2 (11.5)
Sex, women versus men	15	3 vs 2	3 vs 7
Body mass index, kg/m², mean (SD)	15	0.79 (0.08)	1.01 (0.1)
Peripheral blood eosinophils, /μL, mean (SD)	15	726 (430)	942 (370)
Cumulative PSL dose, g, mean (SD)	15	14.2 (7.6)	11.2 (4.9)
Duration of PSL, mth, mean (SD)	15	67.6 (36.1)	55.0 (24.3)

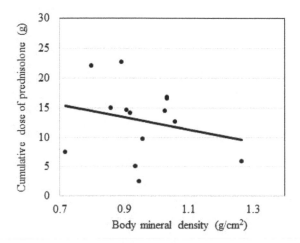

Figure 2. Relationship between cumulative prednisolone (PSL) and body mineral density ($r = -0.028$, $p = 0.434$).

4. Discussion

This study first revealed the prevalence of systemic adverse effects of frequent intermittent courses of oral corticosteroids for the prior 12 months, at least in patients with refractory nasal polyps from eosinophilic CRS. Based on a review of the literature [16], 16 articles were identified that evaluated the use of oral corticosteroids in patients with CRS and nasal polyps. However, no consensus was found to exist regarding the dosage or duration of the use of oral corticosteroids in the management of CRS and nasal polyps. All the studies highlighted benefits with very few adverse effects, and no severe adverse events were reported. We focused on glucose metabolism, suppression of the hypothalamic pituitary adrenal axis, and osteoporosis as adverse events.

Glucocorticoids are the main cause of drug-induced hyperglycemia/diabetes mellitus. The mechanisms that have been proposed to explain glucocorticoid-induced diabetes mellitus include decreased peripheral insulin sensitivity, increased hepatic glucose production, and inhibition of pancreatic insulin production and secretion [26]. Glucocorticoid-induced diabetes mellitus is common, but detection is generally difficult in a clinical setting due to the benign and asymptomatic profile. In the present study, we found only one out of 43 patients (2.3%) with glucocorticoid-induced diabetes mellitus. The frequency of glucocorticoid-induced diabetes mellitus in the present study was apparently lower than in a survey in Japan, which reported an incidence of approximately 6%–9% [27].

The use of corticosteroids is associated with numerous side effects and is considered to be the most common cause of adrenal insufficiency [28]. Chronic use of corticosteroids inhibits the function of the hypothalamic-pituitary-adrenal axis via negative feedback. Adrenal insufficiency is a serious, potentially life-threatening side effect of corticoid use. In asthma patients, the percentage of adrenal insufficiency ranges from 2.4% (low dose corticosteroids) to 21.5% (high dose corticosteroids), and according to treatment duration, from 1.4% (<28 days) to 27.4% (>1 year). These findings suggest that the risk of adrenal insufficiency cannot be excluded regardless of the dose or treatment duration [20]. A previous study [17] of patients with CRS with nasal polyps stated that asymptomatic adrenal insufficiency had a high prevalence of 48.8%. In contrast, in the present study, the use of oral corticosteroids in patients with eosinophilic CRS resulted in negligible adrenal insufficiency. However, oral corticosteroids should be used judiciously, understanding the potential complications of adrenal insufficiency associated with their long-term use.

Oral corticosteroid treatment has been associated with osteoporosis and an increased risk of fracture [29]. Bonfils et al. [17] reported a high prevalence of osteoporosis and osteopenia (12.2% and 48.8%, respectively) compared with the normal population. Patients with CRS with nasal polyps had taken at least four courses of oral steroid during the previous 12 months. Each course included PSL at 1 mg/kg body weight/day for 6–10 days. Rajasekaran et al. [18] evaluated the degree of osteoporosis in patients with CRS with and without nasal polyps, who had taken oral steroid (>5 mg daily) for at least three months. The overall prevalence of low bone density or osteopenia or osteoporosis was 38.6%. The cumulated steroid correlated strongly with bone density. In this study, we evaluated the effect of a short-course of 5–10 days of oral corticosteroids for at least 12 months based upon the bone metabolism assessed by objective measures of BMD. Approximately 30% of our subjects had a diagnosis of osteoporosis, but no subject had a vertebral fracture. No relationship was found between the cumulative PSL dose and BMD. Thus, long-term oral corticosteroid use, either short-course or daily-course, had an osteoporosis prevalence of 10%–30% in eosinophilic CRS. In patients taking long-term oral corticosteroids for chronic lung diseases, 58% had osteoporosis and 61% had a vertebral fracture. Furthermore, a high cumulative PSL dose is related to a low BMD [12]. Thus, the prevalence of osteoporosis in eosinophilic CRS is comparable to that in lung diseases, whereas the presence of vertebral fracture is completely different between upper and lower airway disorders. Nevertheless, the present study, a limited number of patients showed a trend of reduced BMD in relation to PSL use. Notably, low BMD is a risk factor for future fractures and appropriate treatment for osteoporosis is required.

This study has several limitations that need further investigation. First, the present study is a retrospective analysis of a series of cases. A case/control study with odds ratio calculation or a cohort study with relative risk calculation would be necessary to confirm our preliminary findings. Second, the present study evaluated the relationship between the adverse effects and cumulative dose of corticosteroid. However, the adverse effects of oral corticosteroid may depend on the daily dose, regimen of administration (continuous or frequent intermittent), or duration, which were not evaluated here. A larger sample size sufficient to classify differences in the types of dose and duration of oral corticosteroid therapy will allow the determination of the ideal dose with minimal adverse effects. Third, bone metabolism may be influenced by lifetime cigarette consumption, alcohol intake, calcium intake, age at menopause, exercise, glucose metabolism, and hypothalamic pituitary adrenal axis. Considering these multifactorial causes of the adverse effects may be necessary using a multivariable analysis including other variables that can influence the results.

5. Conclusions

Patients taking long-term and repeated short-course oral corticosteroids for refractory nasal polyps of eosinophilic CRS are likely to show a potentially increased risk for osteoporosis. However, no consensus exists on the dose and duration of oral corticosteroids prescription. Future research, including randomized controlled trials, registry studies, and prospective evaluations, are required to clarify the risk of osteoporosis in eosinophilic CRS patients.

Author Contributions: K.I. was involved in all stages of the study. R.M., S.I., H.H., N.O., H.O., Y.K., and A.S. were involved in data collection and laboratory examination. R.M. was involved in drafting the manuscript. All authors provided final approval for the publication of this manuscript. All authors read and approved the final manuscript.

Acknowledgments: This study was funded by a Grant-in-Aid (S1311011) from MEXT (Ministry of Education, Culture, Sports, Science and Technology) Supported Program for the Strategic Research Foundation at Private University.

Conflicts of Interest: The authors declare no conflict of interest. The founding sponsors had no role in the design of the study; in the collection, analyses, or interpretation of data; in the writing of the manuscript, and in the decision to publish the results.

References

1.   Bachert, C.; Zhang, N.; Hellings, P.W.; Bousquet, J. Endotype-driven care pathways in patients with chronic rhinosinusitis. *Allergy Clin. Immunol.* **2018**, *141*, 1543–1551. [CrossRef] [PubMed]

2.   Schleimer, R.P. Immunopathogenesis of Chronic Rhinosinusitis and Nasal Polyposis. *Annu. Rev. Pathol.* **2017**, *12*, 331–357. [CrossRef] [PubMed]

3.   Saitoh, T.; Kusunoki, T.; Yao, T.; Kawano, K.; Kojima, Y.; Miyahara, K.; Onoda, J.; Yokoi, H.; Ikeda, K. Role of interleukin-17A in the eosinophil accumulation and mucosal remodeling in chronic rhinosinusitis with nasal polyps associated with asthma. *Int. Arch. Allergy Immunol.* **2009**, *151*, 8–16. [CrossRef] [PubMed]

4.   Ikeda, K.; Shiozawa, A.; Ono, N.; Kusunoki, T.; Hirotsu, M.; Homma, H.; Saitoh, T.; Murata, J. Subclassification of chronic rhinosinusitis with nasal polyp based on eosinophil and neutrophil. *Laryngoscope* **2013**, *123*, E1–E9. [CrossRef] [PubMed]

5.   Van Zele, T.; Claeys, S.; Gevaert, P.; Van Maele, G.; Holtappels, G.; Van Cauwenberge, P.; Bachert, C. Differentiation of chronic sinus disease by measurement of inflammatory mediators. *Allergy* **2006**, *61*, 1280–1289. [CrossRef] [PubMed]

6.   Mygind, N.; Lildholdt, T. Nasal polyps treatment: Medical management. *Allergy Asthma Proc.* **1996**, *17*, 275–282. [CrossRef] [PubMed]

7.   Badia, L.; Lund, V. Topical corticosteroids in nasal polyposis. *Drugs* **2001**, *61*, 573–578. [CrossRef] [PubMed]

8.   Fokkens, W.J.; Lund, V.J.; Mullol, J.; Bachert, C.; Alobid, I.; Baroody, F.; Cohen, N.; Cervin, A.; Douglas, R.; Gevaert, P.; et al. EPOS 2012: European position paper on rhinosinusitis and nasal polyps 2012. A summary for otorhinolaryngologists. *Rhinology* **2012**, *50*, 1–12. [PubMed]

9. Stjarne, P.; Olsson, P.; Alenius, M. Use of mometasone furoate to prevent polyp relapse after endoscopic sinus surgery. *Arch. Otolaryngol. Head Neck Surg.* **2009**, *135*, 296–302. [CrossRef] [PubMed]

10. Dingsor, G.; Kramer, J.; Olsholt, R.; Soderstrom, T. Flunisolide nasal spray 0.025% in the prophylactic treatment of nasal polyposis after polypectomy. A randomized, double blind, parallel, placebo controlled study. *Rhinology* **1985**, *23*, 49–58. [PubMed]

11. Hissaria, P.; Smith, W.; Wormald, P.J.; Taylor, J.; Vadas, M.; Gillis, D.; Kette, F. Short course of systemic corticosteroids in sinonasal polyposis: A double-blind, randomized, placebo-controlled trial with evaluation of outcome measures. *J. Allergy Clin. Immunol.* **2006**, *118*, 128–133. [CrossRef] [PubMed]

12. Walsh, L.J.; Lewis, S.A.; Wong, C.A.; Cooper, S.; Oborne, J.; Cawte, S.A.; Harrison, T.; Green, D.J.; Pringle, M.; Hubbard, R.; et al. The impact of oral corticosteroid use on bone mineral density and vertebral fracture. *Am. J. Respir. Crit. Care Med.* **2002**, *166*, 691–695. [CrossRef] [PubMed]

13. Van Zele, T.; Gevaert, P.; Holtappels, G.; Beule, A.; Wormald, P.J.; Mayr, S.; Hens, G.; Hellings, P.; Ebbens, F.A.; Fokkens, W.; et al. Oral steroids and doxycycline: Two different approaches to treat nasal polyps. *J. Allergy Clin. Immunol.* **2010**, *125*, 1069–1076. [CrossRef] [PubMed]

14. Kirtsreesakul, V.; Wongsritrang, K.; Ruttanaphol, S. Clinical efficacy of a short course of systemic steroids in nasal polyposis. *Rhinology* **2011**, *49*, 525–532. [PubMed]

15. Vaidyanathan, S.; Barnes, M.; Williamson, P.; Hopkinson, P.; Donnan, P.T.; Lipworth, B. Treatment of chronic rhinosinusitis with nasal polyposis with oral steroids followed by topical steroids: A randomized trial. *Ann. Intern. Med.* **2011**, *154*, 293–302. [CrossRef] [PubMed]

16. Poetker, D.M. Oral corticosteroids in the management of chronic rhinosinusitis with and without nasal polyps: Risks and benefits. *Am. J. Rhinol. Allergy* **2015**, *29*, 339–342. [CrossRef] [PubMed]

17. Bonfils, P.; Halimi, P.; Malinvaud, D. Adrenal suppression and osteoporosis after treatment of nasal polyposis. *Acta Otolaryngol.* **2006**, *126*, 1195–1200. [CrossRef] [PubMed]

18. Rajasekaran, K.; Seth, R.; Abelson, A.; Betra, P.S. Prevalence of metabolic bone disease among chronic rhinosinusitis patients treated with oral glucorticoids. *Am. J. Rhinol. Allergy* **2010**, *24*, 215–219. [CrossRef] [PubMed]

19. Kapucu, B.; Cekin, E.; Erkul, B.E.; Cincik, H.; Gungor, A.; Berber, U. The effects of systemic, topical, and intralesional steroid treatments on apoptosis level of nasal polyps. *Otolaryngol. Head Neck Surg.* **2012**, *147*, 563–567. [CrossRef] [PubMed]

20. Broersen, L.H.A.; Pereira, A.M.; Jorgensen, J.O.L.; Dekkers, O.M. Adrenal insufficiency in corticosteroids use: Systemic review and meta-analysis. *J. Clin. Endocrinol. Metab.* **2015**, *100*, 2171–2180. [CrossRef] [PubMed]

21. Mullol, J.; Obando, A.; Pujols, L.; Alobid, I. Corticosteroid treatment in chronic rhinosinusitis: The possibilities and the limits. *Immunol. Allergy Clin. N. Am.* **2009**, *29*, 657–668. [CrossRef] [PubMed]

22. Tokunaga, T.; Sakashita, M.; Haruna, T.; Asaka, D.; Takeno, S.; Ikeda, H.; Nakayama, T.; Seki, N.; Ito, S.; Murata, J.; et al. Novel scoring system and algorithm for classifying chronic rhinosinusitis: The JESREC Study. *Allergy* **2015**, *70*, 995–1003. [CrossRef] [PubMed]

23. Ikeda, K.; Kondo, Y.; Sunose, H.; Hirano, K.; Oshima, T.; Shimomura, A.; Suzuki, H.; Takasaka, T. Subjective and objective evaluation in endoscopic sinus surgery. *Am. J. Rhinol.* **1996**, *10*, 217–220. [CrossRef]

24. Seino, Y.; Nanjo, K.; Tajima, N.; Kadowaki, T.; Kashiwagi, A.; Araki, E.; Ito, C.; Inagaki, N.; Iwamoto, Y.; Kasuga, M. Report of the committee on the classification and diagnostic criteria of diabetes mellitus. *J. Diabetes Investig.* **2010**, *1*, 212–228. [CrossRef] [PubMed]

25. Altman, D.G. *Practical Statistics for Medical Research*; Chapman and Hall: London, UK, 1996; pp. 299–303.

26. Delaunay, F.; Khan, A.; Cintra, A.; Davani, B.; Ling, Z.C.; Andersson, A.; Ostenson, C.G.; Gustafsson, J.A.; Efendic, S.; Okret, S. Pancreatic beta cells are important targets for the diabetogenic effects of glucocorticoids. *J. Clin. Investig.* **1997**, *100*, 2094–2098. [CrossRef] [PubMed]

27. Imatoh, T.; Sai, K.; Hori, K.; Segawa, K.; Kawakami, J.; Kimura, M.; Saito, Y. Development of a novel algorithm for detecting glucocorticoid-induced diabetes mellitus using a medical information database. *J. Clin. Pharm. Ther.* **2017**, *42*, 215–220. [CrossRef] [PubMed]

28. Arlt, W.; Allolio, B. Adrenal insufficiency. *Lancet* **2003**, *361*, 1881–1893. [CrossRef]

29. Adinoff, A.D.; Hollister, J.R. Steroid induced fractures and bone loss in patients with asthma. *N. Engl. J. Med.* **1983**, *309*, 265–268. [CrossRef] [PubMed]

17

The Role of Taste Receptors in Airway Innate Immune Defense

Alan D. Workman [1],* (iD), Neil N. Patel [1], Ryan M. Carey [1], Edward C. Kuan [1] and Noam A. Cohen [1,2,3]

[1] Department of Otorhinolaryngology, Head and Neck Surgery, University of Pennsylvania, Philadelphia, PA 19104, USA; neilnpatel89@gmail.com (N.N.P.); ryancarey91@gmail.com (R.M.C.); edwardkuan81@gmail.com (E.C.K.); noam.cohen@uphs.upenn.edu (N.A.C.)
[2] Monell Smell and Taste Center, Philadelphia, PA 19104, USA
[3] Philadelphia Veterans Affairs Medical Center, Philadelphia, PA 19104, USA
* Correspondence: WorkmanA@pennmedicine.upenn.edu

Abstract: Bitter (T2R) and sweet (T1R) taste receptors are expressed in the upper airway, where they play key roles in antimicrobial innate immune defense. Bitter bacterial products are detected by taste receptors on ciliated cells and solitary chemosensory cells, resulting in downstream nitric oxide and antimicrobial peptide release, respectively. Genetic polymorphisms in taste receptors contribute to variations in T1R and T2R functionality, and phenotypic differences correlate with disease status and disease severity in chronic rhinosinusitis (CRS). Correspondingly, there are also subjective bitter and sweet taste differences between patients with CRS and individuals without CRS across a number of compounds. The ability to capture these differences with a simple and inexpensive taste test provides a potentially useful diagnostic tool, while bitter compounds themselves could potentially serve as therapeutic agents. The present review examines the physiology of airway taste receptors and the recent literature elucidating the role taste receptors play in rhinologic disease.

Keywords: taste receptors; solitary chemosensory cell; taste test; T2R; T1R

1. Introduction

Taste receptors are typically associated with oral sensory perception as an adaptive mechanism for detecting energy rich foods as well as poisons and other unpalatable compounds. Bitter taste receptors are a specific subset of taste receptors that classically respond to toxins, chemicals, and other aversive products that can be detrimental to organismal health. However, recent research has identified taste receptors in many other anatomic compartments of the body with a variety of functions extending far beyond the canonical sensory capacity of the tongue [1–6]. Taste receptors have been found in the brain, pancreas, testicles, bladder, and gastrointestinal tract [1–4,7]. This review will examine the role of bitter and sweet taste receptors that are expressed in the airway, and the important roles that these taste receptors play in innate immune defense [8,9].

2. Taste Receptor Physiology

Bitter and sweet taste receptors, unlike the ion-sensitive salt and sour taste receptors, are G-protein coupled receptors (GPCRs) [10,11]. The sweet taste receptor (T1R) family responds to sugars, including sucrose, glucose, and fructose, and T1Rs are classified as a part of taste receptor family 1 subtype 2 and 3 (TAS1R2/TAS1R3) [5,12,13]. A wider variety of bitter taste receptors exist in taste receptor family 2 (T2Rs), and these diverse receptors respond to an assortment of bitter compounds [14], including sesquiterpene lactones, strychnine, and denatonium [15]. Each bitter taste receptor can respond to a multitude of chemically similar compounds, and each compound can stimulate more than one taste receptor. Humans have at least 25 T2R subtypes, reflecting a broad perceptual range [12,16]. There is also a high degree of genetic diversity in T2Rs. On a phenotypic level, this results in differing sensitivity to specific bitter compounds among individuals, both on the tongue and in the airway. This diversity partially explains variation in taste preferences between groups and within groups [17,18]. For example, certain individuals find some bitter foods, such as coffee, to be aversive, while others are less sensitive.

The mechanisms involved in taste receptor activation are relatively conserved and follow similar pathways in the tongue and airway. However, while the expression of taste receptors in the sinonasal epithelium is ubiquitous on disparate cell types, including ciliated cells and solitary chemosensory cells, in the tongue taste receptor expression is confined to type II cells within the taste buds. Furthermore, while some bitter taste receptors in the airway are upstream of a nervous signaling cascade, others act in a cell-autonomous fashion only [8,19,20]. When a ligand binds to a taste GPCR, there is activation of phospholipase C isoform β2 (PLCB2), which triggers downstream inositol 1,4,5-trisphosphate (IP3) production. The IP3 receptor on the endoplasmic reticulum releases calcium in response to this increase in IP3 [21]. Simultaneously, there is also an activation of phosphodiesterases (PDEs) that attenuate cyclic adenosine monophosphate (cAMP) levels and protein kinase A (PKA) activity. As PKA is an inhibitor of an IP3 receptor isoform, removal of this inhibition causes further release of calcium from the endoplasmic reticulum [22]. Calcium ultimately activates the non-selective cation channel, TRPM5, that causes cellular depolarization, activates voltage-gated sodium (Na^+) channels, and ultimately results in an action potential that causes ATP release through CALHM1, a large pore channel [5,22–25]. In the tongue, this ATP activates receptors on taste cells and sensory fibers that transmit sensations to the central nervous system [5,25,26].

3. Bitter Taste Receptors in the Airway

Many different bitter taste receptors are expressed in the rodent and human airways [9,27–30] and in these locations, they respond to bitter bacterial products that are produced. One example of this is the lactone class of bitter compounds, which includes acyl-homoserine lactones (AHLs) that are produced by many gram-negative bacteria [31,32]. These lactones serve as biofilm "quorum-sensing molecules"; bacteria will initiate biofilm formation when a high enough concentration of AHLs is reached in a localized area. Biofilms can provide protection for bacteria from host innate immune defenses as well as antibiotics [33]. It is hypothesized that bitter taste receptors attempt to "spy" on these bacterial communications, effectively detecting AHLs before a sufficient concentration is reached for biofilm formation [8]. The bitter taste receptors themselves elicit innate immune responses that can eradicate bacteria before pathogenic levels are achieved.

This highlights a critical component of upper airway immunity: recognition of foreign bacteria, viruses, fungi, or toxins, followed by prompt reduction in pathogenic biomass. Toll-like receptors (TLRs) respond to pathogen-associated molecular patterns (PAMPs), which include foreign cellular components. However, TLR signaling is gradual, taking up to 12 h to exert an immune response through changes in expression of genes that play a role in innate immunity [34]. Conversely, bitter taste receptors can detect bacterial products, such as AHLs, and elicit downstream increases in immune defenses in a much more expedient fashion (seconds to minutes).

3.1. Bitter Taste Receptors on Ciliated Cells

Bitter taste receptors on ciliated cells respond to bacterial compounds and elicit a potent downstream response of nitric oxide (NO) production [35,36] (Figure 1). Nitric oxide diffuses quickly into bacteria, where it participates in destruction of cellular components [9,37]. Some bacteria, such as *Pseudomonas aeruginosa*, are highly sensitive to NO, while others are more resistant [38]. In addition to this antimicrobial activity, NO also activates protein kinase G (PKG) and guanylyl cyclase to directly speed up ciliary beat frequency (CBF), increasing mucociliary clearance [39]. Rapid ciliary beating can clear bacteria and mucus to the nasopharynx or oropharynx, where they can be eliminated by swallowing. Additionally, released innate immune products are spread out across the airway surface by ciliary beating [40]. These compounds—including lactoferrin, lysozyme, and defensins—act in concert with NO and other reactive oxygen species to create a potent antimicrobial response [41].

T2R38 is a bitter taste receptor located on ciliated cells in humans, and it responds to at least three AHLs produced by *P. aeruginosa*: *N*-butyryl-L-homoserine lactone, *N*-hexanoyl-L-homoserine lactone and *N*-3-oxo-dodecanoyl-L-homoserine lactone [9]. In addition to its response to bacterial compounds, T2R38 reacts in a similar fashion to the compounds phenylthiocarbamide (PTC) and propylthiouracil (PROP) [42]. In response to PTC stimulation, sinonasal epithelial cells expressing a functional T2R38 receptor demonstrate a substantial increase in NO production. Importantly, the TRPM5 channel and PLCβ2 are necessary for this NO response, and these are two canonical components of taste signaling. Interestingly, the taste G-protein gustducin does not appear to be involved [9]. The resultant NO production following PTC stimulation is sufficient for a highly bactericidal response.

Just as the genetic variation in T2Rs can cause differences in taste preferences on the tongue, receptor variation in the airway also appears to play a key role in the ability to mount a respiratory defense in response to bitter compounds. The genetic locus for T2R38, *TAS2R38*, has common polymorphisms that can render the receptor non-functional. Individuals with a proline-alanine-valine (PAV) amino acid sequence at a key portion of the taste receptor are able to respond to T2R38 agonists, while individuals with an alanine-valine-isoleucine (AVI) sequence at this same locus possess a non-functional receptor variant [18]. Cells isolated from individuals with an AVI/AVI genotype show highly attenuated NO production in response to AHLs, PTC, or PROP stimulation, compared to cells isolated from individuals with a PAV/PAV genotype. Downstream reductions in mucociliary clearance and bacterial killing are correspondingly observed [9]. As would be expected, AVI/AVI individuals also do not taste PTC or PROP when presented with an oral taste test challenge [43].

This reduction in responsiveness observed in AVI-expressing individuals has clinical consequences. Several studies in the past five years have highlighted a potential relevance of T2R38 in chronic rhinosinusitis (CRS). Individuals who express the fully functional, PAV/PAV genotype are less likely to require surgical intervention for CRS symptoms than patients with an AVI/AVI genotype [43,44]. Additionally, levels of gram-negative infection are lower in PAV/PAV patients [43–46], confirming that the NO-dependent response of T2R38 acts as a critical defense for this class of bacteria. A hallmark of CRS is mucociliary stasis, in which bacteria are inadequately cleared. At pathogenic levels of proliferation, bacterial toxins can be destructive to cells and cilia, perpetuating the process of impaired mucociliary function [47]. It is known that sinonasal explants from patients with CRS have an attenuated response to a variety of compounds (bitter and non-bitter) that stimulate ciliary beating in control tissue [48]. Other studies, while part of an inconclusive set of literature, have shown differences in NO levels in patients with airway diseases [49]. Without the action of NO to kill bacteria and increase ciliary beating in response to AHLs, it appears that the non-functional T2R38 polymorphism has a phenotypic effect on upper airway disease [9].

Other bitter taste receptors on ciliated cells, such as T2R4 and T2R14 [50], respond to different bitter agonists, such as quinine hydrochloride. Quinine is an alkaloid derivative that is isolated from the cinchona tree, and is found in several medicinal and commercial products [51]. Recent work shows that quinine stimulates a rapid T2R-dependent NO response from ciliated cells in the airway [52]. While quinine is a more promiscuous bitter taste receptor agonist than PTC or PROP, there are common genetic variants in bitter taste receptor genes on chromosome 12 that strongly contribute to the perception of quinine taste intensity [53]. Quinine taste sensitivity has also been selected independently in some world populations, especially for low concentrations of quinine [54]. Concentrations of bitter microbial products in the airway are also at low concentrations [9], and these differences in taste perception of dilute quinine solutions may be reflective of varying responses of these bitter taste receptors in both the airway and on the tongue. Allele expression studies have shown that patients with CRS differ from control patients at several genetic loci for taste receptors, including TAS2R14 and TAS2R49 [45].

3.2. Taste Receptors on Solitary Chemosensory Cells

Solitary chemosensory cells (SCCs) are a non-ciliated airway cell type that is relatively rare, representing approximately 1% of the total upper airway epithelial cell population [55]. These cells are immunoreactive with α-gustducin, a taste signalling component, and they share many similarities with taste bud cells [28]. Because of their rarity, they are difficult to isolate experimentally [19]. Solitary chemosensory cells express both sweet and bitter taste receptors that are capable of responding to a variety of compounds [8,20,27,56,57]. In response to bitter stimulation, these cells do not activate NO production, but instead mediate a separate cohort of responses. In mouse SCCs, the calcium response resulting from bitter taste receptor stimulation causes acetylcholine (ACh) release that has breath holding effects and also results in downstream inflammatory mediator release [8,19,20]. Both of these responses are at least partially immunomodulatory in nature: breath holding limits toxin or organism aspiration, while inflammatory mediators often participate in a larger immune signaling cascade. In the human upper airway, SCC stimulation results in the calcium-mediated release of antimicrobial peptides from adjacent ciliated cells, including β-defensin 1 (DEFB1) and β-defensin 2 (DEFB2) [29,58] (Figure 1). These defensins are potently antimicrobial and have effects on both gram-positive and gram-negative bacteria, including methicillin-resistant *Staphylococcus aureus* and *P. aeruginosa* [59]. Unlike the antimicrobial peptide release observed with TLR stimulation, which occurs over several hours as a result of changes in messenger RNA [34], bitter taste receptor stimulation causes release of pre-formed stores of antimicrobial peptides. Denatonium is a specific bitter compound that has agonist properties for bitter taste receptors on SCCs, and application of denatonium to airway epithelial cells from mouse and human cultures stimulates calcium responses that spread to adjacent cells via gap junctions [29]. Similar to the cascades observed in bitter taste receptor stimulation in ciliated cells, the calcium responses from SCC stimulation also require canonical components of taste signaling, such as TRPM5, PLCβ2, and gustducin [29].

In addition to expressing bitter taste receptors, SCCs also express sweet taste receptors, the T1Rs [27,29,60]. These receptors are sensitive to sweet compounds, such as glucose, in concentrations far lower than those detected orally [61]. Typically, airway surface liquid (ASL) glucose levels are maintained at a homeostatic level of approximately 0.5 mM; there is a physiologic leak and continuous reuptake of glucose from the adjacent basolateral serum that maintains this concentration [29]. At this physiologic level of glucose, T1R2 and T1R3 receptors are tonically activated. The activation of sweet taste receptors on SCCs appears to antagonize the action of bitter taste receptor cascades through activation of cAMP and phosphodiesterase which subsequently block activation of the IP3 receptor [29]. During bacterial infection, there is a reduction in ASL glucose due to increased bacterial consumption. It is hypothesized that it is this reduction in glucose that causes a reduction in sweet taste receptor activation, resulting in a corresponding increase in bitter taste receptor activity and responsivity to microbial bitter products [29]. Thus, the balance tips in favor of T2R responses and mobilization of innate immune defenses, theoretically restoring the balance towards airway microbial homeostasis and normalized glucose concentrations.

Several experiments have been conducted to support this hypothesis of antagonistic actions of bitter and sweet taste receptors. When glucose or sucrose is added to airway surface liquid of in vitro mouse cultures, calcium responses to denatonium are greatly diminished. Mice that were genetically modified to not express sweet taste receptors showed a normal SCC response to denatonium under the same conditions [29,62]. Additional experiments have shown that T1Rs can also be activated by D-amino acids produced by bacteria. Lee et al. demonstrated that at least two T1R-activating D-amino acids produced by *S. aureus* suppress SCC calcium responses, with corresponding decreases in antimicrobial peptide secretion [58]. These D-amino acids may be produced by the bacteria for protection from host innate immune responses and may allow for increased colonization and potential opportunistic infection. Just as observed with T2Rs, there is *TAS1R* genetic variation that contributes to preferences in oral sweet taste perception [63]. Several allelic variations in *TAS1R* genes demonstrate frequency differences of greater than 10% when comparing CRS patients and control individuals [45]. Just as is the case with bitter receptors, there is genetic variation in *TAS1R* genes that manifests as individual preference in sweet taste [63]. While no single locus has yet been identified, there are allele variations among the *TAS1R* genes that show frequency differences of >10% in 16 loci between patients with CRS and controls [45].

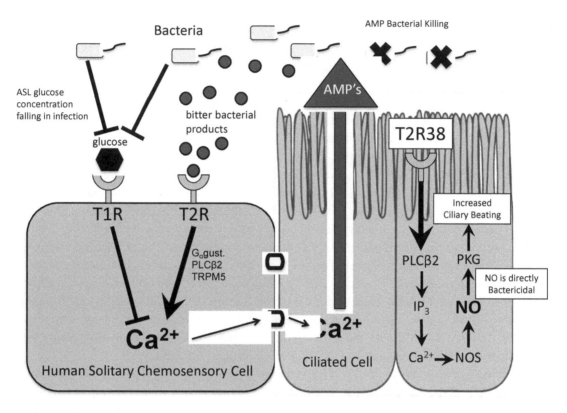

Figure 1. Bitter and sweet taste receptor-induced innate immune defenses in ciliated and solitary chemosensory cells in the human upper airway. ASL: airway surface liquid; AMP: anti-microbial peptide; NOS: nitric oxide synthase; NO: nitric oxide; PKG: protein kinase G.

3.3. Bitter and Sweet Taste Testing

Based on the existing evidence that genetic variation in bitter and sweet taste receptors is correlated with disease status and disease severity, phenotypic oral taste tests may be clinically useful to assess taste receptor variation. On a broad level, individuals with insensitive bitter taste receptors or hypersensitive sweet taste receptors would be expected to be overrepresented in a cohort of individuals with CRS. Two recent papers report on taste testing results in hundreds of patients with CRS as well as propensity matched control individuals without rhinologic disease [52,64]. Patients with CRS without nasal polyps perceived denatonium, an SCC T2R agonist, as having lower subjective intensity, while patients with CRS with nasal polyps perceived quinine, a ciliated cell T2R agonists, as having lower subjective intensity as well (Table 1). All CRS patients rated sucrose, a T1R agonist, as having higher subjective intensity. There was no difference in taste sensitivity to a neutral compound, sodium chloride, between CRS and control patients [52,64]. When bitter and sweet taste ratings were aggregated into an overall "score" that took into account the opposing physiologic effects of bitter and sweet taste receptor stimulation in SCCs, there were even more highly significant differences between CRS and control subjects. Some of these subjective taste differences also appear to be reflected at the physiologic level; experiments have shown an inverse association between in vitro biofilm formation and PTC taste intensity ratings [65]. The implications for these differences are broad. Physiologically, this may reflect a less active SCC response to bitter microbial products in the airway of CRS patients, with an additional compounding effect of an increased sensitivity to glucose. This increased glucose sensitivity would perhaps inhibit SCC T2R immunomodulatory function even with intact T2R responses, due to the relative T1R affinity. These phenotypic differences can also help explain why CRS tends to run in families, suggesting a critical genetic influence in the disease [66]. Furthermore, the stratification of patient sensitivity in ciliated and SCCs T2Rs based on CRS polyp status is additionally interesting, as this may demonstrate unique T2R contributions to different types of CRS.

Table 1. Subjective taste intensity ratings in patients with chronic rhinosinusitis (CRS) without nasal polyps (CRSsNP) and with nasal polyps (CRSwNP), relative to control patient taste intensity ratings.

	Bitter Perception		Sweet Perception	Salt Perception
	Quinine	Denatonium	Sucrose	NaCl
CRSsNP	No difference	Decreased	Increased	No difference
CRSwNP	Decreased	No difference	Increased	No difference

3.4. Diagnostics and Therapeutics

Oral taste tests are inexpensive to produce and administer, and the ability to assess variations in airway taste receptor functionality could help predict impaired innate immunity or predisposition to respiratory disease. Bitter taste testing with specific agonists, such as PTC, could potentially be used to stratify surgical candidates or identify individuals who should receive more aggressive management. With optimized taste testing compound concentrations that reflect respiratory tract affinity levels, improved patient stratification for CRS and control patients could be achieved. Additionally, the utilization of multiple bitter and sweet compounds for taste testing could improve performance parameters with an overall "taste score". Beyond the diagnostic realm, bitter taste receptor agonists may have therapeutic potential as topical agents in harnessing potent innate immune defenses as an alternative to more conventional treatments, such as antibiotics. T1R antagonists, such as lactisole and amiloride, could also release the inhibition of T1Rs on antimicrobial responses [29,67].

4. Conclusions

Bitter and sweet taste receptors play important roles in the regulation of innate immune defenses in the upper respiratory tract. Bitter taste receptors mediate rapid antimicrobial nitric oxide or β-defensin responses in the presence of bacterial compounds, while sweet taste receptors attenuate these responses at higher levels of glucose. There is a high degree of genetic variation in airway taste receptors, and genetic polymorphisms can predispose people to recalcitrant CRS and create an increased susceptibility to infection. Phenotypic oral taste tests can capture some of this taste receptor variation, correlating with disease status in CRS. Further, bitter taste receptor agonists and sweet taste receptor antagonists can potentially serve as alternative therapies for respiratory disease that harness endogenous immune defenses.

Author Contributions: A.D.W., N.N.P., R.M.C., and E.C.K. drafted the manuscript, N.A.C. conceived and designed many experiments described and critically reviewed the manuscript.

Funding: This work was supported by a grant from the RLG Foundation, In, and USPHS grant R01DC013588.

Conflicts of Interest: The authors declare no conflict of interest.

References

1. Laffitte, A.; Neiers, F.; Briand, L. Functional roles of the sweet taste receptor in oral and extraoral tissues. *Curr. Opin. Clin. Nutr. Metab. Care* **2014**, *17*, 379–385. [CrossRef] [PubMed]

2. Clark, A.A.; Liggett, S.B.; Munger, S.D. Extraoral bitter taste receptors as mediators of off-target drug effects. *FASEB J.* **2012**, *26*, 4827–4831. [CrossRef] [PubMed]

3. Depoortere, I. Taste receptors of the gut: Emerging roles in health and disease. *Gut* **2014**, *63*, 179–190. [CrossRef] [PubMed]

4. Behrens, M.; Meyerhof, W. Oral and extraoral bitter taste receptors. *Results Probl. Cell Differ.* **2010**, *52*, 87–99. [PubMed]

5. Kinnamon, S.C. Taste receptor signalling—From tongues to lungs. *Acta Physiol.* **2012**, *204*, 158–168. [CrossRef] [PubMed]

6. Sternini, C.; Anselmi, L.; Rozengurt, E. Enteroendocrine cells: A site of 'taste' in gastrointestinal chemosensing. *Curr. Opin. Endocrinol. Diabetes Obes.* **2008**, *15*, 73–78. [CrossRef] [PubMed]

7. Malki, A.; Fiedler, J.; Fricke, K.; Ballweg, I.; Pfaffl, M.W.; Krautwurst, D. Class I odorant receptors, TAS1R and TAS2R taste receptors, are markers for subpopulations of circulating leukocytes. *J. Leukoc. Biol.* **2015**, *97*, 533–545. [CrossRef] [PubMed]

8. Tizzano, M.; Gulbransen, B.D.; Vandenbeuch, A.; Clapp, T.R.; Herman, J.P.; Sibhatu, H.M.; Churchill, M.E.; Silver, W.L.; Kinnamon, S.C.; Finger, T.E. Nasal chemosensory cells use bitter taste signaling to detect irritants and bacterial signals. *Proc. Natl. Acad. Sci. USA* **2010**, *107*, 3210–3215. [CrossRef] [PubMed]

9. Lee, R.J.; Xiong, G.; Kofonow, J.M.; Chen, B.; Lysenko, A.; Jiang, P.; Abraham, V.; Doghramji, L.; Adappa, N.D.; Palmer, J.N.; et al. T2R38 taste receptor polymorphisms underlie susceptibility to upper respiratory infection. *J. Clin. Invest.* **2012**, *122*, 4145–4159. [CrossRef] [PubMed]

10. Zhang, Y.; Hoon, M.A.; Chandrashekar, J.; Mueller, K.L.; Cook, B.; Wu, D.; Zuker, C.S.; Ryba, N.J. Coding of sweet, bitter, and umami tastes: Different receptor cells sharing similar signaling pathways. *Cell* **2003**, *112*, 293–301. [CrossRef]

11. Iwata, S.; Yoshida, R.; Ninomiya, Y. Taste transductions in taste receptor cells: Basic tastes and moreover. *Curr. Pharm. Des.* **2014**, *20*, 2684–2692. [CrossRef] [PubMed]

12. Margolskee, R.F. Molecular mechanisms of bitter and sweet taste transduction. *J. Biol. Chem.* **2002**, *277*, 1–4. [CrossRef] [PubMed]

13. Treesukosol, Y.; Smith, K.R.; Spector, A.C. The functional role of the T1R family of receptors in sweet taste and feeding. *Physiol. Behav.* **2011**, *105*, 14–26. [CrossRef] [PubMed]

14. Adler, E.; Hoon, M.A.; Mueller, K.L.; Chandrashekar, J.; Ryba, N.J.; Zuker, C.S. A novel family of mammalian taste receptors. *Cell* **2000**, *100*, 693–702. [CrossRef]

15. Brockhoff, A.; Behrens, M.; Massarotti, A.; Appendino, G.; Meyerhof, W. Broad tuning of the human bitter taste receptor hTAS2R46 to various sesquiterpene lactones, clerodane and labdane diterpenoids, strychnine, and denatonium. *J. Agric. Food Chem.* **2007**, *55*, 6236–6243. [CrossRef] [PubMed]

16. Chandrashekar, J.; Mueller, K.L.; Hoon, M.A.; Adler, E.; Feng, L.; Guo, W.; Zuker, C.S.; Ryba, N.J. T2Rs function as bitter taste receptors. *Cell* **2000**, *100*, 703–711. [CrossRef]

17. Hayes, J.E.; Wallace, M.R.; Knopik, V.S.; Herbstman, D.M.; Bartoshuk, L.M.; Duffy, V.B. Allelic variation in TAS2R bitter receptor genes associates with variation in sensations from and ingestive behaviors toward common bitter beverages in adults. *Chem. Senses* **2011**, *36*, 311–319. [CrossRef] [PubMed]

18. Bufe, B.; Breslin, P.A.; Kuhn, C.; Reed, D.R.; Tharp, C.D.; Slack, J.P.; Kim, U.K.; Drayna, D.; Meyerhof, W. The molecular basis of individual differences in phenylthiocarbamide and propylthiouracil bitterness perception. *Curr. Biol.* **2005**, *15*, 322–327. [CrossRef] [PubMed]

19. Saunders, C.J.; Christensen, M.; Finger, T.E.; Tizzano, M. Cholinergic neurotransmission links solitary chemosensory cells to nasal inflammation. *Proc. Natl. Acad. Sci. USA* **2014**, *111*, 6075–6080. [CrossRef] [PubMed]

20. Gulbransen, B.; Silver, W.; Finger, T.E. Solitary chemoreceptor cell survival is independent of intact trigeminal innervation. *J. Comp. Neurol.* **2008**, *508*, 62–71. [CrossRef] [PubMed]

21. Giovannucci, D.R.; Groblewski, G.E.; Sneyd, J.; Yule, D.I. Targeted phosphorylation of inositol 1,4,5-trisphosphate receptors selectively inhibits localized Ca^{2+} release and shapes oscillatory Ca^{2+} signals. *J. Biol. Chem.* **2000**, *275*, 33704–33711. [CrossRef] [PubMed]

22. Taruno, A.; Matsumoto, I.; Ma, Z.; Marambaud, P.; Foskett, J.K. How do taste cells lacking synapses mediate neurotransmission? CALHM1, a voltage-gated ATP channel. *Bioessays* **2013**, *35*, 1111–1118. [CrossRef] [PubMed]

23. Zhang, Z.; Zhao, Z.; Margolskee, R.; Liman, E. The transduction channel TRPM5 is gated by intracellular calcium in taste cells. *J. Neurosci.* **2007**, *27*, 5777–5786. [CrossRef] [PubMed]

24. Miyoshi, M.A.; Abe, K.; Emori, Y. IP(3) receptor type 3 and PLCβ2 are co-expressed with taste receptors T1R and T2R in rat taste bud cells. *Chem. Senses* **2001**, *26*, 259–265. [CrossRef] [PubMed]

25. Taruno, A.; Vingtdeux, V.; Ohmoto, M.; Ma, Z.; Dvoryanchikov, G.; Li, A.; Adrien, L.; Zhao, H.; Leung, S.; Abernethy, M.; et al. CALHM1 ion channel mediates purinergic neurotransmission of sweet, bitter and umami tastes. *Nature* **2013**, *495*, 223–226. [CrossRef] [PubMed]

26. Behrens, M.; Born, S.; Redel, U.; Voigt, N.; Schuh, V.; Raguse, J.D.; Meyerhof, W. Immunohistochemical detection of TAS2R38 protein in human taste cells. *PLoS ONE* **2012**, *7*, e40304. [CrossRef] [PubMed]

27. Barham, H.P.; Cooper, S.E.; Anderson, C.B.; Tizzano, M.; Kingdom, T.T.; Finger, T.E.; Kinnamon, S.C.; Ramakrishnan, V.R. Solitary chemosensory cells and bitter taste receptor signaling in human sinonasal mucosa. *Int. Forum Allergy Rhinol.* **2013**, *3*, 450–457. [CrossRef] [PubMed]

28. Tizzano, M.; Cristofoletti, M.; Sbarbati, A.; Finger, T.E. Expression of taste receptors in solitary chemosensory cells of rodent airways. *BMC Pulm. Med.* **2011**, *11*, 3. [CrossRef] [PubMed]

29. Lee, R.J.; Kofonow, J.M.; Rosen, P.L.; Siebert, A.P.; Chen, B.; Doghramji, L.; Xiong, G.; Adappa, N.D.; Palmer, J.N.; Kennedy, D.W.; et al. Bitter and sweet taste receptors regulate human upper respiratory innate immunity. *J. Clin. Investig.* **2014**, *124*, 1393–1405. [CrossRef] [PubMed]

30. Shah, A.S.; Ben-Shahar, Y.; Moninger, T.O.; Kline, J.N.; Welsh, M.J. Motile cilia of human airway epithelia are chemosensory. *Science* **2009**, *325*, 1131–1134. [CrossRef] [PubMed]

31. Jimenez, P.N.; Koch, G.; Thompson, J.A.; Xavier, K.B.; Cool, R.H.; Quax, W.J. The multiple signaling systems regulating virulence in *Pseudomonas aeruginosa*. *Microbiol. Mol. Biol. Rev.* **2012**, *76*, 46–65. [CrossRef] [PubMed]

32. Li, Z.; Nair, S.K. Quorum sensing: How bacteria can coordinate activity and synchronize their response to external signals? *Protein Sci.* **2012**, *21*, 1403–1417. [CrossRef] [PubMed]

33. Parsek, M.R.; Greenberg, E.P. Acyl-homoserine lactone quorum sensing in gram-negative bacteria: A signaling mechanism involved in associations with higher organisms. *Proc. Natl. Acad. Sci. USA* **2000**, *97*, 8789–8793. [CrossRef] [PubMed]

34. Hume, D.A.; Underhill, D.M.; Sweet, M.J.; Ozinsky, A.O.; Liew, F.Y.; Aderem, A. Macrophages exposed continuously to lipopolysaccharide and other agonists that act via toll-like receptors exhibit a sustained and additive activation state. *BMC Immunol.* **2001**, *2*, 11. [CrossRef]

35. Carey, R.M.; Workman, A.D.; Chen, B.; Adappa, N.D.; Palmer, J.N.; Kennedy, D.W.; Lee, R.J.; Cohen, N.A. *Staphylococcus aureus* triggers nitric oxide production in human upper airway epithelium. *Int. Forum Allergy Rhinol.* **2015**, *5*, 808–813. [CrossRef] [PubMed]

36. Carey, R.M.; Workman, A.D.; Yan, C.H.; Chen, B.; Adappa, N.D.; Palmer, J.N.; Kennedy, D.W.; Lee, R.J.; Cohen, N.A. Sinonasal T2R-mediated nitric oxide production in response to *Bacillus cereus*. *Am. J. Rhinol. Allergy* **2017**, *31*, 211–215. [CrossRef] [PubMed]

37. Barraud, N.; Hassett, D.J.; Hwang, S.H.; Rice, S.A.; Kjelleberg, S.; Webb, J.S. Involvement of nitric oxide in biofilm dispersal of *Pseudomonas aeruginosa*. *J. Bacteriol.* **2006**, *188*, 7344–7353. [CrossRef] [PubMed]

38. Workman, A.D.; Carey, R.M.; Kohanski, M.A.; Kennedy, D.W.; Palmer, J.N.; Adappa, N.D.; Cohen, N.A. Relative susceptibility of airway organisms to antimicrobial effects of nitric oxide. *Int. Forum Allergy Rhinol.* **2017**, *7*, 770–776. [CrossRef] [PubMed]

39. Salathe, M. Regulation of mammalian ciliary beating. *Annu. Rev. Physiol.* **2007**, *69*, 401–422. [CrossRef] [PubMed]

40. Sleigh, M.A.; Blake, J.R.; Liron, N. The propulsion of mucus by cilia. *Am. Rev. Respir. Dis.* **1988**, *137*, 726–741. [CrossRef] [PubMed]

41. Parker, D.; Prince, A. Innate immunity in the respiratory epithelium. *Am. J. Respir. Cell Mol. Biol.* **2011**, *45*, 189–201. [CrossRef] [PubMed]

42. Kim, U.K.; Drayna, D. Genetics of individual differences in bitter taste perception: Lessons from the *PTC* gene. *Clin. Genet.* **2005**, *67*, 275–280. [CrossRef] [PubMed]

43. Adappa, N.D.; Zhang, Z.; Palmer, J.N.; Kennedy, D.W.; Doghramji, L.; Lysenko, A.; Reed, D.R.; Scott, T.; Zhao, N.W.; Owens, D.; et al. The bitter taste receptor T2R38 is an independent risk factor for chronic rhinosinusitis requiring sinus surgery. *Int. Forum Allergy Rhinol.* **2014**, *4*, 3–7. [CrossRef] [PubMed]

44. Adappa, N.D.; Howland, T.J.; Palmer, J.N.; Kennedy, D.W.; Doghramji, L.; Lysenko, A.; Reed, D.R.; Lee, R.J.; Cohen, N.A. Genetics of the taste receptor T2R38 correlates with chronic rhinosinusitis necessitating surgical intervention. *Int. Forum Allergy Rhinol.* **2013**, *3*, 184–187. [CrossRef] [PubMed]

45. Mfuna Endam, L.; Filali-Mouhim, A.; Boisvert, P.; Boulet, L.P.; Bosse, Y.; Desrosiers, M. Genetic variations in taste receptors are associated with chronic rhinosinusitis: A replication study. *Int. Forum Allergy Rhinol.* **2014**, *4*, 200–206. [CrossRef] [PubMed]

46. Adappa, N.D.; Workman, A.D.; Hadjiliadis, D.; Dorgan, D.J.; Frame, D.; Brooks, S.; Doghramji, L.; Palmer, J.N.; Mansfield, C.; Reed, D.R.; et al. T2R38 genotype is correlated with sinonasal quality of life in homozygous ΔF508 cystic fibrosis patients. *Int. Forum Allergy Rhinol.* **2016**, *6*, 356–361. [CrossRef] [PubMed]

47. Min, Y.G.; Oh, S.J.; Won, T.B.; Kim, Y.M.; Shim, W.S.; Rhee, C.S.; Min, J.Y.; Dhong, H.J. Effects of staphylococcal enterotoxin on ciliary activity and histology of the sinus mucosa. *Acta Otolaryngol.* **2006**, *126*, 941–947. [CrossRef] [PubMed]

48. Chen, B.; Shaari, J.; Claire, S.E.; Palmer, J.N.; Chiu, A.G.; Kennedy, D.W.; Cohen, N.A. Altered sinonasal ciliary dynamics in chronic rhinosinusitis. *Am. J. Rhinol.* **2006**, *20*, 325–329. [CrossRef] [PubMed]

49. Naraghi, M.; Deroee, A.F.; Ebrahimkhani, M.; Kiani, S.; Dehpour, A. Nitric oxide: A new concept in chronic sinusitis pathogenesis. *Am. J. Otolaryngol.* **2007**, *28*, 334–337. [CrossRef] [PubMed]

50. Yan, C.H.; Hahn, S.; McMahon, D.; Bonislawski, D.; Kennedy, D.W.; Adappa, N.D.; Palmer, J.N.; Jiang, P.; Lee, R.J.; Cohen, N.A. Nitric oxide production is stimulated by bitter taste receptors ubiquitously expressed in the sinonasal cavity. *Am. J. Rhinol. Allergy* **2017**, *31*, 85–92. [CrossRef] [PubMed]

51. Upadhyaya, J.D.; Chakraborty, R.; Shaik, F.A.; Jaggupilli, A.; Bhullar, R.P.; Chelikani, P. The Pharmacochaperone Activity of Quinine on Bitter Taste Receptors. *PLoS ONE* **2016**, *11*, e0156347. [CrossRef] [PubMed]

52. Workman, A.D.; Maina, I.W.; Brooks, S.G.; Kohanski, M.A.; Cowart, B.J.; Mansfield, C.; Kennedy, D.W.; Palmer, J.N.; Adappa, N.D.; Reed, D.R.; et al. The Role of Quinine-Responsive Taste Receptor Family 2 in Airway Immune Defense and Chronic Rhinosinusitis. *Front. Immunol.* **2018**, *9*, 624. [CrossRef] [PubMed]

53. Reed, D.R.; Zhu, G.; Breslin, P.A.; Duke, F.F.; Henders, A.K.; Campbell, M.J.; Montgomery, G.W.; Medland, S.E.; Martin, N.G.; Wright, M.J. The perception of quinine taste intensity is associated with common genetic variants in a bitter receptor cluster on chromosome 12. *Hum. Mol. Genet.* **2010**, *19*, 4278–4285. [CrossRef] [PubMed]

54. Ledda, M.; Kutalik, Z.; Souza Destito, M.C.; Souza, M.M.; Cirillo, C.A.; Zamboni, A.; Martin, N.; Morya, E.; Sameshima, K.; Beckmann, J.S.; et al. GWAS of human bitter taste perception identifies new loci and reveals additional complexity of bitter taste genetics. *Hum. Mol. Genet.* **2014**, *23*, 259–267. [CrossRef] [PubMed]

55. Zancanaro, C.; Caretta, C.M.; Merigo, F.; Cavaggioni, A.; Osculati, F. α-Gustducin expression in the vomeronasal organ of the mouse. *Eur. J. Neurosci.* **1999**, *11*, 4473–4475. [CrossRef] [PubMed]

56. Osculati, F.; Bentivoglio, M.; Castellucci, M.; Cinti, S.; Zancanaro, C.; Sbarbati, A. The solitary chemosensory cells and the diffuse chemosensory system of the airway. *Eur. J. Histochem.* **2007**, *51*, 65–72. [PubMed]

57. Lin, W.; Ezekwe, E.A.; Zhao, Z., Jr.; Liman, E.R.; Restrepo, D. TRPM5-expressing microvillous cells in the main olfactory epithelium. *BMC Neurosci.* **2008**, *9*, 114. [CrossRef] [PubMed]

58. Lee, R.J.; Hariri, B.M.; McMahon, D.B.; Chen, B.; Doghramji, L.; Adappa, N.D.; Palmer, J.N.; Kennedy, D.W.; Jiang, P.; Margolskee, R.F.; et al. Bacterial D-amino acids suppress sinonasal innate immunity through sweet taste receptors in solitary chemosensory cells. *Sci. Signal.* **2017**, *10*, eaam7703. [CrossRef] [PubMed]

59. Selsted, M.E.; Tang, Y.Q.; Morris, W.L.; McGuire, P.A.; Novotny, M.J.; Smith, W.; Henschen, A.H.; Cullor, J.S. Purification, primary structures, and antibacterial activities of β-defensins, a new family of antimicrobial peptides from bovine neutrophils. *J. Biol. Chem.* **1993**, *268*, 6641–6648. [CrossRef] [PubMed]

60. Braun, T.; Mack, B.; Kramer, M.F. Solitary chemosensory cells in the respiratory and vomeronasal epithelium of the human nose: A pilot study. *Rhinology* **2011**, *49*, 507–512. [PubMed]

61. Kalsi, K.K.; Baker, E.H.; Fraser, O.; Chung, Y.L.; Mace, O.J.; Tarelli, E.; Philips, B.J.; Baines, D.L. Glucose homeostasis across human airway epithelial cell monolayers: Role of diffusion, transport and metabolism. *Pflugers Arch.* **2009**, *457*, 1061–1070. [CrossRef] [PubMed]

62. Lemon, C.H.; Margolskee, R.F. Contribution of the T1R3 taste receptor to the response properties of central gustatory neurons. *J. Neurophysiol.* **2009**, *101*, 2459–2471. [CrossRef] [PubMed]

63. Bachmanov, A.A.; Bosak, N.P.; Lin, C.; Matsumoto, I.; Ohmoto, M.; Reed, D.R.; Nelson, T.M. Genetics of taste receptors. *Curr. Pharm. Des.* **2014**, *20*, 2669–2683. [CrossRef] [PubMed]

64. Workman, A.D.; Brooks, S.G.; Kohanski, M.A.; Blasetti, M.T.; Cowart, B.J.; Mansfield, C.; Kennedy, D.W.; Palmer, J.N.; Adappa, N.D.; Reed, D.R.; et al. Bitter and sweet taste tests are reflective of disease status in chronic rhinosinusitis. *J. Allergy Clin. Immunol. Pract.* **2017**, *6*, 1078–1080. [CrossRef] [PubMed]

65. Adappa, N.D.; Truesdale, C.M.; Workman, A.D.; Doghramji, L.; Mansfield, C.; Kennedy, D.W.; Palmer, J.N.; Cowart, B.J.; Cohen, N.A. Correlation of T2R38 taste phenotype and in vitro biofilm formation from nonpolypoid chronic rhinosinusitis patients. *Int. Forum Allergy Rhinol.* **2016**, *6*, 783–791. [CrossRef] [PubMed]

66. Cohen, N.A.; Widelitz, J.S.; Chiu, A.G.; Palmer, J.N.; Kennedy, D.W. Familial aggregation of sinonasal polyps correlates with severity of disease. *Otolaryngol. Head Neck Surg.* **2006**, *134*, 601–604. [CrossRef] [PubMed]

67. Jiang, P.; Cui, M.; Zhao, B.; Liu, Z.; Snyder, L.A.; Benard, L.M.; Osman, R.; Margolskee, R.F.; Max, M. Lactisole interacts with the transmembrane domains of human T1R3 to inhibit sweet taste. *J. Biol. Chem.* **2005**, *280*, 15238–15246. [CrossRef] [PubMed]

18

Medical Management of Chronic Rhinosinusitis in Adults

John Malaty

Department of Community Health and Family Medicine, University of Florida, Gainesville, FL 32609, USA; malaty@ufl.edu

Academic Editor: Claudina A. Pérez Novo

Abstract: Chronic rhinosinusitis can be refractory and has detrimental effects not only on symptoms, but also on work absences, work productivity, annual productivity costs, and disease-specific quality of life measures. The pathophysiology of chronic rhinosinusitis continues to evolve. There is evidence that it is driven by various inflammatory pathways and host factors and is not merely an infectious problem, although pathogens, including bacterial biofilms, may certainly contribute to this inflammatory cascade and to treatment resistance. Given this, medical management should be tailored to the specific comorbidities and problems in an individual patient. In addition to treating acute exacerbations of chronic rhinosinusitis with amoxicillin-clavulanate, second or third generation cephalosporins, or fluoroquinolones, one must consider if nasal polyps are present, when symptoms and disease severity correlate to mucosal eosinophilia, and there is the best evidence for intranasal corticosteroids and saline irrigation. Asthma worsens severity of chronic rhinosinusitis and it is felt to be mediated by increased leukotrienes, when leukotriene antagonists may be utilized. Cystic fibrosis has a genetic defect and increased mucin, which are potential treatment targets with dornase alfa showing efficacy. Other comorbidities that may impact treatment include allergies, ciliary dyskinesia, immunodeficiency, and possibly allergic fungal rhinosinusitis.

Keywords: treatment; medical; management; chronic; sinusitis; rhinosinusitis; adult; polyps

1. Introduction

Chronic rhinosinusitis affects all races to a significant extent. Prevalence within the United States in one study was 13.8% in African Americans, 13% in Caucasians, 8.8% in Hispanics, and 7% in Asians [1]. In another cross-sectional study in the United States, data examining 215 million adults demonstrated the prevalence of chronic rhinosinusitis was approximately 5%. It was associated with one lost workday per year, increased activity limitation (OR 1.54), work limitation (OR 1.50), and social limitation (OR 1.49) [2]. However, when looking at refractory chronic rhinosinusitis, mean lost work days per year was significantly worse at 25 when absent from work and 39 when considering absences from work, in addition to reduced performance at work. Overall, reduced annual productivity cost from refractory chronic rhinosinusitis was $10,077 per patient and it increased with worsening disease-specific quality of life measures [3]. This emphasizes that chronic rhinosinusitis has a significant impact on all ethnicities and has a large economic impact. Furthermore, the total annual cost of chronic rhinosinusitis in the United States was estimated to be $22 billion in 2014 (both direct and indirect costs) [4]. This highlights the importance of effective treatment. Unfortunately, it is evident that there are substantial disparities in the volume of research published on chronic rhinosinusitis over the past forty-five years when compared to other prevalent problems, such as asthma or diabetes mellitus [5]. Thus, we must carefully examine the currently available literature to enhance our treatment approach.

2. Definition and Classification

Rhinosinusitis is defined as inflammation of the paranasal sinuses and nasal cavity that causes symptoms. It may be classified as acute rhinosinusitis (ARS) when it lasts less than four weeks' duration or as chronic rhinosinusitis (CRS) when it lasts more than 12 weeks. During this time, patients may have acute exacerbations, superimposed on their chronic rhinosinusitis. Rhinosinusitis may be caused by viruses, bacteria, fungi, and noninfectious causes, although primary emphasis has recently been placed on noninfectious and bacterial causes [6].

3. Diagnosis and Assessment

Clinicians should assess for nasal obstruction, facial pain/pressure/fullness, purulent nasal discharge, and hyposmia, with two or more symptoms for greater than 12 weeks being highly sensitive for CRS. However, since these symptoms are also nonspecific, it is also recommended that patients have objective evidence of sinonasal inflammation, which can be visualized during anterior rhinoscopy, nasal endoscopy, or on computed tomography. Inflammation is documented when one visualizes purulent rhinorrhea or edema in the middle meatus or anterior ethmoid region, polyps in the nasal cavity or middle meatus, and/or radiographic findings of inflammation. These findings and the patient's symptoms should be persistent for greater than 12 weeks despite adequate treatment for ARS, in order to diagnose CRS [6–9].

In addition, clinicians should assess for other factors that may affect treatment in CRS: the presence or absence of nasal polyps, asthma, cystic fibrosis, ciliary dyskinesia, and an immunocompromised state. One may also consider obtaining testing for allergy and immune function [6,10–14].

4. Treatment

4.1. Acute Exacerbations of CRS and Biofilms

It is widely accepted that acute exacerbations of CRS should be treated with oral antibiotics and this is recommended by American, European, and Canadian guidelines/position papers [15–18]. It is well accepted that bacteria trigger ARS and there has been concern that inadequately treated ARS could cause CRS but this is currently unclear. Many reports show increased rates of *Staphylococcus aureus*, Gram-negative rods, and anaerobes in CRS [19–27]. However, some studies have not shown differences in microbiology between patients with CRS and controls, and it has also been shown that there are similar bacteria in the diseased and non-diseased contralateral sides of the same patient, which raises the question of bacterial colonization *versus* pathologic involvement in CRS [28–30]. It is also possible that these studies may have methodological differences, including performing cultures after antibiotic treatment, patients may have comorbidities affecting these patients' symptoms that were not identified (*i.e.*, allergies), and there is some evidence that bacterial biofilms and bacteria within epithelial cells contribute to inflammatory cascades, but these are not readily detected via standard techniques [31–33].

Biofilms including *Streptococcus pneumonia*, *Haemophilus influenzae*, *Moraxella catarrhalis*, *S. aureus*, and *Pseudomonas aeruginosa* have been commonly identified in CRS patients both with and without nasal polyps [34–38]. There is evidence that epithelial disruption can be present in CRS and this may contribute to biofilm formation [39]. It is clear that bacteria causing an acute exacerbation should be treated, but eradication of possibly colonizing bacteria is not advocated at this time. However, bacterial biofilms raise the concern that pathologic bacteria are present and evading host defenses that are not identified in traditional cultures. These are not felt to be colonizing bacteria. Furthermore, they have shown to be involved in both Th1 and Th2 immune responses [40,41]. In addition, patients with biofilms have more severe preoperative sinus disease, persistence of postoperative symptoms after sinus surgery, ongoing mucosal inflammation, and infections [42–45]. Effective treatments targeting biofilms merit further study. *In vitro*, photodynamic therapy has shown promise at eradicating *P. aeruginosa* and methicillin-resistant *S. aureus*, without causing abnormalities of the epithelium or respiratory cilia [46–48]. Clinical studies of this therapy are needed to determine if it is efficacious in patients.

In general, empiric oral antibiotics are used to treat acute exacerbations and antibiotic coverage can potentially be narrowed when positive cultures are available. Empiric antibiotic coverage targets common bacteria found in CRS: *S. pneumonia*, *H. influenzae*, *M. catarrhalis*, *S. aureus*, *P. aeruginosa*, and anaerobes [27]. Antibiotics should be prescribed after considering local antibiotic sensitivity patterns. In general, some effective options include amoxicillin-clavulanate, second or third generation cephalosporins, and respiratory fluoroquinolones [49].

4.2. Chronic Rhinosinusitis with Nasal Polyps

There is a lot of evidence emerging that *S. aureus* is implicated in at least a subset of patients with CRS with nasal polyps. There has been a suggestion this may be occurring because colonizing staphylococcal bacteria are producing superantigenic toxins (Sags) that increase eosinophilic inflammation and promote the formation of nasal polyps, in addition to evidence of B and T cell responses in local tissues to these staph superantigens [50,51]. This has not been found uniformly in patients with nasal polyps and it is felt to be a contributor, as opposed to a single etiology. At this time, acute exacerbations in CRS with nasal polyps should include treatment for *S. aureus* [52].

The inflammatory cascade has been demonstrated to be active in a variety of different ways in CRS with nasal polyps. There has been evidence of local eosinophilic infiltration (mediated by increased GM-CSF), mast cell degranulation, interleukin upregulation (*i.e.*, including but not limited to IL-4, IL-5, IL-8, IL-13, IL-32), VPF/VEGF upregulation, increase in T lymphocytes, increase in dendritic cells, and other pro-inflammatory activity [53–60]. Sinus mucosal eosinophilia (>5/hpf) in histologic samples of patients with CRS correlated with worse CRS disease severity on CT, endoscopy, and smell identification test (hyposmia), whereas the total eosinophil counts correlated with the presence of nasal polyps, asthma, and aspirin intolerance [61].

When nasal polyps are present in CRS, patients should be treated with intranasal therapy, including topical intranasal steroids and/or saline nasal irrigation for symptomatic relief, in addition to long-term management of the nasal polyps themselves with intranasal glucocorticoids which decrease polyp size, polyp recurrence, decrease nasal symptoms, and improve nasal airflow [6,62–70]. Glucocorticoids have been shown to impact epithelial GM-CSF and prolong eosinophil survival [71]. Topical intranasal corticosteroids are more effective when administered with correct technique but there does not appear to be a significant difference between corticosteroids. Oral corticosteroids are effective in decreasing polyp size and nasal symptoms in the short term, but this must be balanced with the risks of oral corticosteroids [72,73]. It may be useful for planned short-term improvement. Long-term oral macrolides may be beneficial because of their anti-inflammatory effects, but this needs to be further elucidated through further study of randomized placebo-controlled trials to better assess the benefits *versus* risks [15,74–77]. Intranasal saline irrigation should be used, as opposed to intranasal saline spray because of increased effectiveness on symptom relief and improving quality of life [68,78].

Endoscopic sinus surgery is safe and effective in patients with CRS with nasal polyps and is typically recommended when patients' signs and symptoms are refractory to medical therapy. In one randomized study, endoscopic sinus surgery was shown to have equivalent efficacy to medical management [79,80].

4.3. Chronic Rhinosinusitis without Nasal Polyps

Intranasal steroids and/or nasal saline irrigation have been shown to be beneficial in CRS without nasal polyps with improved symptom scores [81–86]. This improvement did not seem to be significantly related to a specific corticosteroid. Subgroup analysis suggests that sinus delivery methods may be more effective than nasal delivery.

Additions to nasal saline irrigation that have shown benefit include sodium hypochlorite 0.05% in patients with *S. aureus* [87]. This is also felt to have possible effects on *P. aeruginosa* although further trials need to be done to better evaluate this. Using xylitol in water as a sinonasal irrigation improved symptom control compared to saline irrigation and can potentially be a useful adjunctive treatment [88].

There is inadequate data to promote the use of oral steroids in CRS without nasal polyps [89]. Topical antibiotics do not show benefit in CRS without nasal polyps [90–93]. Long-term antibiotics, primarily macrolides (azithromycin 500 g weekly or roxithromycin 150 g daily), have shown possible therapeutic response after treatment for 12 weeks, but the evidence is very limited and subject to bias [75–77,94–97]. Further study with placebo-controlled randomized controlled trials is needed to make further conclusions. In addition, as in other conditions that use low-dose long-term antibiotics, there is concern for development of antibiotic resistant bacteria with subsequent infections.

Endoscopic sinus surgery in CRS without nasal polyps has been shown to be safe and effective when medical treatment has failed.

4.4. Allergy

Allergic rhinitis is present in 40%–84% of patients with CRS [98,99]. Patients with allergies and CRS are also more symptomatic than those that have CRS without allergic rhinitis, despite similar CT findings [100,101]. Allergy testing is an option for patients with CRS, with allergy skin testing being the preferred method to evaluate for IgE-mediated sensitivity [102]. There is some, albeit limited, evidence that allergen avoidance or immunotherapy improves CRS [15,103]. Intranasal glucocorticoids and/or nasal irrigation can be beneficial. It is felt that allergic rhinitis is a superimposed exacerbating factor of CRS.

4.5. Asthma and Aspirin Sensitivity

There is a high prevalence of CRS in patients with asthma and they have found that asthma severity directly correlates with the severity of sinus disease on imaging [11,12,104]. When CRS is treated (medically or surgically), asthma symptoms improve and the need for asthma medications decreases [105–108].

Some patients may also have aspirin sensitivity (in the presence or absence of asthma) which has been found to be secondary to upregulation of eicosanoids, mediated by oxidative metabolism of arachidonic acid, with a specific increase of leukotrienes (LTB4, LTC4, LTD4, and LTE4). Leukotrienes in airway mucosa are primarily released by mast cells and eosinophils. These leukotrienes bind to receptors CYSLTR1 and CYSLTR2. In aspirin-tolerant patients with asthma or allergic rhinitis, leukotriene inhibitors that antagonize CYSLTR1 can be potentially beneficial (montelukast and zafirlukast). There has been a study that combined treatment with intranasal fluticasone and montelukast and demonstrated decreased peripheral blood eosinophil counts that correlated with improvement of nasal polyp size and CT findings, in addition to others that demonstrate montelukast is better than placebo in CRS with nasal polyps [109,110]. The studies to date do not elucidate how much improvement you get in CRS beyond the effect of intranasal corticosteroids, but its use in patients with concomitant asthma would provide additional benefit in controlling asthma. The strongest association with leukotriene levels, aside from aspirin sensitivity, is present with nasal polyps. Leukotriene levels were found to be highest in aspirin-sensitive polyps, followed by CRS with nasal polyps (without aspirin sensitivity), CRS without nasal polyps, and then normal mucosa [111–115]. In aspirin sensitive patients, aspirin avoidance is an important part of the management plan. One may also consider aspirin desensitization.

4.6. Cystic Fibrosis (CF)

CRS is reported in 30 to 67% of patients with CF (within all age groups) [116–119]. Some studies have suggested that this may be because of genetic mutation, such as the ΔF508 and 394delTT mutation in Finland [120]. It is clearer that similar bacteria occupy the upper and lower airways of these CF patients, suggesting a possible spread from the upper to lower airways [121–124]. In addition, COX-1 and COX-2 are upregulated in CF patients with CRS leading to increased prostaglandin levels and there is an increase in mucus gland proliferation, surfactant gene expression, and MUC mucin gene expression. These findings suggest that inflammatory pathways may be treatment targets, in addition to gene therapy and treatment of their microbiology. More aggressive combined medical and surgical treatment demonstrates improved control of CRS in CF patients [125–128]. A mucolytic, dornase alfa, once daily (2.5 mg) administered intranasally either one month after endoscopic sinus surgery, or without surgery in another trial, has been found to be improve nasal symptoms, endoscopic appearance, CT findings, forced expiratory volume in 1 s, and quality of life compared to hypotonic saline or normal saline [129,130]. It is also used for lower airway disease in these patients, but with different dosing regimens and administration route (oral inhalation). Reviews of topical antimicrobials show that they should not be first-line therapies in CF patients for CRS [131]. Nasal irrigation or nebulization was more effective than when applied by nasal spray. Initial attempts to use gene therapy via a viral vector (transmembrane conductance regulator) has been tried in CF patients but has not yet been found to be effective, although it was safely administered to the sinuses [132]. There was a case report of successful use of ivacaftor in refractory CRS in a patient that had the related CF gene defect. Ivacaftor, a CF transmembrane conductance regulator (CFTR) potentiator, targets the G55ID-CFTR mutation in CF [133]. Limited data demonstrates that endoscopic sinus surgery results in similar improvement in CF *versus* non-CF patients with CRS. In addition, patients with CF that have endoscopic sinus surgery with serial antimicrobial lavage had better outcomes than surgery alone [126,134].

4.7. Ciliary Dyskinesia

Decreased mucociliary clearance from ciliary dyskinesia impacts a small percentage of patients with CRS (aside from CF). Mucociliary transit time (MTT) is prolonged when patients have underlying genetic-related ciliary dyskinesia [135–137]. However, there are conflicting results regarding decreased ciliary beat frequency as part of the pathogenesis of CRS and it is still not well understood [136]. Effective treatments need to be further elucidated.

4.8. Immunodeficiency

Some immunodeficient states are found in patients with CRS, including selective IgA deficiency, specific antibody deficiency, common variable immunodeficiency, and human immunodeficiency virus infection (HIV) [138]. Testing for these immunodeficiencies is important to consider in these CRS patients, especially in those with refractory CRS to aggressive treatment or if they have associated otitis media, bronchiectasis, or pneumonia. Testing may demonstrate low serum IgA, low serum IgG, functional abnormalities of IgG to polysaccharide vaccines (based on pre-immunization and post-immunization antibody responses to pneumococcal polysaccharide vaccines or tetanus toxoid), abnormal CH50, decreased measurement of T-cell number and function (tested via delayed hypersensitivity skin testing and flow cytometry analysis of T cells), and positive HIV testing [139–142]. Treatment with intravenous immunoglobulins (IVIG) and/or prophylactic antibiotics is indicated in those with immunoglobulin deficiency, which can improve survival and decrease life-threatening infections [143]. However, it does not appear to affect radiologic appearance of CRS and it is unclear that this clinically improves CRS [144]. Those with immunosuppression from HIV infection should be treated for HIV to raise their CD4 count.

4.9. Fungal

Fungi have been found to be prevalent in patients with CRS and local nasal tissue samples exhibit increased eosinophils, but without increased IgE to indicate a mold allergy. There have been concerns that the eosinophilic response in these patients may be secondary to other underlying etiologies. For instance, the majority of these patients had concomitant asthma that could explain the eosinophilic response. It is recommended not to use oral or topical antifungals given greater risk of harm over potential benefit based on systematic reviews of randomized controlled trials, in addition to their high cost [6,64,69,74,145–147]. One area that remains less clear is allergic fungal rhinosinusitis which appears to be a clinically distinct entity. It demonstrates a Th2 immune response and also has specific IgE in eosinophilic mucin and mucosa [148–150]. Treatment impact of this needs to be further elucidated. Surgery with and without concomitant medical management has been beneficial in allergic fungal rhinosinusitis [151].

5. Conclusions

Chronic rhinosinusitis presents with uniform signs and symptoms, but should be medically managed according to the medical comorbidities and clinical features present in an individual patient. Inflammatory pathways and host factors continue to be elucidated and treatments will likely continue to evolve as these are better understood, including the potential treatment of bacterial biofilms and modification of the inflammatory cascade in subsets of chronic rhinosinusitis patients.

Conflicts of Interest: The author declares no conflict of interest.

References

1. Soler, Z.M.; Mace, J.C.; Litvack, J.R.; Smith, T.L. Chronic rhinosinusitis, race, and ethnicity. *Am. J. Rhinol. Allergy* **2012**, *26*, 110–116. [CrossRef] [PubMed]
2. Bhattacharyya, N. Functional limitations and workdays lost associated with chronic rhinosinusitis and allergic rhinitis. *Am. J. Rhinol. Allergy* **2012**, *26*, 120–122. [CrossRef] [PubMed]
3. Rudmik, L.; Smith, T.L.; Schlosser, R.J.; Hwang, P.H.; Mace, J.C.; Soler, Z.M. Productivity costs in patients with refractory chronic rhinosinusitis. *Laryngoscope* **2014**, *124*, 2007–2012. [CrossRef] [PubMed]
4. Smith, K.A.; Orlandi, R.R.; Rudmik, L. Cost of adult chronic rhinosinusitis: A systematic review. *Laryngoscope* **2015**, *125*, 1547–1556. [CrossRef] [PubMed]
5. Rudmik, L. Chronic rhinosinusitis: An under-researched epidemic. *J. Otolaryngol. Head Neck Surg.* **2015**, *44*, 11. [CrossRef] [PubMed]
6. Rosenfeld, R.M.; Piccirillo, J.F.; Chandrasekhar, S.S.; Brook, I.; Kumar, K.A.; Kramper, M.; Orlandi, R.R.; Palmer, J.N.; Patel, Z.M.; Peters, A.; et al. Clinical practice guideline (update): Adult sinusitis executive summary. *Otolaryngol. Head Neck Surg.* **2015**, *152*, 598–609. [CrossRef] [PubMed]
7. Bhattacharyya, N. Clinical and symptom criteria for the accurate diagnosis of chronic rhinosinusitis. *Laryngoscope* **2006**, *116*, 1–22. [CrossRef] [PubMed]
8. Hwang, P.H.; Irwin, S.B.; Griest, S.E.; Caro, J.E.; Nesbit, G.M. Radiologic correlates of symptom-based diagnostic criteria for chronic rhinosinusitis. *Otolaryngol. Head Neck Surg.* **2003**, *128*, 489–496. [CrossRef]
9. Stankiewicz, J.A.; Chow, J.M. Nasal endoscopy and the definition and diagnosis of chronic rhinosinusitis. *Otolaryngol. Head Neck Surg.* **2002**, *126*, 623–627. [CrossRef] [PubMed]
10. Lanza, D.C.; Kennedy, D.W. Adult rhinosinusitis defined. *Otolaryngol. Head Neck Surg.* **1997**, *117*, S1–S7. [CrossRef]
11. Ten Brinke, A.; Grootendorst, D.C.; Schmidt, J.T.; De Bruine, F.T.; van Buchem, M.A.; Sterk, P.J.; Rabe, K.F.; Bel, E.H. Chronic sinusitis in severe asthma is related to sputum eosinophilia. *J. Allergy Clin. Immunol.* **2002**, *109*, 621–626. [CrossRef] [PubMed]
12. Lin, D.C.; Chandra, R.K.; Tan, B.K.; Zirkle, W.; Conley, D.B.; Grammer, L.C.; Kern, R.C.; Schleimer, R.P.; Peters, A.T. Association between severity of asthma and degree of chronic rhinosinusitis. *Am. J. Rhinol. Allergy* **2011**, *25*, 205–208. [CrossRef] [PubMed]
13. Wang, L.; Freedman, S.D. Laboratory tests for the diagnosis of cystic fibrosis. *Am. J. Clin. Pathol.* **2002**, *117*, S109–S115. [CrossRef] [PubMed]
14. Cowan, M.J.; Gladwin, M.T.; Shelhamer, J.H. Disorders of ciliary motility. *Am. J. Med. Sci.* **2001**, *321*, 3–10. [CrossRef] [PubMed]
15. Fokkens, W.J.; Lund, V.J.; Mullol, J.; Bachert, C.; Alobid, I.; Baroody, F.; Cohen, N.; Cervin, A.; Douglas, R.; Gevaert, P.; et al. European position paper on rhinosinusitis and nasal polyps 2012. *Rhinol. Suppl.* **2012**, *23*, 1–298.
16. Kaplan, A. Canadian guidelines for chronic rhinosinusitis: Clinical summary. *Can. Fam. Phys.* **2013**, *59*, 1275–1281.

17. Rosenfeld, R.M.; Piccirillo, J.F.; Chandrasekhar, S.S.; Brook, I.; Ashok Kumar, K.; Kramper, M.; Orlandi, R.R.; Palmer, J.N.; Patel, Z.M.; Peters, A.; et al. Clinical practice guideline (update): Adult sinusitis. *Otolaryngol. Head Neck Surg.* **2015**, *152*, S1–S39. [CrossRef] [PubMed]

18. Thomas, M.; Yawn, B.P.; Price, D.; Lund, V.; Mullol, J.; Fokkens, W.; European Position Paper on Rhinosinusitis and Nasal Polyps Group. Epos primary care guidelines: European position paper on the primary care diagnosis and management of rhinosinusitis and nasal polyps 2007—A summary. *Prim. Care Respir. J.* **2008**, *17*, 79–89. [CrossRef] [PubMed]

19. Meltzer, E.O.; Hamilos, D.L.; Hadley, J.A.; Lanza, D.C.; Marple, B.F.; Nicklas, R.A.; Bachert, C.; Baraniuk, J.; Baroody, F.M.; Benninger, M.S.; et al. Rhinosinusitis: Establishing definitions for clinical research and patient care. *J. Allergy Clin. Immunol.* **2004**, *114*, 155–212. [CrossRef] [PubMed]

20. Brook, I. Microbiology of sinusitis. *Proc. Am. Thorac. Soc.* **2011**, *8*, 90–100. [CrossRef] [PubMed]

21. Doyle, P.W.; Woodham, J.D. Evaluation of the microbiology of chronic ethmoid sinusitis. *J. Clin. Microbiol.* **1991**, *29*, 2396–2400. [PubMed]

22. Finegold, S.M.; Flynn, M.J.; Rose, F.V.; Jousimies-Somer, H.; Jakielaszek, C.; McTeague, M.; Wexler, H.M.; Berkowitz, E.; Wynne, B. Bacteriologic findings associated with chronic bacterial maxillary sinusitis in adults. *Clin. Infect. Dis.* **2002**, *35*, 428–433. [CrossRef] [PubMed]

23. Hoyt, W.H., 3rd. Bacterial patterns found in surgery patients with chronic sinusitis. *J. Am. Osteopath. Assoc.* **1992**, *92*, 209–212.

24. Hsu, J.; Lanza, D.C.; Kennedy, D.W. Antimicrobial resistance in bacterial chronic sinusitis. *Am. J. Rhinol.* **1998**, *12*, 243–248. [CrossRef] [PubMed]

25. Jiang, R.S.; Lin, J.F.; Hsu, C.Y. Correlation between bacteriology of the middle meatus and ethmoid sinus in chronic sinusitis. *J. Laryngol. Otol.* **2002**, *116*, 443–446. [CrossRef] [PubMed]

26. Kim, H.J.; Lee, K.; Yoo, J.B.; Song, J.W.; Yoon, J.H. Bacteriological findings and antimicrobial susceptibility in chronic sinusitis with nasal polyp. *Acta Otolaryngol.* **2006**, *126*, 489–497. [PubMed]

27. Mantovani, K.; Bisanha, A.A.; Demarco, R.C.; Tamashiro, E.; Martinez, R.; Anselmo-Lima, W.T. Maxillary sinuses microbiology from patients with chronic rhinosinusitis. *Braz. J. Otorhinolaryngol.* **2010**, *76*, 548–551. [CrossRef] [PubMed]

28. Bhattacharyya, N. Bacterial infection in chronic rhinosinusitis: A controlled paired analysis. *Am. J. Rhinol.* **2005**, *19*, 544–548. [PubMed]

29. Niederfuhr, A.; Kirsche, H.; Deutschle, T.; Poppert, S.; Riechelmann, H.; Wellinghausen, N. *Staphylococcus aureus* in nasal lavage and biopsy of patients with chronic rhinosinusitis. *Allergy* **2008**, *63*, 1359–1367. [CrossRef] [PubMed]

30. Niederfuhr, A.; Kirsche, H.; Riechelmann, H.; Wellinghausen, N. The bacteriology of chronic rhinosinusitis with and without nasal polyps. *Arch. Otolaryngol. Head Neck Surg.* **2009**, *135*, 131–136. [CrossRef] [PubMed]

31. Palmer, J.N. Bacterial biofilms: Do they play a role in chronic sinusitis? *Otolaryngol. Clin. N. Am.* **2005**, *38*, 1193–1201. [CrossRef] [PubMed]

32. Clement, S.; Vaudaux, P.; Francois, P.; Schrenzel, J.; Huggler, E.; Kampf, S.; Chaponnier, C.; Lew, D.; Lacroix, J.S. Evidence of an intracellular reservoir in the nasal mucosa of patients with recurrent *Staphylococcus aureus* rhinosinusitis. *J. Infect. Dis.* **2005**, *192*, 1023–1028. [CrossRef] [PubMed]

33. Plouin-Gaudon, I.; Clement, S.; Huggler, E.; Chaponnier, C.; Francois, P.; Lew, D.; Schrenzel, J.; Vaudaux, P.; Lacroix, J.S. Intracellular residency is frequently associated with recurrent *Staphylococcus aureus* rhinosinusitis. *Rhinology* **2006**, *44*, 249–254. [PubMed]

34. Foreman, A.; Psaltis, A.J.; Tan, L.W.; Wormald, P.J. Characterization of bacterial and fungal biofilms in chronic rhinosinusitis. *Am. J. Rhinol. Allergy* **2009**, *23*, 556–561. [CrossRef] [PubMed]

35. Prince, A.A.; Steiger, J.D.; Khalid, A.N.; Dogrhamji, L.; Reger, C.; Eau Claire, S.; Chiu, A.G.; Kennedy, D.W.; Palmer, J.N.; Cohen, N.A. Prevalence of biofilm-forming bacteria in chronic rhinosinusitis. *Am. J. Rhinol.* **2008**, *22*, 239–245. [CrossRef] [PubMed]

36. Sanderson, A.R.; Leid, J.G.; Hunsaker, D. Bacterial biofilms on the sinus mucosa of human subjects with chronic rhinosinusitis. *Laryngoscope* **2006**, *116*, 1121–1126. [CrossRef] [PubMed]

37. Suh, J.D.; Cohen, N.A.; Palmer, J.N. Biofilms in chronic rhinosinusitis. *Curr. Opin. Otolaryngol. Head Neck Surg.* **2010**, *18*, 27–31. [CrossRef] [PubMed]

38. Suh, J.D.; Ramakrishnan, V.; Palmer, J.N. Biofilms. *Otolaryngol. Clin. No. Am.* **2010**, *43*, 521–530. [CrossRef] [PubMed]

39. Wood, A.J.; Fraser, J.; Swift, S.; Amirapu, S.; Douglas, R.G. Are biofilms associated with an inflammatory response in chronic rhinusitis? *Int. Forum Allergy Rhinol.* **2011**, *1*, 335–339. [CrossRef] [PubMed]

40. Foreman, A.; Jervis-Bardy, J.; Wormald, P.J. Do biofilms contribute to the initiation and recalcitrance of chronic rhinusitis? *Laryngoscope* **2011**, *121*, 1085–1091. [CrossRef] [PubMed]

41. Hekiert, A.M.; Kofonow, J.M.; Doghramji, L.; Kennedy, D.W.; Chiu, A.G.; Palmer, J.N.; Leid, J.G.; Cohen, N.A. Biofilms correlate with Th1 inflammation in the sinonasal tissue of patients with chronic rhinosinusitis. *Otolaryngol. Head Neck Surg.* **2009**, *141*, 448–453. [CrossRef] [PubMed]

42. Psaltis, A.J.; Weitzel, E.K.; Ha, K.R.; Wormald, P.J. The effect of bacterial biofilms on post-sinus surgical outcomes. *Am. J. Rhinol.* **2008**, *22*, 1–6. [CrossRef] [PubMed]

43. Singhal, D.; Foreman, A.; Jervis-Bardy, J.; Wormald, P.J. *Staphylococcus aureus* biofilms: Nemesis of endoscopic sinus surgery. *Laryngoscope* **2011**, *121*, 1578–1583. [CrossRef] [PubMed]

44. Singhal, D.; Psaltis, A.J.; Foreman, A.; Wormald, P.J. The impact of biofilms on outcomes after endoscopic sinus surgery. *Am. J. Rhinol. Allergy* **2010**, *24*, 169–174. [CrossRef] [PubMed]

45. Zhang, Z.; Linkin, D.R.; Finkelman, B.S.; O'Malley, B.W., Jr.; Thaler, E.R.; Doghramji, L.; Kennedy, D.W.; Cohen, N.A.; Palmer, J.N. Asthma and biofilm-forming bacteria are independently associated with revision sinus surgeries for chronic rhinosinusitis. *J. Allergy Clin. Immunol.* **2011**, *128*, 221–223. [CrossRef] [PubMed]

46. Biel, M.A.; Jones, J.W.; Pedigo, L.; Gibbs, A.; Loebel, N. The effect of antimicrobial photodynamic therapy on human ciliated respiratory mucosa. *Laryngoscope* **2012**, *122*, 2628–2631. [CrossRef] [PubMed]

47. Biel, M.A.; Pedigo, L.; Gibbs, A.; Loebel, N. Photodynamic therapy of antibiotic-resistant biofilms in a maxillary sinus model. *Int. Forum Allergy Rhinol.* **2013**, *3*, 468–473. [CrossRef] [PubMed]

48. Biel, M.A.; Sievert, C.; Usacheva, M.; Teichert, M.; Balcom, J. Antimicrobial photodynamic therapy treatment of chronic recurrent sinusitis biofilms. *Int. Forum Allergy Rhinol.* **2011**, *1*, 329–334. [CrossRef] [PubMed]

49. Anon, J.B.; Jacobs, M.R.; Poole, M.D.; Ambrose, P.G.; Benninger, M.S.; Hadley, J.A.; Craig, W.A.; Sinus And Allergy Health Partnership. Antimicrobial treatment guidelines for acute bacterial rhinosinusitis. *Otolaryngol. Head Neck Surg.* **2004**, *130*, 1–45. [PubMed]

50. Bachert, C.; Gevaert, P.; Holtappels, G.; Johansson, S.G.; van Cauwenberge, P. Total and specific ige in nasal polyps is related to local eosinophilic inflammation. *J. Allergy Clin. Immunol.* **2001**, *107*, 607–614. [CrossRef] [PubMed]

51. Bachert, C.; Zhang, N.; Patou, J.; van Zele, T.; Gevaert, P. Role of staphylococcal superantigens in upper airway disease. *Curr. Opin. Allergy Clin. Immunol.* **2008**, *8*, 34–38. [CrossRef] [PubMed]

52. Tan, N.C.; Foreman, A.; Jardeleza, C.; Douglas, R.; Vreugde, S.; Wormald, P.J. Intracellular *Staphylococcus aureus*: The trojan horse of recalcitrant chronic rhinosinusitis? *Int. Forum Allergy Rhinol.* **2013**, *3*, 261–266. [CrossRef] [PubMed]

53. Ayers, C.M.; Schlosser, R.J.; O'Connell, B.P.; Atkinson, C.; Mulligan, R.M.; Casey, S.E.; Bleier, B.S.; Wang, E.W.; Sansoni, E.R.; Kuhlen, J.L.; *et al.* Increased presence of dendritic cells and dendritic cell chemokines in the sinus mucosa of chronic rhinosinusitis with nasal polyps and allergic fungal rhinosinusitis. *Int. Forum Allergy Rhinol.* **2011**, *1*, 296–302. [CrossRef] [PubMed]

54. Van Zele, T.; Claeys, S.; Gevaert, P.; Van Maele, G.; Holtappels, G.; Van Cauwenberge, P.; Bachert, C. Differentiation of chronic sinus diseases by measurement of inflammatory mediators. *Allergy* **2006**, *61*, 1280–1289. [CrossRef] [PubMed]

55. Aaseth, K.; Grande, R.B.; Kvaerner, K.; Lundqvist, C.; Russell, M.B. Chronic rhinosinusitis gives a ninefold increased risk of chronic headache. The akershus study of chronic headache. *Cephalalgia* **2010**, *30*, 152–160. [CrossRef] [PubMed]

56. Jankowski, R. Eosinophils in the pathophysiology of nasal polyposis. *Acta Otolaryngol.* **1996**, *116*, 160–163. [CrossRef] [PubMed]

57. Drake-Lee, A.; Price, J. Mast cell ultrastructure in the inferior turbinate and stroma of nasal polyps. *J. Laryngol. Otol.* **1997**, *111*, 340–345. [CrossRef] [PubMed]

58. Jahnsen, F.L.; Brandtzaeg, P.; Haye, R.; Haraldsen, G. Expression of functional vcam-1 by cultured nasal polyp-derived microvascular endothelium. *Am. J. Pathol.* **1997**, *150*, 2113–2123. [PubMed]

59. Lloyd, G.A. Ct of the paranasal sinuses: Study of a control series in relation to endoscopic sinus surgery. *J. Laryngol. Otol.* **1990**, *104*, 477–481. [CrossRef] [PubMed]

60. Orlandi, R.R.; Marple, B.F. The role of fungus in chronic rhinosinusitis. *Otolaryngol. Clin. N. Am.* **2010**, *43*, 531–537. [CrossRef] [PubMed]

61. Soler, Z.M.; Sauer, D.A.; Mace, J.; Smith, T.L. Relationship between clinical measures and histopathologic findings in chronic rhinosinusitis. *Otolaryngol. Head Neck Surg.* **2009**, *141*, 454–461. [CrossRef] [PubMed]

62. Joe, S.A.; Thambi, R.; Huang, J. A systematic review of the use of intranasal steroids in the treatment of chronic rhinosinusitis. *Otolaryngol. Head Neck Surg.* **2008**, *139*, 340–347. [CrossRef] [PubMed]

63. Kalish, L.; Snidvongs, K.; Sivasubramaniam, R.; Cope, D.; Harvey, R.J. Topical steroids for nasal polyps. *Cochrane Database Syst. Rev.* **2012**, *12*. [CrossRef]

64. Wei, C.C.; Adappa, N.D.; Cohen, N.A. Use of topical nasal therapies in the management of chronic rhinosinusitis. *Laryngoscope* **2013**, *123*, 2347–2359. [CrossRef] [PubMed]

65. Lildholdt, T.; Rundcrantz, H.; Lindqvist, N. Efficacy of topical corticosteroid powder for nasal polyps: A double-blind, placebo-controlled study of budesonide. *Clin. Otolaryngol. Allied Sci.* **1995**, *20*, 26–30. [CrossRef] [PubMed]

66. Aukema, A.A.; Mulder, P.G.; Fokkens, W.J. Treatment of nasal polyposis and chronic rhinosinusitis with fluticasone propionate nasal drops reduces need for sinus surgery. *J. Allergy Clin. Immunol.* **2005**, *115*, 1017–1023. [CrossRef] [PubMed]

67. Harvey, R.; Hannan, S.A.; Badia, L.; Scadding, G. Nasal saline irrigations for the symptoms of chronic rhinosinusitis. *Cochrane Database Syst. Rev.* **2007**. [CrossRef]

68. Van den Berg, J.W.; de Nier, L.M.; Kaper, N.M.; Schilder, A.G.; Venekamp, R.P.; Grolman, W.; van der Heijden, G.J. Limited evidence: Higher efficacy of nasal saline irrigation over nasal saline spray in chronic rhinosinusitis—An update and reanalysis of the evidence base. *Otolaryngol. Head Neck Surg.* **2014**, *150*, 16–21. [CrossRef] [PubMed]

69. Rudmik, L.; Hoy, M.; Schlosser, R.J.; Harvey, R.J.; Welch, K.C.; Lund, V.; Smith, T.L. Topical therapies in the management of chronic rhinosinusitis: An evidence-based review with recommendations. *Int. Forum Allergy Rhinol.* **2013**, *3*, 281–298. [CrossRef] [PubMed]

70. Snidvongs, K.; Kalish, L.; Sacks, R.; Craig, J.C.; Harvey, R.J. Topical steroid for chronic rhinosinusitis without polyps. *Cochrane Database Syst. Rev.* **2011**. [CrossRef]

71. Watanabe, K.; Shirasaki, H.; Kanaizumi, E.; Himi, T. Effects of glucocorticoids on infiltrating cells and epithelial cells of nasal polyps. *Ann. Otol. Rhinol. Laryngol.* **2004**, *113*, 465–473. [CrossRef] [PubMed]

72. Benitez, P.; Alobid, I.; de Haro, J.; Berenguer, J.; Bernal-Sprekelsen, M.; Pujols, L.; Picado, C.; Mullol, J. A short course of oral prednisone followed by intranasal budesonide is an effective treatment of severe nasal polyps. *Laryngoscope* **2006**, *116*, 770–775. [CrossRef] [PubMed]

73. Martinez-Anton, A.; de Bolos, C.; Alobid, I.; Benitez, P.; Roca-Ferrer, J.; Picado, C.; Mullol, J. Corticosteroid therapy increases membrane-tethered while decreases secreted mucin expression in nasal polyps. *Allergy* **2008**, *63*, 1368–1376. [CrossRef] [PubMed]

74. Soler, Z.M.; Oyer, S.L.; Kern, R.C.; Senior, B.A.; Kountakis, S.E.; Marple, B.F.; Smith, T.L. Antimicrobials and chronic rhinosinusitis with or without polyposis in adults: An evidenced-based review with recommendations. *Int. Forum Allergy Rhinol.* **2013**, *3*, 31–47. [CrossRef] [PubMed]

75. Hashiba, M.; Baba, S. Efficacy of long-term administration of clarithromycin in the treatment of intractable chronic sinusitis. *Acta Otolaryngol. Suppl.* **1996**, *525*, 73–78. [PubMed]

76. Kimura, N.; Nishioka, K.; Nishizaki, K.; Ogawa, T.; Naitou, Y.; Masuda, Y. Clinical effect of low-dose, long-term roxithromycin chemotherapy in patients with chronic sinusitis. *Acta Med. Okayama* **1997**, *51*, 33–37. [PubMed]

77. Ragab, S.M.; Lund, V.J.; Scadding, G. Evaluation of the medical and surgical treatment of chronic rhinosinusitis: A prospective, randomised, controlled trial. *Laryngoscope* **2004**, *114*, 923–930. [CrossRef] [PubMed]

78. Pynnonen, M.A.; Mukerji, S.S.; Kim, H.M.; Adams, M.E.; Terrell, J.E. Nasal saline for chronic sinonasal symptoms: A randomized controlled trial. *Arch. Otolaryngol. Head Neck Surg.* **2007**, *133*, 1115–1120. [CrossRef] [PubMed]

79. Hopkins, C.; Browne, J.P.; Slack, R.; Lund, V.; Topham, J.; Reeves, B.; Copley, L.; Brown, P.; van der Meulen, J. The national comparative audit of surgery for nasal polyposis and chronic rhinosinusitis. *Clin. Otolaryngol.* **2006**, *31*, 390–398. [CrossRef] [PubMed]

80. Ragab, S.M.; Lund, V.J.; Scadding, G.; Saleh, H.A.; Khalifa, M.A. Impact of chronic rhinosinusitis therapy on quality of life: A prospective randomized controlled trial. *Rhinology* **2010**, *48*, 305–311. [CrossRef] [PubMed]

81. Kosugi, E.M.; Moussalem, G.F.; Simoes, J.C.; de Souza, R.P.; Chen, V.G.; Saraceni Neto, P.; Mendes Neto, J.A. Topical therapy with high-volume budesonide nasal irrigations in difficult-to-treat chronic rhinosinusitis. *Braz. J. Otorhinolaryngol.* **2015**. [CrossRef] [PubMed]

82. Furukido, K.; Takeno, S.; Ueda, T.; Yajin, K. Cytokine profile in paranasal effusions in patients with chronic sinusitis using the yamik sinus catheter with and without betamethasone. *Eur. Arch. Otorhinolaryngol.* **2005**, *262*, 50–54. [CrossRef] [PubMed]

83. Lavigne, F.; Cameron, L.; Renzi, P.M.; Planet, J.F.; Christodoulopoulos, P.; Lamkioued, B.; Hamid, Q. Intrasinus administration of topical budesonide to allergic patients with chronic rhinosinusitis following surgery. *Laryngoscope* **2002**, *112*, 858–864. [CrossRef] [PubMed]

84. Lund, V.J.; Black, J.H.; Szabo, L.Z.; Schrewelius, C.; Akerlund, A. Efficacy and tolerability of budesonide aqueous nasal spray in chronic rhinosinusitis patients. *Rhinology* **2004**, *42*, 57–62. [PubMed]

85. Parikh, A.; Scadding, G.K.; Darby, Y.; Baker, R.C. Topical corticosteroids in chronic rhinosinusitis: A randomized, double-blind, placebo-controlled trial using fluticasone propionate aqueous nasal spray. *Rhinology* **2001**, *39*, 75–79. [PubMed]

86. Jorissen, M.; Bachert, C. Effect of corticosteroids on wound healing after endoscopic sinus surgery. *Rhinology* **2009**, *47*, 280–286. [CrossRef] [PubMed]

87. Raza, T.; Elsherif, H.S.; Zulianello, L.; Plouin-Gaudon, I.; Landis, B.N.; Lacroix, J.S. Nasal lavage with sodium hypochlorite solution in *Staphylococcus aureus* persistent rhinosinusitis. *Rhinology* **2008**, *46*, 15–22. [PubMed]

88. Weissman, J.D.; Fernandez, F.; Hwang, P.H. Xylitol nasal irrigation in the management of chronic rhinosinusitis: A pilot study. *Laryngoscope* **2011**, *121*, 2468–2472. [CrossRef] [PubMed]

89. Lal, D.; Hwang, P.H. Oral corticosteroid therapy in chronic rhinosinusitis without polyposis: A systematic review. *Int. Forum Allergy Rhinol.* **2011**, *1*, 136–143. [CrossRef] [PubMed]

90. Chiu, A.G.; Antunes, M.B.; Palmer, J.N.; Cohen, N.A. Evaluation of the *in vivo* efficacy of topical tobramycin against pseudomonas sinonasal biofilms. *J. Antimicrob. Chemother.* **2007**, *59*, 1130–1134. [CrossRef] [PubMed]

91. Desrosiers, M.Y.; Salas-Prato, M. Treatment of chronic rhinosinusitis refractory to other treatments with topical antibiotic therapy delivered by means of a large-particle nebulizer: Results of a controlled trial. *Otolaryngol. Head Neck Surg.* **2001**, *125*, 265–269. [CrossRef] [PubMed]

92. Videler, W.J.; van Drunen, C.M.; Reitsma, J.B.; Fokkens, W.J. Nebulized bacitracin/colimycin: A treatment option in recalcitrant chronic rhinosinusitis with staphylococcus aureus? A double-blind, randomized, placebo-controlled, cross-over pilot study. *Rhinology* **2008**, *46*, 92–98. [PubMed]

93. Sykes, D.A.; Wilson, R.; Chan, K.L.; Mackay, I.S.; Cole, P.J. Relative importance of antibiotic and improved clearance in topical treatment of chronic mucopurulent rhinosinusitis. A controlled study. *Lancet* **1986**, *2*, 359–360. [CrossRef]

94. Pynnonen, M.A.; Venkatraman, G.; Davis, G.E. Macrolide therapy for chronic rhinosinusitis: A meta-analysis. *Otolaryngol. Head Neck Surg.* **2013**, *148*, 366–373. [CrossRef] [PubMed]

95. Piromchai, P.; Thanaviratananich, S.; Laopaiboon, M. Systemic antibiotics for chronic rhinosinusitis without nasal polyps in adults. *Cochrane Database Syst. Rev.* **2011**. [CrossRef]

96. Videler, W.J.; Badia, L.; Harvey, R.J.; Gane, S.; Georgalas, C.; van der Meulen, F.W.; Menger, D.J.; Lehtonen, M.T.; Toppila-Salmi, S.K.; Vento, S.I.; *et al.* Lack of efficacy of long-term, low-dose azithromycin in chronic rhinosinusitis: A randomized controlled trial. *Allergy* **2011**, *66*, 1457–1468. [CrossRef] [PubMed]

97. Wallwork, B.; Coman, W.; Mackay-Sim, A.; Greiff, L.; Cervin, A. A double-blind, randomized, placebo-controlled trial of macrolide in the treatment of chronic rhinosinusitis. *Laryngoscope* **2006**, *116*, 189–193. [CrossRef] [PubMed]

98. Emanuel, I.A.; Shah, S.B. Chronic rhinosinusitis: Allergy and sinus computed tomography relationships. *Otolaryngol. Head Neck Surg.* **2000**, *123*, 687–691. [CrossRef] [PubMed]

99. Tan, B.K.; Zirkle, W.; Chandra, R.K.; Lin, D.; Conley, D.B.; Peters, A.T.; Grammer, L.C.; Schleimer, R.P.; Kern, R.C. Atopic profile of patients failing medical therapy for chronic rhinosinusitis. *Int. Forum Allergy Rhinol.* **2011**, *1*, 88–94. [CrossRef] [PubMed]

100. Krouse, J.H. Computed tomography stage, allergy testing, and quality of life in patients with sinusitis. *Otolaryngol. Head Neck Surg.* **2000**, *123*, 389–392. [CrossRef] [PubMed]

101. Stewart, M.G.; Donovan, D.T.; Parke, R.B., Jr.; Bautista, M.H. Does the severity of sinus computed tomography findings predict outcome in chronic sinusitis? *Otolaryngol. Head Neck Surg.* **2000**, *123*, 81–84. [CrossRef] [PubMed]

102. Wilson, K.F.; McMains, K.C.; Orlandi, R.R. The association between allergy and chronic rhinosinusitis with and without nasal polyps: An evidence-based review with recommendations. *Int. Forum Allergy Rhinol.* **2014**, *4*, 93–103. [CrossRef] [PubMed]

103. Slavin, R.G.; Spector, S.L.; Bernstein, I.L.; Kaliner, M.A.; Kennedy, D.W.; Virant, F.S.; Wald, E.R.; Khan, D.A.; Blessing-Moore, J.; Lang, D.M.; *et al.* The diagnosis and management of sinusitis: A practice parameter update. *J. Allergy Clin. Immunol.* **2005**, *116*, S13–S47. [CrossRef] [PubMed]

104. Bresciani, M.; Paradis, L.; Des Roches, A.; Vernhet, H.; Vachier, I.; Godard, P.; Bousquet, J.; Chanez, P. Rhinosinusitis in severe asthma. *J. Allergy Clin. Immunol.* **2001**, *107*, 73–80. [CrossRef] [PubMed]

105. Ikeda, K.; Tanno, N.; Tamura, G.; Suzuki, H.; Oshima, T.; Shimomura, A.; Nakabayashi, S.; Takasaka, T. Endoscopic sinus surgery improves pulmonary function in patients with asthma associated with chronic sinusitis. *Ann. Otol. Rhinol. Laryngol.* **1999**, *108*, 355–359. [CrossRef] [PubMed]

106. Palmer, J.N.; Conley, D.B.; Dong, R.G.; Ditto, A.M.; Yarnold, P.R.; Kern, R.C. Efficacy of endoscopic sinus surgery in the management of patients with asthma and chronic sinusitis. *Am. J. Rhinol.* **2001**, *15*, 49–53. [CrossRef] [PubMed]

107. Ragab, S.; Scadding, G.K.; Lund, V.J.; Saleh, H. Treatment of chronic rhinosinusitis and its effects on asthma. *Eur. Respir. J.* **2006**, *28*, 68–74. [CrossRef] [PubMed]

108. Vashishta, R.; Soler, Z.M.; Nguyen, S.A.; Schlosser, R.J. A systematic review and meta-analysis of asthma outcomes following endoscopic sinus surgery for chronic rhinosinusitis. *Int. Forum Allergy Rhinol.* **2013**, *3*, 788–794. [CrossRef] [PubMed]

109. Nonaka, M.; Sakanushi, A.; Kusama, K.; Ogihara, N.; Yagi, T. One-year evaluation of combined treatment with an intranasal corticosteroid and montelukast for chronic rhinosinusitis associated with asthma. *J. Nippon Med. Sch.* **2010**, *77*, 21–28. [CrossRef] [PubMed]

110. Wentzel, J.L.; Soler, Z.M.; DeYoung, K.; Nguyen, S.A.; Lohia, S.; Schlosser, R.J. Leukotriene antagonists in nasal polyposis: A meta-analysis and systematic review. *Am. J. Rhinol. Allergy* **2013**, *27*, 482–489. [CrossRef] [PubMed]

111. Funk, C.D. Prostaglandins and leukotrienes: Advances in eicosanoid biology. *Science* **2001**, *294*, 1871–1875. [CrossRef] [PubMed]

112. Perez-Novo, C.A.; Watelet, J.B.; Claeys, C.; van Cauwenberge, P.; Bachert, C. Prostaglandin, leukotriene, and lipoxin balance in chronic rhinosinusitis with and without nasal polyposis. *J. Allergy Clin. Immunol.* **2005**, *115*, 1189–1196. [CrossRef] [PubMed]

113. Steinke, J.W.; Bradley, D.; Arango, P.; Crouse, C.D.; Frierson, H.; Kountakis, S.E.; Kraft, M.; Borish, L. Cysteinyl leukotriene expression in chronic hyperplastic sinusitis-nasal polyposis: Importance to eosinophilia and asthma. *J. Allergy Clin. Immunol.* **2003**, *111*, 342–349. [CrossRef] [PubMed]

114. Perez-Novo, C.A.; Claeys, C.; Van Cauwenberge, P.; Bachert, C. Expression of eicosanoid receptors subtypes and eosinophilic inflammation: Implication on chronic rhinosinusitis. *Respir. Res.* **2006**, *7*, 75. [CrossRef] [PubMed]

115. Van Crombruggen, K.; Van Bruaene, N.; Holtappels, G.; Bachert, C. Chronic sinusitis and rhinitis: Clinical terminology "chronic rhinosinusitis" further supported. *Rhinology* **2010**, *48*, 54–58. [CrossRef] [PubMed]

116. Babinski, D.; Trawinska-Bartnicka, M. Rhinosinusitis in cystic fibrosis: Not a simple story. *Int. J. Pediatr. Otorhinolaryngol.* **2008**, *72*, 619–624. [CrossRef] [PubMed]

117. Gysin, C.; Alothman, G.A.; Papsin, B.C. Sinonasal disease in cystic fibrosis: Clinical characteristics, diagnosis, and management. *Pediatr. Pulmonol.* **2000**, *30*, 481–489. [CrossRef]

118. Marshak, T.; Rivlin, Y.; Bentur, L.; Ronen, O.; Uri, N. Prevalence of rhinosinusitis among atypical cystic fibrosis patients. *Eur. Arch. Otorhinolaryngol.* **2011**, *268*, 519–524. [CrossRef] [PubMed]

119. Slavin, R.G. Resistant rhinosinusitis: What to do when usual measures fail. *Allergy Asthma Proc.* **2003**, *24*, 303–306. [PubMed]

120. Hytonen, M.; Patjas, M.; Vento, S.I.; Kauppi, P.; Malmberg, H.; Ylikoski, J.; Kere, J. Cystic fibrosis gene mutations deltaf508 and 394deltt in patients with chronic sinusitis in finland. *Acta Otolaryngol.* **2001**, *121*, 945–947. [CrossRef] [PubMed]

121. Berkhout, M.C.; Rijntjes, E.; El Bouazzaoui, L.H.; Fokkens, W.J.; Brimicombe, R.W.; Heijerman, H.G. Importance of bacteriology in upper airways of patients with cystic fibrosis. *J. Cyst. Fibros.* **2013**, *12*, 525–529. [CrossRef] [PubMed]

122. Bonestroo, H.J.; de Winter-de Groot, K.M.; van der Ent, C.K.; Arets, H.G. Upper and lower airway cultures in children with cystic fibrosis: Do not neglect the upper airways. *J. Cyst. Fibros.* **2010**, *9*, 130–134. [CrossRef] [PubMed]

123. Godoy, J.M.; Godoy, A.N.; Ribalta, G.; Largo, I. Bacterial pattern in chronic sinusitis and cystic fibrosis. *Otolaryngol. Head Neck Surg.* **2011**, *145*, 673–676. [CrossRef] [PubMed]

124. Mainz, J.G.; Naehrlich, L.; Schien, M.; Kading, M.; Schiller, I.; Mayr, S.; Schneider, G.; Wiedemann, B.; Wiehlmann, L.; Cramer, N.; *et al.* Concordant genotype of upper and lower airways *P. aeruginosa* and *S. aureus* isolates in cystic fibrosis. *Thorax* **2009**, *64*, 535–540. [CrossRef] [PubMed]

125. Aanaes, K.; von Buchwald, C.; Hjuler, T.; Skov, M.; Alanin, M.; Johansen, H.K. The effect of sinus surgery with intensive follow-up on pathogenic sinus bacteria in patients with cystic fibrosis. *Am. J. Rhinol. Allergy* **2013**, *27*, e1–e4. [CrossRef] [PubMed]

126. Khalid, A.N.; Mace, J.; Smith, T.L. Outcomes of sinus surgery in adults with cystic fibrosis. *Otolaryngol. Head Neck Surg.* **2009**, *141*, 358–363. [CrossRef] [PubMed]

127. Liang, J.; Higgins, T.S.; Ishman, S.L.; Boss, E.F.; Benke, J.R.; Lin, S.Y. Surgical management of chronic rhinosinusitis in cystic fibrosis: A systematic review. *Int. Forum Allergy Rhinol.* **2013**, *3*, 814–822. [CrossRef] [PubMed]

128. Virgin, F.W.; Rowe, S.M.; Wade, M.B.; Gaggar, A.; Leon, K.J.; Young, K.R.; Woodworth, B.A. Extensive surgical and comprehensive postoperative medical management for cystic fibrosis chronic rhinosinusitis. *Am. J. Rhinol. Allergy* **2012**, *26*, 70–75. [CrossRef] [PubMed]

129. Cimmino, M.; Nardone, M.; Cavaliere, M.; Plantulli, A.; Sepe, A.; Esposito, V.; Mazzarella, G.; Raia, V. Dornase alfa as postoperative therapy in cystic fibrosis sinonasal disease. *Arch Otolaryngol. Head Neck Surg.* **2005**, *131*, 1097–1101. [CrossRef] [PubMed]

130. Mainz, J.G.; Schiller, I.; Ritschel, C.; Mentzel, H.J.; Riethmuller, J.; Koitschev, A.; Schneider, G.; Beck, J.F.; Wiedemann, B. Sinonasal inhalation of dornase alfa in cf: A double-blind placebo-controlled cross-over pilot trial. *Auris Nasus Larynx* **2011**, *38*, 220–227. [CrossRef] [PubMed]

131. Lim, M.; Citardi, M.J.; Leong, J.L. Topical antimicrobials in the management of chronic rhinosinusitis: A systematic review. *Am. J. Rhinol.* **2008**, *22*, 381–389. [CrossRef] [PubMed]

132. Wagner, J.A.; Nepomuceno, I.B.; Messner, A.H.; Moran, M.L.; Batson, E.P.; Dimiceli, S.; Brown, B.W.; Desch, J.K.; Norbash, A.M.; Conrad, C.K.; *et al.* A phase ii, double-blind, randomized, placebo-controlled clinical trial of tgaavcf using maxillary sinus delivery in patients with cystic fibrosis with antrostomies. *Hum. Gene Ther.* **2002**, *13*, 1349–1359. [CrossRef] [PubMed]

133. Chang, E.H.; Tang, X.X.; Shah, V.S.; Launspach, J.L.; Ernst, S.E.; Hilkin, B.; Karp, P.H.; Abou Alaiwa, M.H.; Graham, S.M.; Hornick, D.B.; *et al.* Medical reversal of chronic sinusitis in a cystic fibrosis patient with ivacaftor. *Int. Forum Allergy Rhinol.* **2015**, *5*, 178–181. [CrossRef] [PubMed]

134. Moss, R.B.; King, V.V. Management of sinusitis in cystic fibrosis by endoscopic surgery and serial antimicrobial lavage. Reduction in recurrence requiring surgery. *Arch Otolaryngol. Head Neck Surg.* **1995**, *121*, 566–572. [CrossRef] [PubMed]

135. Armengot, M.; Juan, G.; Carda, C.; Montalt, J.; Basterra, J. Young's syndrome: A further cause of chronic rhinosinusitis. *Rhinology* **1996**, *34*, 35–37. [PubMed]

136. Braverman, I.; Wright, E.D.; Wang, C.G.; Eidelman, D.; Frenkiel, S. Human nasal ciliary-beat frequency in normal and chronic sinusitis subjects. *J. Otolaryngol.* **1998**, *27*, 145–152. [PubMed]

137. Mahakit, P.; Pumhirun, P. A preliminary study of nasal mucociliary clearance in smokers, sinusitis and allergic rhinitis patients. *Asian Pac. J. Allergy Immunol.* **1995**, *13*, 119–121. [PubMed]

138. Orange, J.S.; Ballow, M.; Stiehm, E.R.; Ballas, Z.K.; Chinen, J.; De La Morena, M.; Kumararatne, D.; Harville, T.O.; Hesterberg, P.; Koleilat, M.; *et al.* Use and interpretation of diagnostic vaccination in primary immunodeficiency: A working group report of the basic and clinical immunology interest section of the american academy of allergy, asthma & immunology. *J. Allergy Clin. Immunol.* **2012**, *130*, S1–S24. [PubMed]

139. Carr, T.F.; Koterba, A.P.; Chandra, R.; Grammer, L.C.; Conley, D.B.; Harris, K.E.; Kern, R.; Schleimer, R.P.; Peters, A.T. Characterization of specific antibody deficiency in adults with medically refractory chronic rhinosinusitis. *Am. J. Rhinol. Allergy* **2011**, *25*, 241–244. [CrossRef] [PubMed]

140. Chee, L.; Graham, S.M.; Carothers, D.G.; Ballas, Z.K. Immune dysfunction in refractory sinusitis in a tertiary care setting. *Laryngoscope* **2001**, *111*, 233–235. [CrossRef] [PubMed]

141. Cheng, Y.K.; Decker, P.A.; O'Byrne, M.M.; Weiler, C.R. Clinical and laboratory characteristics of 75 patients with specific polysaccharide antibody deficiency syndrome. *Ann. Allergy Asthma Immunol.* **2006**, *97*, 306–311. [CrossRef]

142. Tahkokallio, O.; Seppala, I.J.; Sarvas, H.; Kayhty, H.; Mattila, P.S. Concentrations of serum immunoglobulins and antibodies to pneumococcal capsular polysaccharides in patients with recurrent or chronic sinusitis. *Ann. Otol. Rhinol. Laryngol.* **2001**, *110*, 675–681. [CrossRef] [PubMed]

143. Stevens, W.W.; Peters, A.T. Immunodeficiency in chronic sinusitis: Recognition and treatment. *Am. J. Rhinol. Allergy* **2015**, *29*, 115–118. [CrossRef] [PubMed]

144. Bondioni, M.P.; Duse, M.; Plebani, A.; Soresina, A.; Notarangelo, L.D.; Berlucchi, M.; Grazioli, L. Pulmonary and sinusal changes in 45 patients with primary immunodeficiencies: Computed tomography evaluation. *J. Comput. Assist. Tomogr.* **2007**, *31*, 620–628. [CrossRef] [PubMed]

145. Isaacs, S.; Fakhri, S.; Luong, A.; Citardi, M.J. A meta-analysis of topical amphotericin b for the treatment of chronic rhinosinusitis. *Int. Forum Allergy Rhinol.* **2011**, *1*, 250–254. [CrossRef] [PubMed]

146. Fokkens, W.J.; Lund, V.J.; Mullol, J.; Bachert, C.; Alobid, I.; Baroody, F.; Cohen, N.; Cervin, A.; Douglas, R.; Gevaert, P.; *et al.* Epos 2012: European position paper on rhinosinusitis and nasal polyps 2012. A summary for otorhinolaryngologists. *Rhinology* **2012**, *50*, 1–12. [PubMed]

147. Sacks, P.L.t.; Harvey, R.J.; Rimmer, J.; Gallagher, R.M.; Sacks, R. Antifungal therapy in the treatment of chronic rhinosinusitis: A meta-analysis. *Am. J. Rhinol. Allergy* **2012**, *26*, 141–147. [CrossRef] [PubMed]

148. Ahn, C.N.; Wise, S.K.; Lathers, D.M.; Mulligan, R.M.; Harvey, R.J.; Schlosser, R.J. Local production of antigen-specific ige in different anatomic subsites of allergic fungal rhinosinusitis patients. *Otolaryngol. Head Neck Surg.* **2009**, *141*, 97–103. [CrossRef] [PubMed]

149. Collins, M.; Nair, S.; Smith, W.; Kette, F.; Gillis, D.; Wormald, P.J. Role of local immunoglobulin E production in the pathophysiology of noninvasive fungal sinusitis. *Laryngoscope* **2004**, *114*, 1242–1246. [CrossRef] [PubMed]

150. Luong, A.; Davis, L.S.; Marple, B.F. Peripheral blood mononuclear cells from allergic fungal rhinosinusitis adults express a th2 cytokine response to fungal antigens. *Am. J. Rhinol. Allergy* **2009**, *23*, 281–287. [CrossRef] [PubMed]

151. Ikram, M.; Abbas, A.; Suhail, A.; Onali, M.A.; Akhtar, S.; Iqbal, M. Management of allergic fungal sinusitis with postoperative oral and nasal steroids: A controlled study. *Ear Nose Throat J.* **2009**, *88*, E8–E11. [PubMed]

LTD$_4$ and TGF-β_1 Induce the Expression of Metalloproteinase-1 in Chronic Rhinosinusitis via a Cysteinyl Leukotriene Receptor 1-Related Mechanism

Rogerio Pezato [1,2]**, Cindy Claeys** [1]**, Gabriele Holtappels** [1]**, Claus Bachert** [1] **and Claudina A. Pérez-Novo** [1,3,]*

[1] Upper Airways Research Laboratory, Department of Otorhinolaryngology, Ghent University Hospital, 9000 Ghent, Belgium; pezatobau@ig.com.br (R.P.); Cindy@praet.eu (C.C.); Gabriele.Holtappels@UGent.be (G.H.); Claus.Bachert@UGent.be (C.B.)

[2] Department of Otorhinolaryngology, Head and Neck Surgery, Federal University of São Paulo, 05405-000 São Paulo, Brazil

[3] Laboratory of Protein chemistry, Proteomics & Epigenetic Signaling, Department Biomedical Sciences, University of Antwerp, 2610 Wilrijk, Belgium

* Correspondence: Claudina.pereznovo@ua.ac.be

Academic Editor: César Picado

Abstract: *Background*: Cysteinyl leukotrienes (CysLTs) play a crucial role in the pathogenesis of airway remodeling. The use of CysLTs receptor antagonists has been included in the management of asthma and rhinitis. However, despite the action of these compounds on leukotriene production has been well documented, their role in airway remodeling remains unclear. *Objective*: We aimed to investigate the capability of the leukotriene receptor antagonist Montelukast to inhibit MMPs release after CysLTs stimulation in nasal tissue fibroblasts. *Methods*: Fibroblasts were isolated from sinunasal tissue collected from five patients suffering of chronic rhinosinusitis without nasal polyposis. Cells were cultured and stimulated first with LTC$_4$ and LTD$_4$ (10^{-10}, 10^{-8}, 10^{-6} M) using as pre-stimulus 10 ng/mL of: IL-4, IL-13, or TGF-beta1 and in presence or absence of Montelukast (10^{-10}, 10^{-8}, 10^{-6} M). To evaluate the regulation of MMP-1 and TIMP-1 we used enzyme immunoassays and to evaluate CysLT1 receptor we used real time PCR. *Results*: LTD$_4$ but not LTC$_4$ induced production of mRNA for CysLT1 receptor in a dose dependent manner and with an additive effect when the cells where primed with TGF-β_1. TNF-α, IL-4, and IL-13 did not influence the expression of the receptor. Levels of MMP-1 but not of TIMP-1 were statistically enhanced in cells primed with TGF-β_1 and stimulated with LTD$_4$. Montelukast significantly decreased Cys-LT$_1$ receptor and MMP-1 concentrations in a dose-dependent way in cells stimulated with LTD$_4$ and TGF-β_1 separately and when they were applied together. *Conclusion*: The leukotriene pathway may play an important role in extra-cellular matrix formation in an inflamed environment, such as chronic sinusitis and, consequently, leukotriene receptor antagonists such as Montelukast may be of great benefit in management of this disease.

Keywords: chronic rhinosinusitis; cysteinyl leukotriene receptor 1; fibroblasts; metalloproteinase 1; Montelukast

1. Introduction

Chronic rhinosinusitis (CRS) is a heterogeneous group of diseases characterized by chronic inflammation of the nasal and sinunasal mucosa, persisting longer than 12 weeks. Recent studies have demonstrated that the spectrum of the disease can be differentiated into distinct subgroups based on clinical parameters and on the characterization of the inflammatory response [1]. Although chronic rhinosinusitis without nasal polyps (CRSsNP) shows mainly a neutrophilic, T_H1-driven inflammatory profile, chronic rhinosinusitis with nasal polyps (CRSwNP) is mainly characterized by a T_H2-skewed, eosinophilic inflammation [1]. However, in both CRS phenotypes, the turnover of the extracellular matrix (ECM) is disturbed by the release of inflammatory mediators such as TGF-β_1, MMP-7, MMP-9, and TIMP-1 in nasal secretions. Resulting in an abnormal tissue remodeling characterized by mucosal thickening, fibrosis, and/or edema [2,3].

ECM remodeling processes consist of a complex interaction between various cell types and a large number of enzymes including tissue serine proteases and the family of matrix metalloproteinases (MMPs) [4]. Matrix metalloproteinases (MMPs) are a family of zinc- and calcium-dependent endopeptidases which can collectively degrade almost all ECM components [5]. They are produced by structural (fibroblasts, endothelial, and epithelial cells) and inflammatory cells (eosinophils, macrophages, neutrophils, and lymphocytes) and the gene expression is tightly regulated by cytokines and growth factors.

The role of MMPs in physiology has been implicated in both normal and pathological structural processes, such as embryogenesis, cell migration, tissue repair, and tumor necrosis [6,7]. The increased expression of MMPs in nasal polyps, COPD, and asthma and the correlation with pathological changes of the airways, together with their action in wound repair have been the basis to suggest the possible role of these compounds in microvascular permeability, cell transmigration, and ECM airway remodeling [8]. Although this evidence exists, the *in vivo* function of these MMPs in airway diseases remains partially unclear.

Cysteinyl leukotrienes (CysLTs) are lipid mediators produced after the release of arachidonic acid from cell membrane phospholipids which is then modified by the 5-lipoxygenase (ALOX5) enzyme to yield LTB_4 or to the cysteinyl-leukotrienes (CysLTs) LTC_4, LTD_4, and LTE_4 [9]. These compounds are released by cells involved in the inflammatory response (mast cells, basophils, eosinophils, neutrophils, and macrophages) and constitute important pro-inflammatory mediators in asthma and other chronic inflammatory diseases [9,10]. Their action is mediated by the binding to CysLTs receptors (CysLT1 and CysLT2 receptors), which are expressed not only in inflammatory and immune cells, but also in structural cells. Binding of CysLTs on their receptors on structural cells results in tissue edema, mucus secretion, bronchoconstriction, and severe impairment in tissue remodeling [11].

In nasal tissue of CRSsNP patients, levels of the CysLTs, the enzymes involved in their synthesis (ALOX5 and LTC_4S), and both CysLT1 and CysLT2 receptors are significantly upregulated compared to controls [12,13]. Several *in vitro* experiments have suggested that CysLTs may induce airway smooth muscle proliferation [14,15], alter fibroblast function [16,17] and induce extracellular matrix [18,19].

Taking into account the important role of leukotrienes in airway inflammation, and especially in asthma, several anti-LTs modifiers have been evaluated in the management of this pathology [20–22]. Leukotriene modifiers include three different groups of drugs: (i) specific inhibitors of FLAP; (ii) inhibitors of ALOX5; and (iii) CysLT1 receptor inhibitors. However, the role of these compounds in upper airway remodeling remains unclear. In this study we evaluated the capability of exogenous CysLTs (LTC_4 and LTD_4) to influence the expression of MMPs in nasal tissue fibroblasts isolated from patients with chronic rhinosinusitis without nasal polyposis (CRSsNP) and evaluate if the leukotriene receptor antagonist Montelukast may modify this effect and, consequently, may have a potential role in regulation upper airway tissue remodeling.

2. Materials and Methods

2.1. Patients

Fibroblasts were isolated from nasal mucosa tissue obtained from CRSsNP patients ($n = 5$) who were scheduled for functional endoscopic sinus surgery at the Department of Otorhinolaryngology at Ghent University Hospital. The diagnosis of CRSsNP was based on history, clinical examination, nasal endoscopy, and computed tomography (CT-Scan) of the paranasal cavities according to the EPOS guidelines [23]. None of the patients had asthma or allergies as assessed by the guidelines (GINA) for the diagnosis and management of asthma [24] and results of a skin prick test. The study was approved by the ethical committee of Ghent University Hospital and all patients gave informed consent before their participation.

2.2. Reagents

Dulbecco's PBS, penicillin-streptomycin (penicillin, 5000 IU/mL; streptomycin, 50 μg/mL), and trypan blue (0.4% solution in PBS) were obtained from Invitrogen (Paisley, UK). Minimum essential medium (MEM), Opti-MEM I reduced serum medium, L-glutamine (200 mM), trypsin-EDTA (1X), and fetal bovine serum (FBS) (qualified; origin, Thermo Fisher Scientific, Waltham, MA, USA) were purchased from Gibco (Life Technologies, Carlsbad, CA, USA). Ultroser™ G serum substitute (5%) was obtained from BioSepra (Port Washington, New York, NY, USA). Interleukin-4 (IL-4) and interleukin—13 (IL-13) were obtained from R and D Systems (Minneapolis, MN, USA). SYBR Green I qPCR Master mix, Aurum Total RNA, and Script cDNA synthesis kits were obtained from Bio-Rad Laboratories (Berkeley, CA, USA). Cysteinyl leukotrienes C_4, $-D_4$ (LTC_4, LTD_4) and the cysteinyl leukotriene receptor 1 (CysLT1) inhibitor Montelukast were purchased from Cayman Chemicals (Ann Arbor, MI, USA).

2.3. Isolation of Nasal Mucosa Fibroblasts

Nasal sinus tissues, obtained from patients with chronic rhinosinusitis, during surgical operations were rinsed several times with Opti-MEM I supplemented with 5% FBS, 5% Ultroser G, 2 mmol/L glutamine, and penicillin (50 IU/mL)–streptomycin (50 μg/mL), and cut into small pieces (approximately 1 mm^2). Diced specimens were then plated (density, 9 pieces/6-well tissue culture dish) and incubated in a humidified atmosphere containing 5% CO_2 at 37 °C, until a monolayer of fibroblast-like cells was observed to be confluent. Then, the explanted tissues were removed, and cells were trypsinized and re-plated into 250-cm^2 tissue culture Falcon tubes at a final volume of 5 mL. The culture medium was then changed every three days for 2–3 weeks until 90% confluence was obtained. Subsequently, the cells were split and stained with antibodies against vimentine, cytokeratin, and α-smooth muscle actin to exclude contamination with epithelial cells.

2.4. Cell Stimulation

Cells (1 × 10^6) were cultured with 10 ng/mL of IL-4, IL-13, TGF-$β_1$, and TNF-α alone or in combination with (10^{-6}, 10^{-8} and 10^{-10} M) of LTC_4 or LTD_4 independently during 24 h at 37 °C in 5% CO_2. For inhibition experiments, sinunasal fibroblasts where first cultured in presence of Montelukast (10^{-8}, 10^{-10}, 10^{-11} M) for 60 min, and after, stimulated with 10 ng/mL of TGF-$β_1$ or in combination with LTD_4 at 10^{-6} M) for 24 h, at 37 °C in 5% CO_2. After all stimulations, supernatants were collected and stored at −20 °C until use. Cells were resuspended in lysis buffer for posterior RNA extraction, and stored at −80 °C.

2.5. Measurement of MMP-1, TIMP-1, and Cysteinyl Leukotrienes

Protein levels of matrix metalloproteinase-1, -2, -3, -7, and -9 (MMP-1, MMP-2, MMP-3, MMP-7, and MMP-9) and TIMP-1 were quantified by the human total MMPs and TIMP-1 Quantikine ELISA kits (R and D Systems) following manufacturer's instructions.

2.6. Real-Time qPCR for CYSLT1 Receptor

Cell pellet was homogenized in Tri-reagent buffer (Sigma-Aldrich, MO, USA), 1 mL per 50–100 mg of tissue and total RNA was isolated using the Aurum total RNA Kit (BioRad Inc. Laboratories) following the manufacturer's instructions. cDNA was synthesized from 2 μg of total RNA using the iScript cDNA synthesis kit Bio-Rad Inc. Laboratories). Amplification reactions were performed on an iQ5 Real-Time PCR Detection System (Bio-Rad Laboratories) using a primer set for human cysteinyl leukotriene receptor 1 (Table 1). PCR reactions contained 20 ng of cDNA (total RNA equivalent) of unknown samples, 1X SYBR Green I Master mix (Bio-Rad Laboratories) and 250 nM of primer pairs in a final volume of 20 μL. PCR protocol consisted of one cycle at 95 °C for 10 min followed by 40 cycles at 95 °C for 15 s and at 60 °C for 1 min. The expression of two housekeeping genes, Beta actin (ACTB) and hydroxymethyl-bilane synthase (HMBS), were used to normalize for transcription and amplification variations among samples. Primer sequences and qPCR conditions are reported previously [25]. Relative normalized quantities were calculated from the obtained Cq values using the qBase software [26].

Table 1. Primer sequence for quantitative real-time PCR.

Gene	Forward Primer $5' \rightarrow 3'$	Reverse Primer $5' \rightarrow 3'$	Amplicon Size (bp)	GenBank Accession Number
CysLT1	TCCTTAGAATGCAGAAGTCCGTG	AAATATAGGAGAGGGTCAAAGCAA	80	NM_001282187
ACTB	CTGGAACGGTGAAGGTGACA	AAGGGACTTCCTGTAACAATGCA	139	NM_001101.3
HMBS	GGCAATGCGGCTGCAA	GGGTACCCACGCGAATCAC	154	NM_000190.3

2.7. Statistical Analysis

The data generated in this study was analyzed using the MedCalc software version 6.0 (Mariakerke, Belgium). To demonstrate statistical differences between the different stimulation conditions we used the Wilcoxon test for paired samples, which is a non-parametric alternative method for the paired-samples *t*-test when the distribution of the samples is not normal, *p* values equal or less than 0.05 was regarded as significant.

3. Results

3.1. Effect of LTC_4, LTD_4, and Cytokines on the Expression of CysLT1 Receptor

Nasal tissue fibroblasts from chronic rhinosinusitis patients were able to express CysLT1 receptor mRNA levels but at very low levels. Stimulation with LTC_4 did not influence the gene expression of the receptor when compared to non-stimulated cells; in contrast to LTD_4 that upregulated the mRNA levels of the receptor in a dose-dependent manner being 10^{-8} M the concentration with the highest effect (Figure 1).

Based on that fribroblasts may change their behaviour and activation profiles when they are under influence of certain cytokine millieu, we decided to study the effect of IL-4, IL-13, TNF-α and TGF-β_1 on the expression of CysLT1 receptor. Results of this stimulation showed that IL-4, IL-13, and TNF-α had no influence on the gene expression of CysLT1 receptor. In contrast, TGF-β_1 significantly increased the expression of the receptor when compared to unstimulated cells (Figure 2).

To evaluate the effect of cytokines on the changes induced by LTD_4 on CySLT1 receptor expression, chronic rhinosinusitis fibroblasts were pre-incubated 24 h with 10 ng/mL of TGF-β_1 and, subsequently, with different concentrations of LTD_4. Of interest, an additive effect on the regulation of CysLT1 receptor was observed. This effect was more pronounced at the LTD_4 concentration of 10^{-8} M as shown in Figure 3.

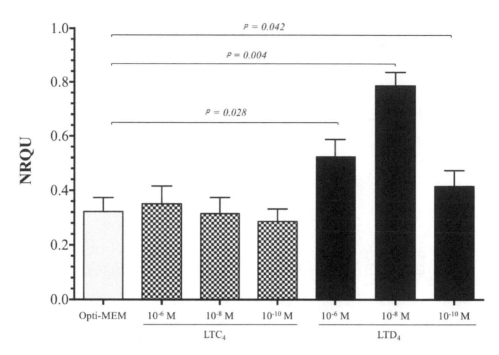

Figure 1. Messenger RNA expression levels of CysLT1 receptor in fibroblasts from chronic rhinosinusitis tissue after stimulation with cysteinyl leukotriene C_4 (LTC$_4$) and D_4 (LTD$_4$). *NRQU:* normalized relative quantification units; *p* value represents the level of significance after a Wilcoxon test for paired samples.

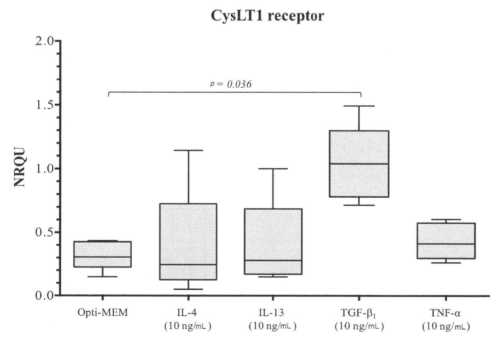

Figure 2. Messenger RNA expression levels of CysLT1 receptor in fibroblasts from chronic rhinosinusitis tissue after stimulation with Interleukin-4 (IL-4), interleukin-13 (IL-13), TNF-α, and TGF-β$_1$. *NRQU:* normalized relative quantification units; *p* value represent the level of significance after a Wilcoxon test for paired samples.

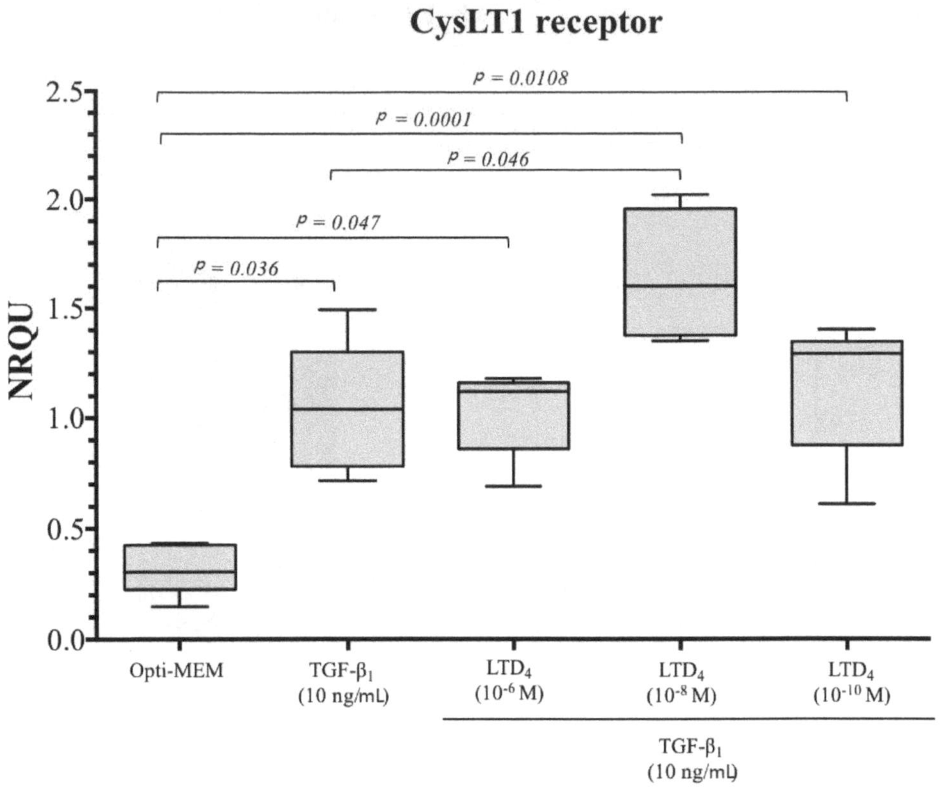

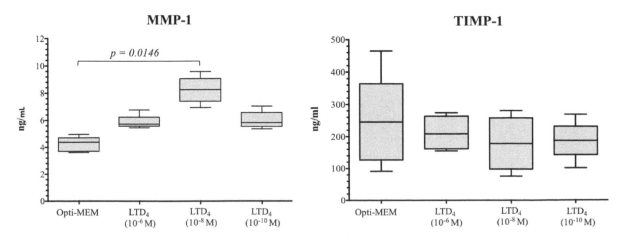

CysLT1 receptor

Figure 3. Messenger RNA expression levels of CysLT1 receptor in fibroblasts from chronic rhinosinusitis tissue after stimulation with TGF-β_1 and LTD$_4$. *NRQU:* normalized relative quantification units; *p* value represents the level of significance after a Wilcoxon test for paired samples.

3.2. Effect of LTC$_4$, LTD$_4$, and Cytokines on the Release of Metalloproteinases

Protein levels of MMP-2, MMP-3, MMP-7, and MMP-9 were below detection limit in all experimental conditions. Only MMP-1 and TIMP-1 were released during basal conditions. Further, LTD$_4$ increased the levels of MMP-1 in a dose-dependent way being the concentration of 10^{-8} M the one showing the best effect (Figure 4). No changes were observed in the expression of TIMP-1 by the addition of LTC$_4$ or LTD$_4$ in the culture medium.

Figure 4. Concentrations of metalloproteinase 1 (MMP-1) and tissue inhibitor of metalloproteinase 1 (TIMP-1) in fibroblasts from chronic rhinosinusitis tissue after stimulation with LTD$_4$. *p* value represents the level of significance after a Wilcoxon test for paired samples.

Pre- incubation of the cells with IL-4, IL-13, TGF-β_1, TNF-α alone or in combination with LTD$_4$ failed to induce changes in TIMP-1 production. Expression of MMP-1 was, however, significantly induced after TGF-β_1 and TNF-α stimulation alone and in combination with 10^{-8} M of LTD$_4$ when compared to non-timulated cells (Figure 5). Addition of TNF-α increased the concentrations of MMP1 but this effect was not related to cytokine concentration, and a non-additive effect was observed after addition of LTD$_4$. The upregulation of MMP-1 levels by TGF-β_1 was more potent than the one observed with LTD$_4$ alone. An additive dose-dependent effect on MMP-1 production was obtained when combined with the two compounds in the culture (Figure 5).

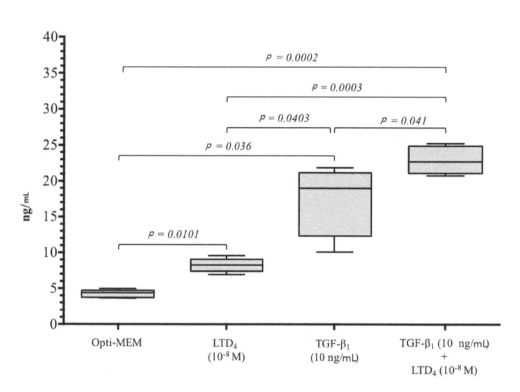

Figure 5. Concentrations of metalloproteinase 1 (MMP-1) in fibroblasts from chronic rhinosinusitis tissue after stimulation with LTD$_4$ and TGF-β_1. p value represents the level of significance after a Wilcoxon test for paired samples.

3.3. Effect of Montelukast on MMP-1 and CysLT1 Receptor Expression Induced by LTD$_4$ and TGF-β_1

Montelukast inhibited the CysLT1 receptor mRNA expression in a dose-dependent manner in fibroblasts stimulated with LTD$_4$, but also attenuated the increase in receptor expression induced by TGF-β_1 alone and in combination with LTD$_4$ (Figure 6). The leukotriene receptor antagonist also restablished in a dose-dependant way the concenrations of MMP1 to baseline levels in fibroblasts stimulated with TGF-β_1 and with LTD$_4$ alone or in combination. However, the lowest concentrations of Montelukast did not diminish the expression of MMP-1 to baseline levels in the cells pre-stimulated with TGF-β_1 (Figure 7).

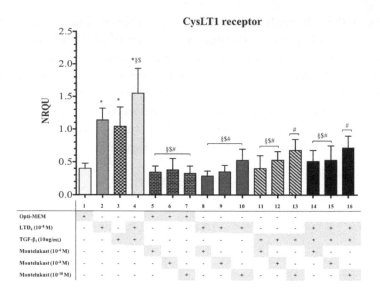

Figure 6. mRNA expression of CYSLT1 receptor in fibroblasts from chronic rhinosinusitis tissue after stimulation with LTD_4 and $TGF-\beta_1$ and in presence or absence of Montelukast. *NRQU:* normalized relative quantification units, *: p value < 0.05 when compared to tissue culture medium (Opti-MEM), §: p value < 0.05 when compared to LTD_4 (10^{-8} M), \$: p value < 0.05 when compared to $TGF-\beta_1$, #: p value < 0.05 when compared to $TGF-\beta_1 + LTD_4$. Tukey's multiple comparisons test for CysLT1 receptor expression in Supplementary Table S1.

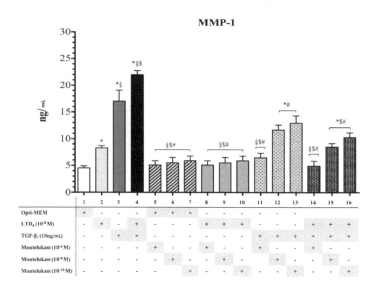

Figure 7. Concentrations of metalloproteinase 1 (MMP-1) in fibroblasts from chronic rhinosinusitis tissue after stimulation with LTD_4 and $TGF-\beta_1$ and in presence or absence of Montelukast. *: p value < 0.05 when compared to tissue culture medium (Opti-MEM), §: p value < 0.05 when compared to LTD_4 (10^{-8} M), \$: p value < 0.05 when compared to $TGF-\beta_1$, #: p value < 0.05 when compared to $TGF-\beta_1 + LTD_4$. Tukey's multiple comparisons test for MMP1 protein concentrations Supplementary Table S2.

4. Discussion

The main finding of this study is that $TGF-\beta_1$ and LTD_4 are potent inducers of MMP-1 protein in chronic rhinosinusitis tissue-derived fibroblasts and that this effect is mediated, in part, by the CysLT1 receptor and, hence, could be attenuated by its antagonist Montelukast. The effect of $TGF-\beta_1$ on MMP-1 production have been reported in lower airways; however, this is the first report in nasal tissue fibroblasts. In CRSsNP tissue, MMP-1 levels are increased when compared to healthy nasal mucosa and it is mainly localized in the nasal epithelium and mucosal and sub-mucosal glands, as well as in some infiltrated inflammatory cells [27]. Further, TGF-β1 and CysLTs are also increased in CRSsNP tissue when compared to non-inflamed nasal mucosa, as reported by Van Bruaene and Perez Novo et al., respectively [12,28]. Balance in collagen degradation MMPs is a crucial mechanism leading to an appropriate tissue wound healing process where fibroblasts represent one of the major cells involved [2].

Leukotrienes play an important role in the regulation of MMP synthesis and, hence, in the remodeling process by enhancing collagenase mRNA expression [29]. Medina et al. demonstrated that LTD4 and IL-1β could induce the secretion of MMP-1 in airway smooth muscle cells resulting in the stimulation of cell proliferation [30]. More recently, it has been suggested that LTD4 has the potential to augment fibroblast chemotaxis, and to contribute to the regulation of the wound healing and remodeling in fibrotic processes of the lung [31,32]. LTD4 may also increase collagen production in activated myofibroblasts by upregulating CysLT1 receptor induced by TGF-β1 [33]. This evidence strongly supports the possible role of lipid mediators, and especially cysteinyl leukotrienes, in airway remodeling and in the regulation of MMP production.

The action of TGF-β1 through the CysLT1 receptor in the regulation of ECM molecules has been previously reported by Asakura et al. [33]. However, in that study LTD4 in combination with TGF-β1 stimulated the production of collagen in a human fetal lung fibroblasts cell line. Our results showed that the same compounds also induced the production of MMP-1, which can induce collagen degradation. This discrepancy can be due to the differences in cell type (lung derived cell line versus primary nasal tissue cells). As stated before MMP-1 degrades collagen. In a previous work we observed that collagen content in CRSsNP is higher than in control and CRSwNP tissues [28]. This is perfectly possible if we take into account that fibroblasts are not the only cells producing MMPs, and in our study we exclude the contribution of these cells. Further the expression of collagen and the influence of other cytokines, which are present in physiological conditions, could not be tested in this study.

It is important to mention that in the study of Steinke et al., [34] the authors failed to show CyLT1 receptor expression in nasal polyp fibroblasts. One explanation for this discrepancy could be the high levels of TGF-β1 present in CRSsNP tissue; this growth factor is an important inducer of CyLT1 receptor as demonstrated by several research works and observed in our study. This factor is also important in the transformation of fibroblasts into myofibroblasts. Fibroblasts isolated from CRSsNP could retain these properties during the seeding procedure and it may be the cause of the low expression of CyLT1 receptor observed. Furthermore, it has been documented from several authors that fibroblast behavior between CRS with and without polyps, and even between polyp subtypes, (for example, with and without asthma or aspirin-exacerbated disease) is different.

To conclude, we can state that the release of cytokines like TGF-β1 and lipid mediators like CysLTs by inflammatory cells can significantly contribute to the regulation of fibroblast CysLT1 receptor and MMP-1 pathways. This is of relevance due to high levels of these molecules observed in chronic rhinosinusitis tissue. Montelukast is a potent and specific CysLT1 receptor inhibitor that has been shown to cause a significant decrease in sputum and peripheral blood eosinophil number, reduce concentrations of eosinophilic cationic protein, of LTC4 and exhaled nitric oxide levels in asthmatic patients [35,36]. However, despite the action of leukotriene modifiers, it has been well documented that its role in upper airways remodeling remains unclear. The findings obtained in this study are in line with previous in vitro and animal studies, suggesting the use of Montelukast as a modifier of lower airway remodeling. Our work involved human nasal fibroblasts from chronic rhinosinusitis patients adding more evidence for the potential role of this LTR antagonist in regulating the remodeling process in upper airways.

Acknowledgments: The study was supported by a grant to Claudina Perez-Novo from the Flemish Research Board (FWO Postdoctoral mandate, Nr. FWO08-PDO-117).

Author Contributions: C.A.P.N. and C.B. conceived and designed the experiments; C.C., G.H. and C.A.P.N. performed the experiments; R.P. and C.A.P.N. analyzed the data; R.P., C.A.P.N. and C.B. wrote the paper.

Conflicts of Interest: The authors declare no conflict of interest.

References

1. Van Zele, T.; Claeys, S.; Gevaert, P.; van Maele, G.; Holtappels, G.; van Cauwenberge, P.; Bachert, C. Differentiation of chronic sinus diseases by measurement of inflammatory mediators. *Allergy Eur. J. Allergy Clin. Immunol.* **2006**, *61*, 1280–1289. [CrossRef] [PubMed]

2. Watelet, J.B.; van Zele, T.; Gjomarkaj, M.; Canonica, G.W.; Dahlen, S.E.; Fokkens, W.; Lund, V.J.; Scadding, G.K.; Mullol, J.; Papadopoulos, N.; *et al.* Tissue remodelling in upper airways: W is the link with lower airway remodelling? *Allergy* **2006**, *61*, 1249–1258. [CrossRef] [PubMed]

3. Kostamo, K.; Toskala, E.; Tervahartiala, T.; Sorsa, T. Role of matrix metalloproteinases in chronic rhinosinusitis. *Curr. Opin. Allergy Clin. Immunol.* **2008**, *8*, 21–27. [CrossRef] [PubMed]

4. Sacco, O.; Silvestri, M.; Sabatini, F.; Sale, R.; Defilippi, A.C.; Rossi, G.A. Epithelial cells and fibroblasts: Structural repair and remodelling in the airways. *Paediatr. Respir. Rev.* **2004**, *5*, S35–S40. [CrossRef]

5. Nagase, H.; Visse, R.; Murphy, G. Structure and function of matrix metalloproteinases and TIMPs. *Cardiovasc. Res.* **2006**, *69*, 562–573. [CrossRef] [PubMed]

6. Murphy, G.; Nagase, H. Progress in matrix metalloproteinase research. *Mol. Asp. Med.* **2009**, *29*, 290–308. [CrossRef] [PubMed]

7. Page-McCaw, A.; Ewald, A.J.; Werb, Z. Matrix metalloproteinases and the regulation of tissue remodelling. *Nat. Rev. Mol. Cell Biol.* **2007**, *8*, 221–233. [CrossRef] [PubMed]

8. Demedts, I.K.; Brusselle, G.G.; Bracke, K.R.; Vermaelen, K.Y.; Pauwels, R.A. Matrix metalloproteinases in asthma and COPD. *Curr. Opin. Pharmacol.* **2005**, *5*, 257–263. [CrossRef] [PubMed]

9. Funk, C.D. Prostaglandins and leukotrienes: Advances in eicosanoid biology. *Science* **2001**, *294*, 1871–1875. [CrossRef] [PubMed]

10. Ogawa, Y.; Calhoun, W.J. The role of leukotrienes in airway inflammation. *J. Allergy Clin. Immunol.* **2006**, *118*, 789–798. [CrossRef] [PubMed]

11. Hui, Y.; Funk, C.D. Cysteinyl leukotriene receptors. *Biochem. Pharmacol.* **2002**, *64*, 1549–1557. [CrossRef]

12. Pérez-Novo, C.A.; Watelet, J.B.; Claeys, C.; Van Cauwenberge, P.; Bachert, C. Prostaglandin, leukotriene, and lipoxin balance in chronic rhinosinusitis with and without nasal polyposis. *J. Allergy Clin. Immunol.* **2005**, *115*, 1189–1196. [CrossRef] [PubMed]

13. Pérez-Novo, C.A.; Claeys, C.; Van Cauwenberge, P.; Bachert, C. Expression of eicosanoid receptors subtypes and eosinophilic inflammation: implication on chronic rhinosinusitis. *Respir. Res.* **2006**, *7*, 75. [CrossRef] [PubMed]

14. Clarke, D.L.; Dakshinamurti, S.; Larsson, A.K.; Ward, J.E.; Yamasaki, A. Lipid metabolites as regulators of airway smooth muscle function. *Pulm. Pharmacol. Ther.* **2009**, *22*, 426–435. [CrossRef] [PubMed]

15. Parameswaran, K.; Radford, K.; Fanat, A.; Stephen, J.; Bonnans, C.; Levy, B.D.; Janssen, L.J.; Cox, P.G. Modulation of human airway smooth muscle migration by lipid mediators and Th-2 cytokines. *Am. J. Respir. Cell Mol. Biol.* **2007**, *37*, 240–247. [CrossRef] [PubMed]

16. Tokuriki, S.; Ohshima, Y.; Yamada, A.; Ohta, N.; Tsukahara, H.; Mayumi, M. Leukotriene D4 enhances the function of endothelin-1-primed fibroblasts. *Clin. Immunol.* **2007**, *125*, 88–94. [CrossRef] [PubMed]

17. Yoshisue, H.; Kirkham-Brown, J.; Healy, E.; Holgate, S.T.; Sampson, A.P.; Davies, D.E. Cysteinyl leukotrienes synergize with growth factors to induce proliferation of human bronchial fibroblasts. *J. Allergy Clin. Immunol.* **2007**, *119*, 132–140. [CrossRef] [PubMed]

18. Gharaee-Kermani, M.; Hu, B.; Thannickal, V.J.; Phan, S.H.; Gyetko, M.R. Current and emerging drugs for idiopathic pulmonary fibrosis. *Expert. Opin. Emerg. Drugs* **2007**, *12*, 627–646. [CrossRef] [PubMed]

19. Potter-Perigo, S.; Baker, C.; Tsoi, C.; Braun, K.R.; Isenhath, S.; Altman, G.M.; Altman, L.C.; Wight, T.N. Regulation of Proteoglycan Synthesis by Leukotriene D4 and Epidermal Growth Factor in Bronchial Smooth Muscle Cells. *Am. J. Respir. Cell Mol. Biol.* **2004**, *30*, 101–108. [CrossRef] [PubMed]

20. Currie, G.P.; McLaughlin, K. The expanding role of leukotriene receptor antagonists in chronic asthma. *Ann. Allergy Asthma Immunol.* **2006**, *97*, 731–742. [CrossRef]

21. Kemp, J.P. Recent advances in the management of asthma using leukotriene modifiers. *Am. J. Respir. Med.* **2003**, *2*, 139–156. [CrossRef] [PubMed]

22. Fukushima, C.; Matsuse, H.; Hishikawa, Y.; Kondo, Y.; Machida, I.; Saeki, S.; Kawano, T.; Tomari, S.; Obase, Y.; Shimoda, T.; Koji, T.; Kohno, S. Pranlukast, a leukotriene receptor antagonist, inhibits interleukin-5 production via a mechanism distinct from leukotriene receptor antagonism. *Int. Arch. Allergy Immunol.* **2005**, *136*, 165–172. [CrossRef] [PubMed]

23. Fokkens, W.J.; Lund, V.J.; Mullol, J.; Bachert, C.; Alobid, I.; Baroody, F.; Cohen, N.; Cervin, A.; Douglas, R.; Gevaert, P.; *et al.* EPOS 2012: European position paper on rhinosinusitis and nasal polyps 2012. A summary for otorhinolaryngologists. *Rhinology* **2012**, *50*, 1–12. [PubMed]

24. Bousquet, J.; Clark, T.J.H.; Hurd, S.; Khaltaev, N.; Lenfant, C.; O'Byrne, P.; Sheffer, A. GINA guidelines on asthma and beyond. *Allergy Eur. J. Allergy Clin. Immunol.* **2007**, *62*, 102–112. [CrossRef] [PubMed]

25. Pérez-Novo, C.A.; Claeys, C.; Speleman, F.; van Cauwenberge, F.; Bachert, C.V.J. Impact of RNA quality on reference gene expression stability. *Biotechniques* **2005**, *39*, 52–56. [CrossRef] [PubMed]

26. Hellemans, J.; Mortier, G.; de Paepe, A.; Speleman, F.; Vandesompele, J. qBase relative quantification framework and software for management and automated analysis of real-time quantitative PCR data. *Genome Biol.* **2007**, *8*, R19. [CrossRef] [PubMed]

27. Eyibilen, A.; Cayli, S.; Aladag, I.; Koç, S.; Gurbuzler, L.; Atay, G.A. Distribution of matrix metalloproteinases MMP-1, MMP-2, MMP-8 and tissue inhibitor of matrix metalloproteinases-2 in nasal polyposis and chronic rhinosinusitis. *Histol. Histopathol.* **2011**, *26*, 615–621. [PubMed]

28. Van Bruaene, N.; Derycke, L.; Perez-Novo, C.A.; Gevaert, P.; Holtappels, G.; de Ruyck, N.; Cuvelier, C.; van Cauwenberge, P.; Bachert, C. TGF-beta signaling and collagen deposition in chronic rhinosinusitis. *J. Allergy Clin. Immunol.* **2009**, *124*, 253–259. [CrossRef] [PubMed]

29. Medina, L.; Pérez-Ramos, J.; Ramírez, R.; Selman, M.; Pardo, A. Leukotriene C4 upregulates collagenase expression and synthesis in human lung fibroblasts. *BBA Mol. Cell Res.* **1994**, *1224*, 168–174. [CrossRef]

30. Rajah, R.; Nunn, S.E.; Herrick, D.J.; Grunstein, M.M.; Cohen, P. Leukotriene D4 induces MMP-1, which functions as an IGFBP protease in human airway smooth muscle cells. *Am. J. Physiol.* **1996**, *271*, L1014–L1022. [PubMed]

31. Kato, J.; Kohyama, T.; Okazaki, H.; Desaki, M.; Nagase, T.; Rennard, S.I.; Takizawa, H. Leukotriene D4 potentiates fibronectin-induced migration of human lung fibroblasts. *Clin. Immunol.* **2005**, *117*, 177–181. [CrossRef] [PubMed]

32. Vannella, K.M.; McMillan, T.R.; Charbeneau, R.P.; Wilke, C.A.; Thomas, P.E.; Toews, G.B.; Peters-Golden, M.; Moore, B.B. Cysteinyl leukotrienes are autocrine and paracrine regulators of fibrocyte function. *J. Immunol.* **2007**, *179*, 7883–7890. [CrossRef] [PubMed]

33. Asakura, T.; Ishii, Y.; Chibana, K.; Fukuda, T. Leukotriene D4 stimulates collagen production from myofibroblasts transformed by TGF-β. *J. Allergy Clin. Immunol.* **2004**, *114*, 310–315. [CrossRef] [PubMed]

34. Steinke, J.W.; Crouse, C.D.; Bradley, D.; Hise, K.; Lynch, K.; Kountakis, S.E.; Borish, L. Characterization of Interleukin-4-Stimulated Nasal Polyp Fibroblasts. *Am. J. Respir. Cell Mol. Biol.* **2004**, *30*, 212–219. [CrossRef] [PubMed]

35. Reiss, T.F.; Chervinsky, P.; Dockhorn, R.J.; Shingo, S.; Seidenberg, B.; Edwards, T.B. Montelukast, a once-daily leukotriene receptor antagonist, in the treatment of chronic asthma: A multicenter, randomized, double-blind trial. Montelukast Clinical Research Study Group. *Arch. Intern. Med.* **1998**, *158*, 1213–1220. [CrossRef] [PubMed]

36. Reiss, T.F.; Sorkness, C.A.; Stricker, W.; Botto, A.; Busse, W.W.; Kundu, S.; Zhang, J. Effects of montelukast (MK-0476); a potent cysteinyl leukotriene receptor antagonist, on bronchodilation in asthmatic subjects treated with and without inhaled corticosteroids. *Thorax* **1997**, *52*, 45–48. [CrossRef] [PubMed]

20

Fatty Acid Composition of Cultured Fibroblasts Derived from Healthy Nasal Mucosa and Nasal Polyps

Suha Jabr Ayyad [1,2], Jordi Roca-Ferrer [1,2,3] and César Picado [1,2,3,]*

[1] Institut d'Investigacions Biomèdiques August Pi y Sunyer (IDIBAPS),08036 Barcelona, Spain; sjayyad@gmail.com (S.J.A.); jrocaferrer@ub.edu (J.R.-F.)
[2] Hospital Clinic, Universitat de Barcelona, 08036 Barcelona, Spain
[3] Centro de Investigaciones Biomédicas en Red de Enfermedades Respiratorias (CIBERES), 08036 Barcelona, Spain
* Correspondence: cpicado@ub.edu

Academic Editor: Claudina A. Pérez Novo

Abstract: Background: Fibroblasts from nasal polyps (NP) of asthma patients have reduced expression of cyclooxygenase 2 (COX-2) and production of prostaglandin E_2 (PGE_2). We hypothesized that the reported alterations are due to alterations in the availability of arachidonic acid (AA). Objective: The objective was to determine the fatty acid composition of airway fibroblasts from healthy subjects and from asthma patients with and without aspirin intolerance. Methods: We analyzed the fatty acid composition of cultured fibroblasts from non-asthmatics ($n = 6$) and from aspirin-tolerant ($n = 6$) and aspirin-intolerant asthmatics ($n = 6$) by gas chromatography-flame ionization detector. Fibroblasts were stimulated with acetyl salicylic acid (ASA). Results: The omega-6 fatty acids dihomo-gamma-linolenic acid (C20:3) and AA (C20:4), and omega-3 fatty acids docosapentaenoic acid (DPA) (C22:5) and docosahexaenoic acid (DHA) (C22:6) were significantly higher in NP fibroblasts than in fibroblasts derived from nasal mucosa. The percentage composition of the fatty acids palmitic acid (C16:0) and palmitoleic acid (C16:1) was significantly higher in fibroblasts from patients with NP and aspirin intolerance than in fibroblasts derived from the nasal NP of aspirin-tolerant patients. ASA did not cause changes in either omega-3 or omega-6 fatty acids. Conclusions. Our data do not support the hypothesis that a reduced production of AA in NP fibroblasts can account for the reported low production of PGE_2 in nasal polyps. Whether the increased proportion of omega-3 fatty acids can contribute to reduced PGE_2 production in nasal polyps by competitively inhibiting COX-2 and reducing the amount of AA available to the COX-2 enzyme remains to be elucidated.

Keywords: arachidonic acid; aspirin intolerance; asthma; cyclooxygenase; eicosanoids; fatty acids; fibroblast; inflammation; nasal mucosa; nasal polyps

1. Introduction

Asthma is a syndrome characterized by the presence of chronic inflammation, resulting in airway obstruction and bronchial hyper-responsiveness that causes wheezing, coughing, and dyspnea [1]. Nasal polyposis (NP) is a chronic inflammatory disease of the sinus mucosa usually seen in association with chronic rhinosinusitis (CRS) and asthma [2]. The pathogenesis of CRS with NP is related to an altered inflammatory state that results in a tissue remodeling process [3].

Aspirin-intolerant asthma (AIA) is a distinct syndrome characterized by asthma, CRS, NP, and aspirin sensitivity. Aspirin sensitivity may be present in 5 to 10% of the asthmatic population [4,5]. The pathophysiological mechanism of AIA is only partially understood and appears to be related to anomalies in the metabolism of arachidonic acid AA [4,5].

AA is produced from membrane phospholipids by the action of phospholipase A2 enzymes; it can then be converted into different eicosanoids. AA can be enzymatically metabolized by three main pathways: P-450 epoxygenase, cyclooxygenases (COXs) and lipoxygenases (LOXs). The LOXs convert AA into leukotriene (LT) A_4, which is the precursor of LTB_4 and cysteinyl leukotrienes (LTC_4, LTD_4 and LTE_4) [6]. The COX pathway produces PGG_2 and PGH_2, which are in turn converted into prostaglandins (PGEs) and thromboxanes. There are two isoforms of the COX enzymes: prostaglandin H synthase-1 (PGHS-1), also known as COX-1, is generally constitutively expressed and is typically considered a "house-keeping" gene; and prostaglandin H synthase-2 (PGHS-2), also known as COX-2, is usually only expressed under inflammatory conditions [7].

Eicosanoids are released from cells during hypersensitivity reactions and are involved in the clinical manifestations of rhinitis and asthma. LTs are potent pro-inflammatory mediators and this can explain why anti-LTs are beneficial in asthma and rhinitis [6]. PGs might act as both pro-inflammatory and anti-inflammatory mediators, depending on the context; this is partly due to the level of expression of the four PG receptors in the cells involved in the response [7]. The COX pathway is the major target for non-steroidal anti-inflammatory drugs (NSAIDs), the most popular medications used to treat fever, pain, and inflammation [7]. However, and in contrast with other inflammatory diseases such as arthritis [7] and cystic fibrosis [8], inhibition of COX with aspirin or NSAIDs does not provide any salutary effect to asthma patients. In fact, for a subset of patients with asthma, ingestion of NSAIDs induces bronchoconstriction and nasal obstruction [4,5]. Interestingly, selective COX-2 inhibitors are usually well tolerated by AIA [4,5].

These observations suggest that eicosanoids can be differentially regulated in asthma, unlike other inflammatory airway diseases [5]. In patients with asthma, and especially in AIA, various data support the existence of an altered regulation of the COX pathway [9–15]. PGE_2 levels have been reported to be low in the nasal polyps of asthma patients, as well as in nasal-polyp and bronchial fibroblasts from asthmatic patients, particularly those with aspirin sensitivity [11,13–15]. As PGE_2 production mostly depends on the level of COX-2 induction under conditions of inflammation, it should be expected that the low production of PGE_2 detected in asthma and nasal polyps would be accompanied by a similar, concomitant alteration in the expression of COX-2. Accordingly, lack of up-regulation of COX-2 in the nasal polyps of asthma patients, both with and without aspirin sensitivity, has been reported in various studies [9–12,15].

The mechanisms involved in the abnormal production of prostaglandin E_2 in nasal polyps, and in particular in those associated with AIA, are still unclear [5]. Various studies have shown that the activity of COX-1 and COX-2 enzymes is controlled differentially by regulating the amount of AA available to the enzymes [6]. As PGE_2 production by COX-1 and COX-2 is dependent, at least in part, on the availability of AA, it could be possible that alterations in the AA supply may account for the anomalies in PGE_2 production reported in nasal polyps and AIA.

A number of observations support the notion that fibroblasts are more than just structural cells with no other physiological or modulator functions [16]. Fibroblasts can contribute to the regulation of inflammatory and immunological responses by producing various growth factors, cytokines and eicosanoids [17].

The hypothesis of the present study establishes that the reported alteration in the production of some prostanoids such as PGE_2 in the nasal polyps of asthma patients, particularly in those with aspirin intolerance, is at least partly due to alterations in the availability of AA.

The main objective of this study is to determine and compare the fatty acid composition of airway fibroblasts from healthy subjects and those from nasal polyps of asthma patients with and without aspirin intolerance.

2. Material and Methods

2.1. Population and Tissue Handling

Nasal polyp tissue was obtained from 12 asthmatic subjects (6 aspirin-tolerant, and 6 aspirin-intolerant) referred to our institution for sinus surgery. The study subjects were selected on the basis of a medical history consistent with severe chronic NP, documented via CT scan [2]. The diagnosis of asthma was established from the clinical history and the demonstration of a reversible bronchial obstruction. Diagnosis of aspirin intolerance was based on a clear-cut history of asthma attacks precipitated by non-steroidal anti-inflammatory drugs (NSAID) and confirmed by aspirin nasal challenge in patients with an isolated episode of NSAID-induced asthma exacerbation [18]. Nasal mucosa from 6 subjects undergoing nasal corrective surgery was used as control. The characteristics of the asthmatic and non-asthmatic patients are shown in Table 1.

Table 1. Characteristics of study subjects.

Variables	Controls	Asthma Aspirin Tolerant	Asthma Aspirin Intolerant
N	6	6	6
Age (years)			
Mean $\pm$ SD	53 $\pm$ 19	60 $\pm$ 16	68 $\pm$ 9
Min.–Max.	28–77	44–87	59–82
Gender (M/F)	(4/2)	(5/1)	(1/5)

Age is expressed as mean $\pm$ standard deviation (SD).

All patients with NP were on intranasal glucocorticoid therapy that was discontinued at least five days before surgery. None of the patients were on oral GC therapy at the time of surgery, nor had they received any systemic GCs for at least one month prior to surgery. No subjects from the nasal mucosa control group had a history of nasal or sinus disease, nor had they received GCs for any reason. None of the subjects had suffered from an upper respiratory infection during the two weeks prior to surgery.

The subjects were asked for their permission and written informed consent was given to study pathological specimens under a protocol approved by the human investigations committee of our hospital.

2.2. Fibroblast Culture

Specimens obtained during nasal endoscopic surgery were cut into 3 × 3 mm fragments and placed in six-well plates containing Dulbecco's modified Eagle's medium (DMEM) supplemented with 10% fetal bovine serum (FBS), 100 IU/mL penicillin, 100 μg/mL streptomycin, and 2 μg/mL amphotericin B. After a period of 3 weeks, when fibroblast growth was established, tissue fragments were removed and the first passage was performed. Cultures were washed three times with phosphate buffered saline (PBS) and incubated for 5 min with 0.05% trypsin and 0.02% EDTA. The reaction was stopped by the addition of growth medium, cells were collected by centrifugation (1800 rpm, 5 min), seeded in two 75-cm^2 flasks and grown up to 90% confluence (duplicate per sample). Cells from the sixth passage were used in the study of fibroblasts' lipid composition. When the confluence reached up to 90%, cells were washed with PBS and incubated with DMEM without FBS for 24 h, then the medium was changed for another quantity of DMEM without FBS, for samples stimulated with aspirin; 0.5 mg/dL of aspirin were added, then the samples were left for 24 h in culture before the lipid extraction.

2.3. Lipid Extraction

Total lipids were extracted from fibroblast cells using methanol-chloroform containing 1% BHT according to the method of Bligh and Dyer [19]. The cells were washed three times with ice-cold Ca^{2+}, Mg^{2+}, and free PBS; it was then left and the cells were harvested by scraping. The cells were pelleted by centrifugation at 1200 rpm at 4 °C for 5 min and the PBS was removed. The cells were washed once with 10 mL ice-cold PBS and centrifuged at 1200 rpm at 4 °C for 5 min, then the PBS was removed. 300 µL of ice-cold PBS was added to the sample, and then an aliquot sample of 50 µL was taken to determine the total protein. The rest of the pellets and PBS were transferred to a glass tube and centrifuged at 2500 rpm at 20 °C for 5 min and the PBS was removed. Two milliliters of distilled water were added, then the sample was sonicated to assure further cell lysis, and then centrifuged at 2500 rpm at 4 °C for 10 min; the supernatant was discarded. The pellets were resuspended by 1 mL of physiological serum then the chloroform-methanol (2:1) were added, then the tube contents were centrifuged and the lower phase was collected and dried under nitrogen. One milliliter of 14% BF3/MeOH reagent was added. The mixture was heated at 100 °C for 1 h. Then it was cooled to room temperature and fatty acid methyl esters (FAMEs) were extracted twice in the hexane phase, following the addition of 1 mL H_2O. The aliquot was evaporated to dryness under nitrogen and re-diluted with 75 µL of n-hexane.

2.4. Analysis of FAMEs

Gas chromatography analyses were performed using an Agilent 7890A system (Agilent Technologies, Barcelona, Spain) equipped with a flame ionization and autosampler. Separation of fatty acid methyl esters was carried out on a SupraWAX-280 capillary column (30 m × 0.25 µm × 0.25 mm I.D.) coated with a stationary phase (polyethylene glycol 100%) from Teknokroma (Barcelona, Spain). The operating conditions were as follows: The split-splitless injector was used in split mode with a split ratio of 1:10. The injection volume of the sample was 1 µL. The injector and detector temperatures were kept at 220 °C and 300 °C, respectively. The temperature program was as follows: initial temperature 120 °C for 1 min., increased at 15 °C/min to 210 °C and held at this temperature for 42 min (total running time: 49 min.). For safety reasons, helium was used as the carrier gas, with a head pressure of 300 kPa that referred to a linear velocity of 27.5 cm/s at 140 °C. Detector gas flows: H_2, 40 mL/min; make-up gas (N_2), 40 mL/min; air, 450 mL/min. Data acquisition processing was performed with HP-chemstation software. Samples were determined in duplicate. The identities of sample methyl ester peaks were determined by comparison of their relative retention times with those of well-known standards. The results are expressed in relative amounts (percentage of total fatty acids).

The same batch of a commercial fetal bovine serum (FBS) was used in all the experiments to prevent any interference of culture procedure in the fatty acid composition of fibroblast. The fatty acid composition of fetal bovine serum was also analyzed.

The protein concentration of the cell lysates was measured using a modified Lowry method, with bovine serum albumin as the protein standard. Absorbencies were read at 630 nm in a spectrophotometer.

2.5. Statistical Analysis

Results were described by means frequencies and percentages for qualitative variables and mean ± Standard Deviation (SD) or Standard Error of mean (SE). Data were analyzed using ANCOVA models, adjusting the effect of studied factor by level of protein. For these inferential analyses, a non-parametrical approach by means rank transformation was applied. Statistical significance was considered at $P < 0.05$. Analyses were carried out using the SPSS program for MS Windows (version 15).

3. Results

3.1. Fatty Acid Composition in Nasal Mucosa and Nasal Polyps

The fatty acid composition of fibroblasts from control nasal mucosa and nasal polyps are shown in Table 2. The omega-6 fatty acids, dihomo-gamma-linolenic acid (C20:3) and AA (C20:4), and the omega-3 fatty acids, DPA (C22:5) and DHA (C22:6), were significantly higher in nasal polyp fibroblasts than in fibroblasts derived from nasal mucosa. In contrast, oleic acid (C18:1), gamma-linolenic acid

(C18:3), and eicosadienoic acid (C20:2) were significantly lower in nasal polyp fibroblasts than in those cultured from nasal mucosa.

Table 2. Fatty acid composition in fibroblasts from the different groups.

| | NM | NP | NP-ATA | NP-AIA |
	N = 6	N = 12	N = 6	N = 6
16:0	17.34 ± 2.53	17.78 ± 2.96	16.74 ± 3.80	18.83 ± 1.11 [f]
16:1	2.87 ± 0.74	3.02 ± 1.06	2.55 ± 1.17	3.50 ± 0.69 [d]
18:0	16.72 ± 0.95	16.80 ± 1.67	17.25 ± 1.87	16.35 ± 1.36
18:1	33.38 ± 2.77	31.83 ± 2.78 [c]	31.80 ± 3.71	31.86 ± 1.45
18:2n6	2.15 ± 1.14	1.80 ± 0.64	1.60 ± 0.53	2.01 ± 0.70
18:3n6	0.63 ± 0.38	0.40 ± 0.20 [c]	0.36 ± 0.21	0.43 ± 0.19
18:3n3	0.24 ± 0.14	0.18 ± 0.10	0.19 ± 0.10	0.16 ± 0.10
20:2n6	2.36 ± 0.56	1.61 ± 0.51 [a]	1.81 ± 0.45	1.41 ± 0.51 [e]
20:3n6	1.50 ± 0.38	1.73 ± 0.35 [a]	1.64 ± 0.40	1.81 ± 0.26
20:4n6	5.97 ± 2.12	7.20 ± 1.55 [a]	7.39 ± 1.91	7.00 ± 1.10
20:3n3	0.16 ± 0.11	0.18 ± 0.19	0.23 ± 0.26	0.14 ± 0.03
20:5n3	0.66 ± 0.24	0.68 ± 0.37	0.76 ± 0.40	0.61 ± 0.34
22:5n3	1.83 ± 0.40	2.11 ± 0.39 [c]	2.11 ± 0.40	2.11 ± 0.39
22:6n3	2.69 ± 0.72	3.41 ± 1.10 [c]	3.44 ± 1.14	3.38 ± 1.10
Omega 3	5.59 ± 1.09	6.56 ± 1.65	6.73 ± 1.78	6.40 ± 1.54
Omega 6	12.61 ± 3.02	12.73 ± 2.14	12.80 ± 2.67	12.66 ± 1.51
ω6/ω3	2.33 ± 0.68	2.05 ± 0.57	2.00 ± 0.56	2.10 ± 0.60

Values given as mean ± standard deviation (SD); NM, nasal mucosa; NP, nasal polyp; NP-ATA, nasal polyp aspirin-tolerant asthma; NP-AIA, nasal polyp aspirin-intolerant asthma; [a] $P < 0.001$, [b] $P < 0.01$, and [c] $P < 0.05$, as compared to mucosa; [d] $P < 0.005$, [e] $P < 0.02$, and [f] $P < 0.05$, as compared to NP-ATA. The sum of fatty acids percentage composition is not equal to 100%, because there are fatty acids that were analyzed but not mentioned here.

The comparison between the fatty acid composition of fibroblasts from aspirin-tolerant and aspirin-intolerant patients is also shown in Table 2. The percentages of fatty acid composition in palmitic acid (C16:0), and palmitoleic acid (C16:1) were significantly higher in fibroblasts from patients with nasal polyps and aspirin intolerance than in fibroblasts derived from nasal polyps of aspirin-tolerant patients. In contrast, the percentage of eicosadienoic acid (C20:2 n6) was significantly lower in fibroblasts from aspirin-intolerant patients, compared with those cultured from aspirin-tolerant subjects.

3.2. Effects of Aspirin on Fatty Acid Composition

The effect of aspirin on the fatty acid composition of fibroblasts from nasal mucosa and nasal polyps is shown in Table 3. There was only one statistically significant difference in the percentage composition of 20:3n6, between the mean of an induced aspirin fibroblast and its basal status in aspirin-tolerant patients.

The lipid changes in fibroblasts from asthmatic and non-asthmatic patients were accompanied by changes in the amount of total proteins used to normalize the fatty acid composition.

Table 3. Differences in fatty acid composition of fibroblast after being stimulated with aspirin.

| | NM | NP | NP-ATA | NP-AIA |
	N = 6	N = 12	N = 6	N = 6
16:0	0.03 ± 1.31	−1.44 ± 1.17	−0. 38 ± 2.30	−0.19 ± 0.43
16:1	−0.16 ± 0.46	−0.14 ± 0.38	−0.04 ± 0.62	−0.08 ± 0.43
18:0	−0.46 ± 0.55	0.47 ± 0.63	0.29 ± 0.91	0.27 ± 0.85
18:1	0.83 ± 1.52	0.96 ± 1.13	2.76 ± 1.83	−0.23 ± 0.90
18:2n6	−0.34 ± 0.70	−0.12 ± 0.24	0.13 ± 0.25	−0.31 ± 0.44

Table 3. *Cont.*

	NM	NP	NP-ATA	NP-AIA
	$N = 6$	$N = 12$	$N = 6$	$N = 6$
18:3n6	-0.09 ± 0.24	-0.09 ± 0.08	-0.13 ± 0.12	-0.03 ± 0.12
18:3n3	0.06 ± 0.08	-0.04 ± 0.04	-0.02 ± 0.06	-0.08 ± 0.06
20:2n6	0.26 ± 0.34	0.13 ± 0.22	0.36 ± 0.23	-0.03 ± 0.32
20:3n6	-0.16 ± 0.20	0.24 ± 0.13	0.55 ± 0.20 [a]	-0.09 ± 0.14
20:4n6	-0.19 ± 1.07	0.88 ± 0.64	1.66 ± 1.13	-0.16 ± 0.63
20:3n3	-0.11 ± 0.06	-0.09 ± 0.08	-0.18 ± 0.15	0.00 ± 0.02
20:5n3	0.12 ± 0.12	0.07 ± 0.14	0.05 ± 0.23	0.08 ± 0.21
22:5n3	-0.08 ± 0.25	0.12 ± 0.15	0.25 ± 0.20	-0.02 ± 0.24
22:6n3	0.06 ± 0.46	0.67 ± 0.46	0.63 ± 0.68	0.55 ± 0.67
Omega 3	0.05 ± 0.70	0.72 ± 0.67	0.72 ± 1.03	0.53 ± 0.99
Omega 6	-1.24 ± 1.55	1.04 ± 0.87	2.57 ± 1.52	-0.62 ± 0.86
$\omega6/\omega3$	0.05 ± 0.07	0.01 ± 0.07	-0.05 ± 0.09	0.07 ± 0.11

Values given as a mean difference of fatty acid composition percentages before and after aspirin stimulation $\pm$ standard error of mean (SEM); NM, nasal mucosa; NP, nasal polyp asthmatics; NP-ATA, nasal polyp aspirin-tolerant asthma; NP-AIA, nasal polyp aspirin-intolerant asthma; [a] $p < 0.05$ as compared to the basal status of the same sample before aspirin stimulation.

The fatty lipid composition of fetal bovine serum is shown in Table 4.

Table 4. Total fatty acid composition of the fetal bovine serum used in fibroblast culture.

Fatty Acid	Mean $\pm$ SD
14:0	2.45 ± 0.45
14:1	0.39 ± 0.05
16:0	24.97 ± 0.14
16:1	2.81 ± 0.09
18:0	14.04 ± 0.08
18:1n9	23.86 ± 1.03
18:1n7	5.44 ± 0.16
18:2n6	6.74 ± 0.18
18:3n6	0.50 ± 0.04
18:3n3	0.53 ± 0.03
20:0	0.41 ± 0.03
20:1n9	0.75 ± 0.04
20:2n6	0.24 ± 0.02
20:3n6	1.81 ± 0.07
20:4n6	5.31 ± 0.20
20:3n3	0.57 ± 0.01
20:5n3	0.97 ± 0.04
22:0	1.07 ± 0.05
22:1n9	0.57 ± 0.02
22:5n3	0.39 ± 0.01
24:0	1.08 ± 0.12
22:6n3	3.48 ± 0.18
24:1	1.54 ± 0.20

The sample was analyzed in triplicate. Data are listed as mean $\pm$ SD.

4. Discussion

The concentration of free AA in resting cells is commonly described as "low". In some inflamed tissues, such as the skin of patients with psoriasis, free AA is abundant, but in healthy skin it is scarcer [20]. Similar results have been reported in fibroblasts from hypertrophic scars as compared to normal dermis [21]. These observations suggest that the level of AA increases under conditions of inflammation and remodeling, thereby facilitating the subsequent synthesis of PGs, leukotrienes and lipoxins.

We used fibroblasts from nasal polyps to study the impact of inflammation and aspirin intolerance in fatty acid composition, because previous studies have shown very low production of PGE_2 in nasal polyps from both aspirin-tolerant and aspirin-intolerant patients [11,14,15]. Similarly, other studies have also shown a significantly low production of PGE_2 in cultured bronchial fibroblasts from AIA [13].

Previous studies have shown that PGE_2 production in inflammatory situations is directly related to the level of expression of COX-2 [6]. Other studies have also reported that the induction of COX-2 by inflammatory mediators in human lung fibroblasts does not simply result in an increase in all the prostanoids that a given cell can produce. Instead, there is a shift in the balance of PGs toward the preferential production of prostacyclin and PGE_2 [22]. Based on these observations, we reasoned that the altered production of PGE_2 in airway fibroblasts from nasal polyps of asthma patients might be due, at least in part, to an insufficient amount of AA available to the COX-2 enzyme.

Our results do no support this hypothesis. In fact, the percentage of AA present in fibroblasts derived from an inflamed tissue (nasal polyps) was significantly higher that in those cultured from non-inflamed nasal mucosa. These results concur with others that show an increased presence of AA in airway inflammatory processes such as cystic fibrosis, a disease characterized by a chronic inflammatory process affecting both the lower (bronchiectasis) and upper airways (chronic rhinosinusitis and nasal polyps). After performing nasal tissue biopsies, Freedman *et al.* [23] reported significantly higher levels of AA in cystic fibrosis and asthma patients compared with healthy control subjects. Interestingly, Roca-Ferrer *et al.* [9] also found that COX-2 mRNA and protein were markedly up-regulated in NP from cystic fibrosis patients; these findings contrast with the lack of expression of COX-2 mRNA and COX-2 protein in NP from asthma patients. As expected, in cystic fibrosis the increased release of AA, together with the up-regulated COX-2, results in an enhanced production of PGE_2, as has been demonstrated in saliva, exhaled air and urine [24–26].

To our knowledge, only one *ex vivo* study has assessed the fatty acid composition in the cells of asthma patients [27]. In contrast with our study, the authors reported significantly lower levels of AA in platelets isolated from asthma patients, compared with those obtained from health subjects. The reasons for this discrepancy are unclear, although it is most probably explained by the differences in the cells that were used: fibroblasts and platelets. Significantly, COX-2 platelets make a very limited contribution to prostanoid production [28].

Our study's second finding was that, in addition to the increased presence of omega-6 fatty acid AA, there were also higher levels of omega-3 fatty acids DPA (C22:5) and DHA (C22:6) in the fibroblast derived from NP. The membranes of most cells contain large amounts of AA, compared with other potential prostaglandin precursors, including eicosapentaenoic acid (EPA); thus, our finding explains why AA is usually the principal precursor of eicosanoid synthesis, and also why the series-3 prostaglandins (PG_3) that have EPA as their precursor are formed at a slower rate than series-2 prostaglandins (PG_2). These differences usually result in an increased production of omega-6, in contrast with the low formation of omega-3 in inflammatory diseases. When omega-3 exists in high amounts in cells, it can decrease the levels of AA in the membranes of inflammatory cells, so there will be less substrate available for the synthesis of pro-inflammatory eicosanoids [6,29]. In addition, EPA competitively inhibits the oxygenation of AA by cyclooxygenases [30]. Overall, by means of various mechanisms, omega-3 fatty acids can reduce the production of prostanoids such as PGE_2.

Based on these observations, several studies have evaluated the effects of diet manipulation in the treatment of inflammatory diseases, including those such as asthma that affect the airways. The metabolism of PUFA is highly dependent on the availability of lipid precursors. The AA pool for eicosanoids can only be slowly influenced by dietary omega-6 PUFA. In contrast, the omega-3 PUFA pool is usually smaller and can be modified more rapidly by dietary omega-3 PUFA supplementation [31].

Various uncontrolled fish oil trials have shown clinical benefits in asthma. However, a more recent report covering a large number of studies concluded that "no definitive conclusion can yet be drawn regarding the efficacy of omega-3 FA supplementation as a treatment for asthma" [32]. Another review and meta-analysis concluded that it is unlikely that supplementation with omega-3 plays an important role in the prevention of asthma and allergic diseases [33].

Our finding of an increased presence of omega-3 DHA fatty acid in fibroblasts coming from an inflamed nasal tissue contrasts with previous studies showing the opposite effect. Freedman *et al.* [23], and Javier de Castro *et al.* [27] reported very low proportion of DHA in the nasal tissue of cystic fibrosis patients and platelets of asthma patients, respectively. Differences in the studied disease (cystic fibrosis *vs.* asthma) and in the cells (fibroblast *vs.* platelets) most probably account for the discrepancies.

Recent studies support the notion that PGE_2 exerts anti-inflammatory rather than pro-inflammatory actions in the lung [34]. We are tempted to speculate that the increased production of omega-3 in nasal polyps competitively inhibits the oxygenation of COX-2 and results in a reduced production of the anti-inflammatory PGE_2. If this hypothesis true, any attempt to increase the amount of cell-membrane omega-3 fatty acids by increasing the dietary intake of EPA would result in deleterious rather than salutary effects in asthma patients, particularly in AIA.

Interestingly enough, a diet supplemented with fish oil for 6 weeks was associated with a reduction in prostanoid production, a mild clinical deterioration and increased bronchial obstruction in a group of aspirin-intolerant asthma patients [35]. This observation concurs with a recent study reporting that fish oil supplementation in a mouse model of asthma led to a significant suppression of the production of PGE_2, associated with both an enhanced lung inflammatory response and an increased release of pro-inflammatory cytokine IL-5 and IL-13 [36]. All in all, these results bring into question the proposed potential protective role of fish oil supplementation in the treatment of airway inflammatory processes such as asthma and chronic rhinosinusitis with nasal polyps.

Aspirin-intolerant asthma is characterized by a persistently elevated production of cysteinyl leukotrienes (Cys-LTs) in a steady state, due to the up-regulation of the 5-lipoxygenase pathway enzymes [4]. The release of Cys-LTs is further enhanced when these patients are challenged with aspirin and suffer an episode of bronchoconstriction [4]. The mechanism responsible for the increased release of Cys-LTs is only partially known, although the inhibition of COX-1 appears to be the crucial precipitating event [4,5]. In contrast, selective COX-2 inhibitors are usually well tolerated, do not increase the release of Cys-LTs, and do not cause bronchoconstriction [4]. Diversion of AA from the COX-1 pathway to the 5-LO pathway has been suggested as an explanation for the increased release of Cys-LTs after aspirin exposure [4]. Whether this AA diversion is also accompanied by an increase in the release of AA from membrane phospholipids is a possibility that has not yet been examined. We assessed the effects of aspirin on fatty acid composition in fibroblasts from aspirin-tolerant and aspirin intolerant patients and could not find any change in the levels of AA. This finding suggests that aspirin does not enhance the release of 5-lipoxygenase metabolites by increasing the amount of AA available to the lipooxygenase enzymes.

We compared the fatty acid composition of fibroblasts derived from NP of aspirin-tolerant and aspirin-intolerant patients and we found an increase in the percentage composition of palmitic acid (C16:0). The significance of this difference remains to be clarified.

In summary, the objective of this study was to investigate whether the previously reported low release of PGE_2 in fibroblasts from asthma patients could be caused by a reduced supply of AA. Our data shows an increased presence of the omega-6 AA and the omega-3 DPA and DHA fatty acids in nasal polyp fibroblasts compared with nasal mucosa fibroblasts. Whether the increased presence of omega-3 fatty acids can contribute to reducing PGE_2 production in nasal polyps by competitively inhibiting COX-2 and reducing the levels of AA available to the COX-2 enzyme in the membranes of the inflammatory and structural cells remains to be elucidated.

Acknowledgments: S.J.A. has been supported by the Spanish Ministry of Foreign Affairs and Cooperation (MAEC) and the Spanish Cooperation Agency (AEIC).

Author Contributions: S.J.A., J.R.-F. and C.P. designed the research; S.J.A. and J.R.-F. performed the experimental work; S.J.A. and C.P. wrote the manuscript. All authors discussed, edited and approved the final version.

Conflicts of Interest: The authors declare no conflict of interest.

References

1. Busse, W.W.; Lemanske, R.F. Asthma. *N. Engl. J. Med.* **2001**, *344*, 350–362. [PubMed]
2. Fokkens, W.J.; Lund, V.; Mullol, J. European position paper on rhinosinusitis and nasal polyps group. *Rhinology* **2007**, *45* (Suppl. S20), 1–136.
3. Pawliczak, R.; Lewandowska-Polak, A.; Kowalski, M.L. Pathogenesis of nasal polyps: An update. *Curr. Allergy Asthma Rep.* **2005**, *5*, 463–471. [CrossRef] [PubMed]
4. Stevenson, D.D.; Sczeklik, A. Clinical and pathologic perspectives on aspirin sensitivity and asthma. *J. Allergy Clin. Immunol.* **2006**, *118*, 773–786. [CrossRef] [PubMed]
5. Picado, C. The role of cyclooxygenases in acetylsalicylic acid sensitivity. *Allergy Clin. Immunol. Int.* **2006**, *18*, 1–4. [CrossRef]
6. Harizi, H.; Corcuff, J.B.; Gualde, N. Arachidonic-acid-dereived eicosanoids: Roles in biology and immunopathology. *Trends Mol. Med.* **2008**, *14*, 461–469. [CrossRef] [PubMed]
7. Simmons, D.L.; Botting, R.M.; Hla, T. Cyclooxygenase isozymes: The biology of prostaglandin synthesis and inhibition. *Pharmacol. Rev.* **2004**, *56*, 387–437. [CrossRef] [PubMed]
8. Konstan, M.W. Ibuprofen therapy for cystic fibrosis lung disease: Revisited. *Curr. Opin. Pulm. Med.* **2008**, *14*, 567–573. [CrossRef] [PubMed]
9. Roca-Ferrer, J.; Pujols, L.; Gartner, S.; Moreno, A.; Pumarola, F.; Mullol, J.; Cobos, N.; Picado, C. Upregulation of COX-1 and COX-2 in nasal polyps in cystic fibrosis. *Thorax* **2006**, *61*, 592–596. [CrossRef] [PubMed]
10. Pujols, L.; Mullol, J.; Alobid, I.; Roca-Ferrer, J.; Xaubet, A.; Picado, C. Dynamics of COX-2 in nasal mucosa and nasal polyps from aspirin-tolerant and aspirin-intolerant patients with asthma. *J. Allergy Clin. Immunol.* **2004**, *114*, 814–819. [CrossRef] [PubMed]
11. Perez-Novo, C.A.; Watelet, J.B.; Claeys, C.; Van Cauwenberge, P.; Bachert, C. Prostaglandin, leukotriene, and lipoxin balance in chronic rhinosinusitis with and without nasal polyposis. *J. Allergy Clin. Immunol.* **2005**, *115*, 1189–1196. [CrossRef] [PubMed]
12. Mullol, J.; Fernandez-Morata, J.C.; Roca-Ferrer, J.; Pujols, L.; Xaubet, A.; Benitez, P.; Picado, C. Cyclooxygenase 1 and cyclooxygenase 2 expression is abnormaly regulated in human nasal polyps. *J. Allergy Clin. Immunol.* **2002**, *109*, 824–830. [CrossRef] [PubMed]
13. Pierzchalska, M.; Szabó, Z.; Sanak, M.; Soja, J.; Szczeklik, A. Deficient prostaglandin E2 production by bronchial fibroblasts of asthmatic patients, with special reference to aspirin-induced asthma. *J. Allergy Clin. Immunol.* **2003**, *111*, 1041–1048. [CrossRef] [PubMed]
14. Kowalski, M.L.; Pawliczak, R.; Wozniak, J.; Siuda, K.; Poniatowska, M.; Iwaszkiewicz, J.; Kornatowski, T.; Kaliner, M.A. Differential Metabolism of Arachidonic Acid in Nasal Polyp Epithelial Cells Cultured from Aspirin-sensitive and Aspirin-tolerant Patients. *Am. J. Respir. Crit. Care Med.* **2000**, *161*, 391–398. [CrossRef] [PubMed]
15. Roca-Ferrer, J.; Garcia-Garcia, F.J.; Pereda, J.; Perez-Gonzalez, M.; Pujols, L.; Alobid, I.; Mullol, J.; Picado, C. Reduced Expression of Cyclooxygenases and Production of Prostaglandin E2 in Patients with Nasal Polyps, With or Without Aspirin-Intolerant Asthma. *J. Allergy Clin. Immunol.* **2011**, *128*, 66–72. [CrossRef] [PubMed]
16. Smith, R.S.; Smith, T.J.; Blieden, T.M.; Phipps, R.P. Fibroblasts as sentinel cells. Synthesis of chemokines and regulation of inflammation. *Am. J. Pathol.* **1997**, *151*, 317–322. [PubMed]
17. Olsson, S.; Cagnoni, F.; Dignetti, P.; Melioli, G.; Canonica, G.W. Low concentrations of cytokines produced by allergen-stimulated peripheral blood mononuclear cells have potent effects on nasal polyp-derived fibroblasts. *Clin. Exp. Immunol.* **2003**, *132*, 254–260. [CrossRef] [PubMed]
18. Casadevall, J.; Ventura, P.; Mullol, J.; Picado, C. Intranasal challenge with aspirin in the diagnosis of aspirin intolerant asthma: Evaluation of nasal response by acoustic rhinometry. *Thorax* **2000**, *55*, 921–924. [CrossRef] [PubMed]
19. Bligh, E.G.; Dyer, W.J. A rapid method of total lipid extraction and purification. *Can. J. Biochem. Physiol.* **1959**, *37*, 911–917. [CrossRef] [PubMed]
20. Ikai, K. Psoriasis and the arachidonic acid cascade. *J. Dermatol. Sci.* **1999**, *21*, 135–146. [CrossRef]

21. Nomura, T.; Terashi, H.; Omori, M.; Sakurai, A.; Sunagawa, T.; Hasegawa, M.; Tahara, S. Lipid analysis of normal dermis and hypertrophic scars. *Wound Repair Regen.* **2007**, *15*, 833–837. [CrossRef] [PubMed]

22. Brock, T.G.; McNish, R.W.; Peters-Golden, M. Arachidonic acid is preferentially metabolized by cyclooxygenase-2 to prostacyclin and prostaglandin E2. *J. Biol. Chem.* **1999**, *274*, 11660–11666. [CrossRef] [PubMed]

23. Freedman, S.D.; Blanco, P.G.; Zaman, M.M.; Shea, J.C.; Ollero, M.; Hopper, I.K.; Weed, D.A.; Gelrud, A.; Regan, M.M.; Laposata, M.; *et al.* Association of cystic fibrosis with abnormalities in fatty acid metabolism. *N. Engl. J. Med.* **2004**, *350*, 560–569. [CrossRef] [PubMed]

24. Lucidi, V.; Ciabattoni, G.; Bela, S.; Barnes, P.J.; Montushi, P. Exhaled 8-isoprostane and prostaglandin E(2) in patients with stable and unstable cystic fibrosis. *Free Radic. Biol. Med.* **2008**, *45*, 913–919. [CrossRef] [PubMed]

25. Strandvik, B.; Svensson, E.; Seyberth, H.W. Prostanoid biosynthesis in patients with cystic fibrosis. *Prostaglandins Leukot. Essent. Fat. Acids* **1996**, *55*, 419–425. [CrossRef]

26. Rigas, B.; Korenberg, J.R.; Merrill, W.W.; Levien, L. Prostaglandin E2 and E2 alpha are elevated in saliva of cystic fibrosis patients. *Am. J. Gastroenterol.* **1989**, *84*, 1408–1412. [PubMed]

27. De Castro, J.; Hernandez-Hernandez, A.; Rodriguez, M.C.; Sardina, J.L.; Llanillo, M.; Sanchez-Yagüe, J. Comparison of changes in erythrocyte and platelet phospholipid and fatty acid composition and protein oxidation in chronic obstructive pulmonary disease and asthma. *Platelets* **2007**, *18*, 43–51. [CrossRef] [PubMed]

28. Riondino, S.; Trifiró, E.; Principessa, L.; Mascioletti, S.; de Renzo, L.; Gaudio, C.; Biasucci, L.M.; Crea, F.; Pulcinelli, F.M. Lack of biological relevance of platelets cyclooxygenase-2 dependent thromboxane A2 production. *Thromb. Res.* **2008**, *122*, 359–365. [CrossRef] [PubMed]

29. Calder, P.C. The relationship between the fatty acid composition of immune cells and their function. *Prostaglandins Leukot. Essent. Fat. Acids* **2008**, *79*, 101–108. [CrossRef] [PubMed]

30. Obata, T.; Nagakura, T.; Masaki, T.; Maekawa, K.; Yamashita, K. Eicosapentaenoic acid inhibits prostaglandin D2 generation by inhibiting cyclooxygenase-2 in culture human mast cells. *Clin. Exp. Allergy* **1999**, *29*, 1129–1135. [CrossRef] [PubMed]

31. Galli, C.; Calder, P.C. Effects of fat and fatty acid intake on inflammatory and immune responses: A critical review. *Ann. Nutr. Metab.* **2009**, *55*, 123–139. [CrossRef] [PubMed]

32. Schachter, H.M.; Reisman, J.; Tran, K.; Dales, B.; Kader, K.K.; Barnes, D.; Sampson, M.; Morrison, A.; Gaboury, I.; Blackman, J.B. Health effects of omega 3 fatty acids on asthma. In *Evidence Reports/Technical Assessment No. 91. AHRQ*; AHRQ Publication No. 04-013-2; Agency for Healthcare Research and Quality: Rockville, MD, USA, 2004.

33. Anandan, C.; Nurmatov, U.; Sheikh, A. Omega 3 and 6 oils for primary prevention of allergic disease: A systematic review and meta-analysis. *Allergy* **2009**, *64*, 840–848. [CrossRef] [PubMed]

34. Vancheri, C.; Mastruzzo, C.; Sortino, M.A.; Crimi, N. The lung as a privileged site for the beneficial actions of PGE2. *Trends Immunol.* **2004**, *25*, 40–46. [CrossRef] [PubMed]

35. Picado, C.; Castillo, J.A.; Schinca, N.; Pujades, M.; Ordinas, A.; Coronas, A.; Agusti-Vidal, A. Effects of fish oil enriched diet on aspirin intolerant asthmatic patients: A pilot study. *Thorax* **1988**, *43*, 93–97. [CrossRef] [PubMed]

36. Yin, H.; Liu, W.; Goleniewska, K.; Porter, N.A.; Morrow, J.D.; Peebles, R.S. Dietary supplementation of omega-3 fatty acid-containing fish oil suppresses F2-isoprostanes but enhances inflammatory cytokine responses in a mouse model of ovalbumin-induced allergic lung inflammation. *Free Radic. Biol. Med.* **2009**, *47*, 622–628. [CrossRef] [PubMed]

21

Chronic Rhinosinusitis as a Crucial Symptom of Cystic Fibrosis—Case Report and Discussion on the Sinonasal Compartment as Site of *Pseudomonas aeruginosa* Acquisition into CF Airways

Jochen G. Mainz [1,*], Christin Arnold [1], Andrea Gerber [1], Jürgen Rödel [2], Nina Cramer [3], Hans-Joachim Mentzel [4], James F. Beck [1] and Burkhard Tümmler [3]

[1] CF Center, Pediatric Pneumology, Jena University Hospital, Jena 07740, Germany; Christin.Arnold@med.uni-jena.de (C.A.); Andrea.Gerber@med.uni-jena.de (A.G.); James.Beck@med.uni-jena.de (J.F.B.)

[2] Institute for Medical Microbiology, Jena University Hospital, Jena 07740, Germany; Juergen.Roedel@med.uni-jena.de

[3] Klinische Forschergruppe, Pediatric Pneumology, Med. Hochschule Hannover, Hannover 30625, Germany; Cramer.Nina@mh-hannover.de (N.C.); Tuemmler.Burkhard@mh-hannover.de (B.T.)

[4] Pediatric Radiology, Jena University Hospital, Jena 07740, Germany; hans-joachim.mentzel@med.uni-jena.de

* Correspondence: Jochen.Mainz@med.uni-jena.de

Academic Editor: Claudina A. Pérez Novo

Abstract: Cystic fibrosis (CF) is the most frequent congenital lethal disease in Caucasians. Impaired mucociliary clearance causes chronic bacterial rhinosinusitis in up to 62% of patients, and almost all patients exhibit sinonasal pathology in CT scans. Pathogens like *Pseudomonas aeruginosa* (*P.a.*) chronically colonize about 70% of the CF adults' lungs and are the major reason for pulmonary destruction and premature death. In our 34-year-old female CF patient, rhinosinusitis caused massive orbital hypertelorism despite three sinonasal operations. Her sputum samples had always been negative for *P.a.* Then, *P.a.* was primarily detected in her sputum and additionally in nasal lavage, which since then persisted in both, her upper and lower airways. The *P.a.* strains turned out to be genetically identical in both airway levels, indicating early colonization of the entire airway system with *P.a.* This first report on simultaneous primary *P.a.* detection in the sinonasal and pulmonary compartments highlights the need to include an assessment of upper airway colonization in the standards of CF care, particularly in patients without chronic *P.a.* colonization. Both airway levels need to be considered as one united system, and a strong cooperation between ENT and CF specialists should be established. Prospective longitudinal studies should assess the upper airways´ role in acquisition and persistence of pathogens and evaluate conservative and surgical therapeutic options.

Keywords: cystic fibrosis; rhinosinusitis; *Pseudomonas aeruginosa*; upper airways; paranasal sinus; nose; sinus surgery

1. Introduction

Previously, sinonasal involvement in cystic fibrosis (CF) did not receive much attention in the patients with the most frequent life threatening congenital disease in Caucasians. Only four decades ago, CF regularly led to premature death in preschool-age by pulmonary destruction.

Due to improved prognosis, upper airway involvement is coming into focus, and it has been found to have a much higher impact on CF overall health than expected [1,2]. Patients carrying the disease causing defective chloride and sodium channels in sinonasal mucosa are reported to suffer from symptoms of rhinosinusitis in up to 62% [3–5]. Thereby, sinonasal involvement can play a relevant and underestimated role in colonization of the airway system with pathogens. In early stages, these are *Staphylococcus aureus* and *Haemophilus influenza*. With disease progression, 70% to 80% of adults with CF are chronically colonized with *Pseudomonas aeruginosa (P.a.)*. This pathogen is ubiquitously present in water and cannot be cleared from CF airways because thick viscous secretions impair mucociliary clearance. With time *P.a.* clones change their phenotype and become mucoid by developing an alginate layer and biofilms that additionally impair eradication by the immune system and antibiotics. In addition to its virulence factors, mucoid *P.a.* stimulates the host to an enhanced but frustrating immune reaction that further damages the airway system. The resulting pulmonary destruction is responsible for 90% of premature death in patients with CF [6].

In this context, evidence of the sinonasal role in airway colonization with pathogens remains scarce as the sampling does not belong to the current standards of CF care [7].

2. Case Report

We present a 34-year-old CF patient with genotype F508del/2789+5G→A who exhibited mild pulmonary disease and pancreatic sufficiency. In her first years of life, chronic rhinosinusitis was her leading early symptom, and she underwent three sinonasal surgeries until 1994. Nevertheless, CF-related chronic sinusitis relapsed soon and led to orbital hypertelorism with a broadening of her nasal bridge (Figures 1 and 2).

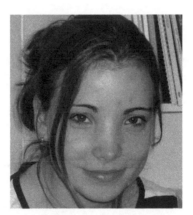

Figure 1. CF patient with massive broadening of the nasal bridge because of chronic rhinosinusitis.

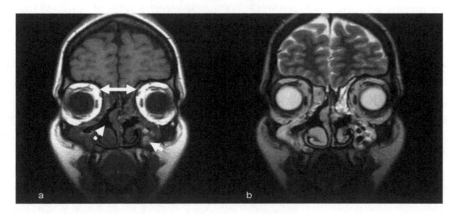

Figure 2. (**a**) T1-weighted MRI sequence: polypous hyperintense structures (arrowhead →) within the left maxillary sinus. Broadening of the ethmoidal segment in correlation to orbital size as cause of hyperteleorism (↔ see Figure 1); (**b**) T2-weighted MRI sequence: thickened mucosa (hyperintense = bright) in maxillary and ethmoidal sinuses; nodular polypous structures in the left maxillary sinus.

In addition to routine sampling of the sputum from the lower airways (LAW), we started including sinonasal sampling by nasal lavage (NL) into our local standards of care in 2005 [8,9]. In our patient LAW and upper airway (UAW) sampling by NL always turned out to be negative for *P.a.* until October 2007. Then, a non-mucoid *P.a.* was detected for the first time in both, sputum and NL, whereas *P.a.*-serum antibodies remained negative. A three-month course with oral ciprofloxacin and bronchial inhalation of colomycin was performed aiming to eradicate the bacterium. Nevertheless, five months later, the sampling of both airways segments again revealed the presence of *P.a.*. UAW and LAW isolates from October 2007, March 2008, and February 2010 were identical in their multi-marker genotype 681A [10], indicating that the patient was chronically carrying the same *P.a.* clone in both airway compartments since the onset of colonization. The genotyping was performed by a microarray for the typing of *P.a.* strains in both the conserved core and the flexible accessory genome.

3. Discussion

Our case report shows to which extent sinonasal involvement in CF influences facial morphology [1], albeit typically in a less severe form than in the presented patient. Our CF patient is an extreme case of chronic sinonasal involvement that is detectable in almost 100% of CF patients by computed tomography or MR imaging [11]. Mucoceles and nasal polyps are very frequent in the disease, occurring even in small children and in more than 50% of adults with CF [1,12]. Therefore, detection of nasal polyps in the first years of life should prompt an evaluation for CF by analysis of chloride in sweat or genetic analysis.

Altogether, our report sheds some doubt on the validity of most of the current standards of airway sampling for CF microbiology. *P.a.* colonization of the patients' upper airways would not have been detected following the current standards of CF care [7]. Thereby, colonization with the bacterium persisted in both airway segments despite anti-pseudomonas therapy, as proven by identical *P.a.* genotypes during a period of currently more than nine years. The initial detection of *P.a.* in both habitats was not accompanied by relevant systemic antibody levels against the pathogen. This indicates that early cross colonization of UAW and LAW segments did not caused a significant systemic humoral response.

The relevance of the UAW concerning *P.a.* persistence has been previously postulated by Walter *et al.* [13], who typed *P.a.* isolates from the lower airways of CF patients prior to and after lung transplantation. It was found that *P.a.* free donor lungs were colonized by *P.a.* belonging to the same genotype as pre-transplant isolates of the CF recipient. The authors concluded that the UAW is the reservoir of the pathogen. These results from end-stage CF pulmonary disease were also seen in adults with less advanced lung destruction [14]. Muhlebach *et al.* [15] also found high concordance of intra-operatively sampled *P.a.* genotypes from both airway segments in children with CF. Prior, we assessed a large cohort of 182 CF patients of all ages non-invasively for upper and lower airway colonization with *P.a.* [8]. During routine outpatient visits, we sampled the UAW by nasal lavage or deep nasal swabs and compared the results to sputa or deep throat swabs from the patients. *P.a.* UAW and LAW isolates from 23 of 24 patients were identical in genotype.

Recently, the Copenhagen CF center [16] published data from longitudinal analysis of sinonasal colonization assessed during surgery or endoscopy guided maxillary swaps. The authors found that the paranasal sinuses can be a site of early colonization with *P.a.*, where the bacteria diversify and evolve pathogenicity, e.g., by antibiotic resistance and adapt to the CF airway. From the sinonasal reservoir, they may intermittently colonize the lungs, ultimately leading to chronic lung infection; thus, sinonasal involvement can be crucial for many CF patients, even those without relevant upper airway symptoms. Repeatedly, sinonasal surgery was discussed as a chance to prevent colonization of the upper airway segment with pathogens such as *P.a.* [4,17]. However, in the presented patient, three sinonasal operations with an establishment of widely patent maxillary ostia (see Figure 2a,b) did not prevent colonization and persistence of pathogens in this habitat. Additionally, sinonasal surgery has recently been reported to represent a risk for pathogen acquisition in a case series of four CF patients with a new *P.a.* colonization after ENT surgery [18].

Whereas the sinonasal niche is not assessed according to most current international standards [7], the very recent German guidelines for prevention of chronic airway colonization with *P.a.* [19] addresses this issue: Additional assessment of the sinonasal niche is recommended at the least when eradication from the LAW does not succeed. Altogether, UAW-sampling in CF patients without chronic *P.a.* colonization can help to prevent or postpone chronic colonization before the pathogen switches to the mucoid persisting phenotype.

After identification of sinonasal pathogen colonization in additional CF patients, we assessed novel therapeutic options: The patients inhaled antibiotics as vibrating aerosols into their paranasal sinuses. Basically, conventional aerosols do not reach the paranasal sinuses when their ostia have not recently been widened by surgery [20]. In contrast, scintigrafic *in vivo* studies proved that vibrating aerosols reach paranasal sinuses [21]. We recently eradicated *P.a.* with such an approach in a CF patient with first-isolated sinonasal colonization with the pathogen [22]. Additionally, we performed a pilot study showing that tobramycin at 1×80 mg a day inhaled with the Pari Sinus™ device can reduce pathogen counts and symptoms in CF patients with sinonasal colonization with *P.a.* [23]. For patients with chronic rhinosinusitis (non-CF) who underwent functional endoscopic sinus surgery with the widening of sinus ostia, Bonfils *et al.* showed that nasal inhalation with tobramycin with a mesh nebulizer can be effective [24]. Furthermore, the Copenhagen CF center brought up a program combining sinonasal surgery with 14 days of intravenous antibiotic treatment (e.g., with tobramycin and ceftazidim), with daily nasal lavages containing antibiotics like colomycin for a period of six months [4]. This approach helped to eradicate *P.a.* from the sinonasal reservoir in a subgroup of the included CF patients. Under the assumption that the sinonasal niche is a site of first and persistent colonization with critical pathogens in CF patients, there is a need for routine sinonasal sampling—at least in the patients who are not yet chronically colonized. Furthermore, prospective investigation is required for better understanding the bidirectional communication between upper and lower airway segments [3] and its conservative [2] and surgical [4] therapy.

Acknowledgments: The authors are grateful to the patient for her support and continuous interest.

Author Contributions: The publication was written by J.G.M., C.A., A.G., J.F.B., and B.T. H.J.M. performed and evaluated the MR, J.R. is responsible for the *P.a.* biobank, B.T. and N.C. genotyped *P.a.* colonies. All authors discussed, edited and approved the final version.

Conflicts of Interest: J.G.M., J.F.B. and C.A. performed investigator initiated studies using vibrating aerosols as cited in References [22] and [23]. Besides, all authors disclose any actual or potential conflict of interest including any financial, personal, or other relationships with other people or organizations that could inappropriately influence the work.

References

1. Gysin, C.; Alothman, G.A.; Papsin, B.C. Sinonasal disease in cystic fibrosis: Clinical characteristics, diagnosis, and management. *Pediatr. Pulmonol.* **2000**, *30*, 481–489. [CrossRef]

2. Mainz, J.G.; Koitschev, A. Management of chronic rhinosinusitis in CF. *J. Cyst. Fibros.* **2009**, *8*, 10–14. [CrossRef]

3. Berkhout, M.C.; Van Rooden, C.J.; Rijntjes, E.; Fokkens, W.J.; el Bouazzaoui, L.H.; Heijerman, H.G. Sinonasal manifestations of cystic fibrosis: A correlation between genotype and phenotype? *J. Cyst. Fibros.* **2014**, *13*, 442–448. [CrossRef] [PubMed]

4. Aanaes, K. Bacterial sinusitis can be a focus for initial lung colonisation and chronic lung infection in patients with cystic fibrosis. *J. Cyst. Fibros.* **2013**, *12*, S1–S20. [CrossRef]

5. Mainz, J.G.; Schien, M.; Naehrlich, L.; Käding, M.; Thoss, K.; Frey, G.; Wiedemann, B.; Beck, J.F. Prevalence of CF-related chronic rhinosinusitis-results from a multicenter interdisciplinary study. *J. Cyst. Fibros.* **2010**, *9*, S118.

6. Hoiby, N. Recent advances in the treatment of *Pseudomonas aeruginosa* infections in cystic fibrosis. *BMC Med.* **2011**, *9*, 32. [CrossRef] [PubMed]

7. Smyth, A.R.; Bell, S.C.; Bojcin, S.; Bryon, M.; Duff, A.; Flume, P.; Nataliya, K.; Anne, M.; Felix, R.; Sarah, J.S.; *et al.* European Cystic Fibrosis Society Standards of Care: Best Practice guidelines. *J. Cyst. Fibros.* **2014**, *13*, S23–S42. [CrossRef] [PubMed]

8. Mainz, J.G.; Nährlich, L.; Schien, M.; Kading, M.; Schiller, I.; Mayr, S.; Schneider, G.; Wiedemann, B.; Wiehlmann, L.; Cramer, N.; *et al.* Concordant genotype of upper and lower airways *P.a.* and *S. aureus* isolates in cystic fibrosis. *Thorax* **2009**, *64*, 535–540. [CrossRef] [PubMed]

9. Hentschel, J.; Muller, U.; Doht, F.; Fischer, N.; Boer, K.; Sonnemann, J.; Hipler, C.; Hünniger, K.; Kurzai, O.; Markert, U.R.; *et al.* Influences of nasal lavage collection-, processing- and storage methods on inflammatory markers–evaluation of a method for non-invasive sampling of epithelial lining fluid in cystic fibrosis and other respiratory diseases. *J. Immunol. Methods* **2014**, *404*, 41–51. [CrossRef] [PubMed]

10. Wiehlmann, L.; Wagner, G.; Cramer, N.; Siebert, B.; Gudowius, P.; Morales, G.; Köhler, T.; van Delden, C.; Weinel, C.; Slickers, P.; *et al.* Population structure of *Pseudomonas aeruginosa. Proc. Natl. Acad. Sci. USA* **2007**, *104*, 8101–8106. [CrossRef] [PubMed]

11. Eggesbo, H.B.; Sovik, S.; Dolvik, S.; Kolmannskog, F. CT characterization of inflammatory paranasal sinus disease in cystic fibrosis. *Acta Radiol.* **2002**, *43*, 21–28. [CrossRef] [PubMed]

12. Schraven, S.P.; Wehrmann, M.; Wagner, W.; Blumenstock, G.; Koitschev, A. Prevalence and histopathology of chronic polypoid sinusitis in pediatric patients with cystic fibrosis. *J. Cyst. Fibros.* **2011**, *10*, 181–186. [CrossRef] [PubMed]

13. Walter, S.; Gudowius, P.; Bosshammer, J.; Romling, U.; Weissbrodt, H.; Schurmann, W.; von der Hardt, H.; Tümmler, B. Epidemiology of chronic *Pseudomonas aeruginosa* infections in the airways of lung transplant recipients with cystic fibrosis. *Thorax* **1997**, *52*, 318–321. [CrossRef] [PubMed]

14. Taylor, R.F.; Morgan, D.W.; Nicholson, P.S.; Mackay, I.S.; Hodson, M.E.; Pitt, T.L. Extrapulmonary sites of *Pseudomonas aeruginosa* in adults with cystic fibrosis. *Thorax* **1992**, *47*, 426–428. [CrossRef] [PubMed]

15. Muhlebach, M.S.; Miller, M.B.; Moore, C.; Wedd, J.P.; Drake, A.F.; Leigh, M.W. Are lower airway or throat cultures predictive of sinus bacteriology in cystic fibrosis? *Pediatr. Pulmonol.* **2006**, *41*, 445–451. [CrossRef] [PubMed]

16. Hansen, S.K.; Rau, M.H.; Johansen, H.K.; Ciofu, O.; Jelsbak, L.; Yang, L.; Folkesson, A.; Jarme, H.S.; Aanæs, K.; von Buchwald, C.; *et al.* Evolution and diversification of *Pseudomonas aeruginosa* in the paranasal sinuses of cystic fibrosis children have implications for chronic lung infection. *ISME J.* **2011**, *6*, 31–45. [CrossRef] [PubMed]

17. Vital, D.; Hofer, M.; Benden, C.; Holzmann, D.; Boehler, A. Impact of Sinus Surgery on Pseudomonal Airway Colonization, Bronchiolitis Obliterans Syndrome and Survival in Cystic Fibrosis Lung Transplant Recipients. *Respiration* **2012**, *86*, 25–36. [CrossRef] [PubMed]

18. Mainz, J.G.; Gerber, A.; Lorenz, M.; Michl, R.; Hentschel, J.; Nader, A.; Beck, J.F.; Pletz, M.W.; Mueller, A.H. *Pseudomonas aeruginosa* Acquisition in Cystic Fibrosis Patients in Context of Otorhinolaryngological Surgery or Dentist Attendance: Case Series and Discussion of Preventive Concepts. *Case Rep. Infect. Dis.* **2015**, *2015*, 9.

19. Muller, F.M.; Bend, J.; Huttegger, I.; Moller, A.; Schwarz, C.; Abele-Horn, M.; Ballmann, M.; Bargon, J.; Baumann, I.; Bremer, W.; *et al.* S3 guidelines on pulmonary disease in cystic fibrosis. Module 1: Diagnostics and therapy after initial detection of *Pseudomonas aeruginosa. Mon. Kinderh.* **2015**, *163*, 590–599.

20. St Martin, M.B.; Hitzman, C.J.; Wiedmann, T.S.; Rimell, F.L. Deposition of aerosolized particles in the maxillary sinuses before and after endoscopic sinus surgery. *Am. J. Rhinol.* **2007**, *21*, 196–197. [CrossRef] [PubMed]

21. Möller, W.; Schuschnig, U.; Khadem Saba, G.; Meyer, G.; Junge-Hulsing, B.; Keller, M.; Häussinger, K. Pulsating aerosols for drug delivery to the sinuses in healthy volunteers. *Otolaryngol. Head Neck Surg.* **2010**, *142*, 382–388. [CrossRef] [PubMed]

22. Mainz, J.G.; Michl, R.; Pfister, W.; Beck, J.F. Cystic fibrosis upper airways primary colonization with *Pseudomonas aeruginosa*: Eradicated by sinonasal antibiotic inhalation. *Am. J. Respir. Crit. Care Med.* **2011**, *184*, 1089–1090. [CrossRef] [PubMed]

23. Mainz, J.G.; Schädlich, K.; Schien, C.; Michl, R.; Schelhorn-Neise, P.; Koitschev, A.; Koitschev, C.; Keller, P.M.; Riethmüller, J.; Wiedemann, B.; *et al.* Sinonasal inhalation of tobramycin vibrating aerosol in cystic fibrosis patients with upper airway *Pseudomonas aeruginosa* colonization: Results of a randomized, double-blind, placebo-controlled pilot study. *Drug Des. Dev. Ther.* **2014**, *8*, 209–217. [CrossRef] [PubMed]

24. Bonfils, P.; Escabasse, V.; Coste, A.; Gilain, L.; Louvrier, C.; Serrano, E.; de Bonnecaze, G.; Mortuaire, G.; Chevalier, D.; Laccourreye, O.; *et al.* Efficacy of tobramycin aerosol in nasal polyposis. *Eur. Ann. Otorhinolaryngol. Head Neck Dis.* **2015**, *132*, 119–123. [CrossRef] [PubMed]

Permissions

List of Contributors

Rosa B. Lipin, Anita Deshpande, Sarah K. Wise and John M. DelGaudio
Department of Otolaryngology—Head and Neck Surgery, Emory University School of Medicine, Atlanta, GA 30308, USA

Zara M. Patel
Department of Otolaryngology—Head and Neck Surgery, Stanford University School of Medicine, Stanford, CA 94305, USA

Francisco Muñoz-López
Pediatric Immunology Center, Barcelona 08028, Spain
Former Head of the Department of Pediatric Immunoallergology, Hospital Clinic, Faculty of Medicine, University of Barcelona, Barcelona 08028, Spain

Michael J. Marino, Charles A. Riley, Eric L. Wu and Jacqueline E. Weinstein
Department of Otolaryngology-Head and Neck Surgery, Tulane University School of Medicine, New Orleans, LA 70112, USA

Edward D. McCoul
Department of Otolaryngology-Head and Neck Surgery, Tulane University School of Medicine, New Orleans, LA 70112, USA
Department of Otorhinolaryngology, Ochsner Clinic Foundation, New Orleans, LA 70121, USA
Ochsner Clinical School, University of Queensland School of Medicine, New Orleans, LA 70121, USA

Angélica Bermúdez
Department of Otorhinolaryngology, Ochsner Clinic Foundation, New Orelans, LA 70121, USA

Amit S. Patel
Department of Otolaryngology, Tulane University School of Medicine, New Orleans, LA 70112, USA

Edward D. McCoul
Department of Otorhinolaryngology, Ochsner Clinic Foundation, New Orelans, LA 70121, USA
Department of Otolaryngology, Tulane University School of Medicine, New Orleans, LA 70112, USA
Ochsner Clinical School, University of Queensland School of Medicine, New Orleans, LA 70121, USA

Jacob P. Brunner and Charles A. Riley
Department of Otolaryngology—Head and Neck Surgery, Tulane University School of Medicine, New Orleans, LA 70112, USA

Edward D. McCoul
Department of Otolaryngology—Head and Neck Surgery, Tulane University School of Medicine, New Orleans, LA 70112, USA
Department of Otorhinolaryngology, Ochsner Clinic Foundation, New Orleans, LA 70121, USA
Ochsner Clinical School, University of Queensland School of Medicine, New Orleans, LA 70121, USA

Amanda E. Dilger, Alexander L. Schneider and John Cramer
Department of Otolaryngology-Head and Neck Surgery, Northwestern University Feinberg School of Medicine, Chicago, IL 60611, USA

Stephanie Shintani Smith
Department of Otolaryngology-Head and Neck Surgery, Northwestern University Feinberg School of Medicine, Chicago, IL 60611, USA
Center for Healthcare Studies, Northwestern University Feinberg School of Medicine, Chicago, IL 60611, USA

Jason D. Pou, Charles A. Riley and Anna K. Bareiss
Department of Otolaryngology, Head and Neck Surgery, Tulane University School of Medicine, New Orleans, LA 70121, USA

Kiranya E. Tipirneni
Ochsner Clinic School, University of Queensland, New Orleans, LA 70121, USA

Edward D. McCoul
Department of Otolaryngology, Head and Neck Surgery, Tulane University School of Medicine, New Orleans, LA 70121, USA
Ochsner Clinic School, University of Queensland, New Orleans, LA 70121, USA
Department of Otorhinolaryngology, Ochsner Clinic Foundation, New Orleans, LA 70121, USA

Basel Al Kadah, Gudrun Helmus and Bernhard Schick
Department of Otorhinolaryngology, University Medical Center Homburg/Saar, D-66424 Homburg, Germany

Quoc Thai Dinh
Department of Pneumology and Experimental Pneumology, University Medical Center Homburg/Saar, D-66424 Homburg, Germany

Michael Smith
Sarah Bush Lincoln Health Center, 1000 Health Center
Dr., Mattoon, IL 61938, USA

Philippe G. Berenger
Department of Pain Management, Cleveland Clinic
Foundation, 9500 Euclid Avenue, Cleveland, OH
44195, USA

**Peter Bonutti, Alisa P. Ramakrishnan and Justin
Beyers**
Bonutti Technologies, 2600 S Raney St., Effingham, IL
62401, USA

Vivek Ramakrishnan
AxioSonic, 2600 S Raney St., Effingham, IL 62401, USA

Russell J. Hopp
Division of Allergy and Immunology, Creighton
University, Omaha, NE 68131, USA
Children's Hospital and Medical Center, Omaha, NE
68131, USA
Department of Pediatrics, Creighton University School
of Medicine, 2500 California Plaza, Omaha, NE 68131,
USA

M. Asghar Pasha
Division of Allergy and Immunology, Albany Medical
College, 176 Washington Avenue Extension, Suite 102,
Albany, NY 12203, USA

Ayami Kajiwara-Morita
Division of Pharmacology and Therapeutics, Graduate
School of Pharmaceutical Sciences, Kumamoto
University, 5-1 Oe-honmachi, Chuo-ku, Kumamoto
862-0973, Japan
Jinnouchi Clinic, Diabetes Care Center, 6-2-3 Kuhonji,
Chuo-ku, Kumamoto 862-0976, Japan

Chandima P. Karunanayake
Canadian Centre for Health and Safety in Agriculture,
University of Saskatchewan, 104 Clinic Place,
Saskatoon, SK S7N 2Z4, Canada

**James A. Dosman, Joshua A. Lawson, Shelley
Kirychuk, Niels Koehncke and Roland F. Dyck**
Canadian Centre for Health and Safety in Agriculture,
University of Saskatchewan, 104 Clinic Place,
Saskatoon, SK S7N 2Z4, Canada
Department of Medicine, University of Saskatchewan,
Royal University Hospital, 103 Hospital Drive,
Saskatoon, SK S7N 0W8, Canada

Donna C. Rennie
Canadian Centre for Health and Safety in Agriculture,
University of Saskatchewan, 104 Clinic Place,
Saskatoon, SK S7N 2Z4, Canada

College of Nursing, University of Saskatchewan, 104
Clinic Place, Saskatoon, SK S7N 2Z4, Canada

Ambikaipakan Senthilselvan
School of Public Health, 3-276 Edmonton Clinic
Health Academy, University of Alberta, 11405-87 Ave,
Edmonton, AB T6G 1C9, Canada

Punam Pahwa
Canadian Centre for Health and Safety in Agriculture,
University of Saskatchewan, 104 Clinic Place,
Saskatoon, SK S7N 2Z4, Canada
Department of Community Health and Epidemiology,
University of Saskatchewan, Health Science Building,
104, Clinic Place, Saskatoon, SK S7N 5E5, Canada

**Amelia Licari, Ilaria Brambilla, Riccardo Castagnoli,
Alessia Marseglia, Valeria Paganelli, Thomas
Foiadelli and Gian Luigi Marseglia**
Pediatric Clinic, University of Pavia, Fondazione
IRCCS Policlinico San Matteo, 27100 Pavia, Italy

Ryan K. Sewell
Department of Otolaryngology-Head and Neck
Surgery, University of Nebraska Medical Center,
981225 UNMC, Omaha, NE 68198-1225, USA

**Remi Motegi, Shin Ito, Hirotomo Homma, Noritsugu
Ono, Hiroko Okada, Yoshinobu Kidokoro, Akihito
Shiozawa and Katsuhisa Ikeda**
Department of Otorhinolaryngology, Juntendo
University Faculty of Medicine, 2-1-1 Hongo, Bunkyo-
ku, Tokyo 113-8421, Japan

**Alan D. Workman, Neil N. Patel, Ryan M. Carey and
Edward C. Kuan**
Department of Otorhinolaryngology, Head and Neck
Surgery, University of Pennsylvania, Philadelphia, PA
19104, USA

Noam A. Cohen
Department of Otorhinolaryngology, Head and Neck
Surgery, University of Pennsylvania, Philadelphia, PA
19104, USA
Monell Smell and Taste Center, Philadelphia, PA
19104, USA
Philadelphia Veterans Affairs Medical Center,
Philadelphia, PA 19104, USA

John Malaty
Department of Community Health and Family Medicine,
University of Florida, Gainesville, FL 32609, USA

Cindy Claeys, Gabriele Holtappels and Claus Bachert
Upper Airways Research Laboratory, Department of
Otorhinolaryngology, Ghent University Hospital, 9000
Ghent, Belgium

Rogerio Pezato
Upper Airways Research Laboratory, Department of Otorhinolaryngology, Ghent University Hospital, 9000 Ghent, Belgium
Department of Otorhinolaryngology, Head and Neck Surgery, Federal University of São Paulo, 05405-000 São Paulo, Brazil

Claudina A. Pérez-Novo
Upper Airways Research Laboratory, Department of Otorhinolaryngology, Ghent University Hospital, 9000 Ghent, Belgium
Laboratory of Protein chemistry, Proteomics & Epigenetic Signaling, Department Biomedical Sciences, University of Antwerp, 2610 Wilrijk, Belgium

Suha Jabr Ayyad
Institut d'Investigacions Biomèdiques August Pi y Sunyer (IDIBAPS),08036 Barcelona, Spain
Hospital Clinic, Universitat de Barcelona, 08036 Barcelona, Spain

Jordi Roca-Ferrer and César Picado
Institut d'Investigacions Biomèdiques August Pi y Sunyer (IDIBAPS),08036 Barcelona, Spain

Hospital Clinic, Universitat de Barcelona, 08036 Barcelona, Spain
Centro de Investigaciones Biomédicas en Red de Enfermedades Respiratorias (CIBERES), 08036 Barcelona, Spain

Jochen G. Mainz, Christin Arnold, Andrea Gerber and James F. Beck
CF Center, Pediatric Pneumology, Jena University Hospital, Jena 07740, Germany

Jürgen Rödel
Institute for Medical Microbiology, Jena University Hospital, Jena 07740, Germany

Nina Cramer and Burkhard Tümmler
Klinische Forschergruppe, Pediatric Pneumology, Med. Hochschule Hannover, Hannover 30625, Germany

Hans-Joachim Mentzel
Pediatric Radiology, Jena University Hospital, Jena 07740, Germany

Index

CPSIA information can be obtained
at www.ICGtesting.com
Printed in the USA
BVHW010154281221
624827BV00014B/19